HEALTH VISITING IN PRACTICE

HEALTH VISITING IN PRACTICE

CAROL ROBERTSON BSc (Hons) RGN RM RHV CHNT RNT

Formerly Lecturer in Health Visiting at the Polytechnic of the South Bank, London

Churchill Livingstone 🏛

EDINBURGH LONDON MELBOURNE AND NEW YORK 1988

CHURCHILL LIVINGSTONE
Medical Division of Longman Group UK Limited

Distributed in the United States of America by
Churchill Livingstone Inc., 1560 Broadway, New York,
N.Y. 10036, and by associated companies, branches
and representatives throughout the world.

First published 1988

ISBN 0-443-03278-5

British Library Cataloguing in Publication Data
Robertson, Carol
    Health visiting in practice.
    1. Visiting nurses
    I. Title
    362.1'4   RT98

Library of Congress Cataloging in Publication Data
Robertson, Carol, RNT.
    Health visiting in practice.
    Includes index.
    1. Community health nursing. I. Title.
[DNLM: 1. Community Health Nursing. WY 106 R649h]
RT98.R63 1988   610.73'43   87–6594

Produced by Longman Singapore Publishers (Pte) Ltd.
Printed in Singapore

Preface

A friend of mine remarked 'What a joy to be able to write whatever you like about health visiting!' and here lies the essential difference between her research and this book! This is, in essence, my opinion: the practice of health visiting as I have seen it and, to a fair extent, as I feel it ought to be. It is inevitable that it is a personal view, as there is very little research into the face-to-face, practical aspects of our work. However, that which is currently available has been incorporated.

Health visiting has remarkably wide potential and aims to accommodate and to provide for enormous variations in people's needs. Hoping to make this complex picture easier to understand, I have tried to muster the description into three main frameworks. They are founded on models which I have used both in practice and in teaching. The challenge of setting them out in print has caused me to refine them in a few small ways.

In essence, these frameworks show 'why', 'what' and 'how' in the work. A prevention model highlights the purpose of health visiting. Another model is one based on family health needs and highlights the various factors covered. The third, the health visitor cycle, outlines the mechanics involved and is derived from the nursing process.

Each model is particularly valuable in certain situations, that is, for considering the work over a period of time, for a particular visit, or for certain aspects of planning the care. After they have been introduced, each is given a chapter or two to show how they can help in thinking about and planning our work. Subsequent chapters continue the theme.

Besides looking at various philosophical aspects of health visiting, it seemed best to try to provide as much practical help as space would allow. Various aspects of the work have received only a cursory mention, others have been left out. It would take a book of encyclopaedic proportions to accommodate a full description. It has proved difficult to become properly informed across such a wide field — but that is a common problem in the practice of health visiting.

Southampton, 1987   C.R.

v

Acknowledgements

I would like to thank:

—my husband John, and Bernadette, Sophie and Jack for their enthusiasm and encouragement over this project;

—the librarians and staff of the District library at the Royal Hampshire County Hospital for the many, many books and papers they made available;

—the people at the South Bank Polytechnic, particularly Frances Appleby, who will recognise some of the ideas for teaching she gave me when I first arrived, and also my first students whose encouragement, support and constructive criticism inspired this book;

—my brave friends, Jean Jones, Debbie Hennessy and Kate Robinson, who valiantly read through the early versions and offered invaluable comment and advice;

—and others, Jean Hooper, Pat Robson, Elizabeth Anionwu, Jean Powell and Wes Hall, who kindly looked through some of the text and made helpful suggestions about particular aspects;

—the health visitors from Teddington and Hampton clinics, who helped me write the circumstances of my imaginary families on to their family records system, and the Richmond, Twickenham and Roehampton Health Authority for permission to reprint the cards (Figs. 8.5a–d).

—and my computer, for its untiring willingness to keep revising the script!

Contents

This chapter gives a brief overview of health visiting and its origins and development. The main models used to describe the work in later chapters are introduced. They are demonstrated through an example of a visit to the home of a young mother.

Health visiting in outline
  Preventive care
  Origins and development

Frameworks for describing the work
  The prevention model
  The family health needs model
  The health visitor cycle

1

Introduction

HEALTH VISITING IN OUTLINE

PREVENTIVE CARE

Health visiting is an aspect of nursing which concentrates upon preventive care. Prerequisites for practice are currently state registration as a nurse and midwifery experience. The year-long course provides an introduction to a wide range of studies, such as psychology, social policy, sociology, and to both the theory and practice of health visiting.

Health Authorities employ health visitors to call on families in their homes, especially where there are small children. The service, which also provides clinics, is mainly educational, aiming to improve community health by informing and encouraging people to remain healthy and by enabling them to make best use of the health and social services.

The caseload is defined by a GP's practice or a geographic area. Health visitors try to select priorities where their preventive health care can have the greatest effect. They tend to concentrate their effort on the under five-year-olds, including the antenatal period, to try to ensure the best foundations for mental and physical health in later years. For some health visitors, this represents the outer limits of their work. Others have time to make regular visits to other groups such as the elderly.

Education, screening and support

Health visitors are mainly concerned with three aspects of community health:

(i) In their educational role, they attempt to prevent the occurrence of disease by increasing people's understanding of healthy ways of living and their awareness of health hazards. For example, they may give advice on child rearing, talks to schools and discussions in young mothers' groups.

(ii) By trying to screen for health defects at an early stage, they hope, through prompt treatment, to prevent irreparable damage.

(iii) Where established conditions already exist, they can help to prevent further deterioration by giving supportive care—often by employing their listening skills to help their clients understand and take a positive approach to their problems. Health visitors can refer people to other health and social services and, sometimes, encourage the establishment of self-help groups.

A few health visitors specialise in the care of a distinct group of clients such as the handicapped or diabetics. Some undertake hospital liaison work.

Health visiting has changed in emphasis and broadened in scope over the years, but its aim has always remained the same: to reduce the incidence of ill-health in the community through anticipatory and supportive care.

ORIGINS AND DEVELOPMENT

Preventive health guidance given in people's homes can be traced back, through the infant welfare movement in the first half of this century, to voluntary work undertaken some fifty years earlier (Robinson, 1982; Connolly, 1980a; 1980b; Owen, 1977; Clark, 1973). Table 1.1 gives a thumbnail sketch of the development of health visiting and the influences that helped shape it.

Mid-19th century—the early days

By the middle of the nineteenth century, Victorian concern with the morality of the poor and the constant threat from epidemics of cholera and typhoid, gave rise to voluntary efforts to take education and relevant help into poor people's homes. In 1861, Manchester and Salford middle class volunteers supervised paid visitors who went from door to door on an organised basis. Similar schemes were set up in a few other towns, some workers being known as 'health missioners' and some as 'sanitary visitors'.

The more pioneering medical officers of health encouraged the idea. With high levels

Table 1.1 Influences in the development of health visiting

Period	Attitudes	Pressures for action	Action	Administration by
Mid-19th century	Paternalistic welfare	Squalid town living Cholera and typhoid	Prevention of acute fatal diseases	Voluntary agencies
Turn of the century	Pragmatic: populate or perish	Infant mortality Boer War World War I	Teaching to prevent disease in the very young	
Post World War II	Egalitarianism: socialised medicine	Wartime experience: separation good nutrition Small family size	Social advice and health education for the whole famiy	
Present day	Cost consciousness; Quality of life	Rising health service costs Increasing public expectations	As above and some: specialisation screening programmes	State

of illiteracy and no mass media, individual tuition provided a useful tool for getting knowledge to the people. Gradually, visitors' training courses were set up. Some of the early visitors included doctors, nurses, people with various degrees and sanitary inspectors. Their work, which brought them into close proximity with social problems, led them to undertake some supportive as well as health educational services.

Turn of the century—infant welfare movement

Robinson described how, with the turn of the century, attention focused on infant care. There was an increase in the already high death rates of the newborn. The poor health of the nation had been exposed, for example, when around half of the Boer War recruits were declared unfit for military service.

Concern about population trends led to the emergence of an influential infant welfare movement. Clinics were set up for the teaching and care of mothers with babies. Local Authorities became increasingly involved. The high death rate in World War I brought more concern. Compulsory notification of birth made it possible to visit all newborn babies. Preventive work was extended to include children under school age, and health visitors also took on work in Child Life Protection (Baly, 1980).

Post World War II

The voluntary element in health visiting disappeared once the welfare state was established after the Second World War. Local Health Authorities continued as the responsible bodies and remained so until 1974. In 1948, some of the health visitors' social service responsibilities, acquired in the previous period, were transferred to Children's Departments.

Ideas were changing. Jane Robinson outlined some of the factors which helped to shape post-war philosophies. Family unity was given high priority. The war had led many families to suffer complete separation through evacuation of children, as well as on account of

military service. Small families had become commonplace. Child health was no longer such a problem, as it had been improved by good nutrition through rationing. It was therefore felt that health visitors should care for the family as a unit and not concentrate only on children. An inquiry in the mid-50s suggested health visitors should undertake 'social advice and health education for the whole family' (Ministry of Health, 1956).

Present day

In the event, a very large proportion of the work still tends to be centred around preventive care for babies and young children, with some supportive care for their parents—especially the mother. But infant mortality figures do not seem to dominate thinking to the same extent as before. Some specialisations have emerged, such as in handicap, the elderly, diabetics and in hospital liaison. The service is now administered by District Health Authorities and, through a recent Act of Parliament (DHSS, 1979), has been drawn even closer to other aspects of nursing. Interprofessional liaison plays an increasingly important role.

The huge costs of the National Health Service are causing increased interest in preventive health care. Screening is one area receiving greater attention (DHSS, 1976). Pressure to justify expenditure seems to be causing an emphasis on the more quantifiable activities in health visiting such as screening and factors like the number of times families are seen, rather than the less easily measured educational and supportive care. Researchers, in the meantime, are gradually finding ways to investigate, and are reporting on qualitative aspects of the work (Luker, 1982; Robinson, 1982; Orr, 1980). It is a difficult task and is only in the early stages, but this and other research will help to show how health visiting should be shaped in the future.

Influence from acute medicine?

From its mid-century beginnings, right through to the current period, few of the major pressures for the preventive work of a health visitor seem to have come directly from the sphere of acute medicine. This may gradually change. Both liaison and attachment to general practice brings an increased possibility of cooperation between acute and preventive care. The current need to contain the costs of acute care may provide a modern stimulus to achieve positive goals in specific fields of preventive work, for example in the care of the elderly.

Health visiting has come a long way, but has had a clearly recognisable structure throughout its development. Health education, the timely discovery of problems and concern for emotional well-being and social support, have been the basis of the work. The profession has been strongly involved in the welfare of the very young, but has also responded to some of the other needs for preventive health in the community.

FRAMEWORKS FOR DESCRIBING THE WORK

A detailed account of health visiting includes an enormously wide and diverse range of factors in family health and social welfare. In this book, certain categorisations or models have been used to bring some order into the description and to help the reader think about the work. The main three are the 'prevention', the 'family health needs' and the 'health visitor cycle' models.

Models simplify and clarify

When trying to describe something complex, it is helpful to find some means of untangling its intricacies to present the information more clearly. Various forms of categorisation and listing may help. There are, of course, limitations on these models or frameworks as they necessarily present a simplistic version. Even though they can only tell part of the story, they are generally easier to remember and to contemplate than the diffuseness and complexity of reality. The reader can benefit by thinking about health visiting through the perspective of several different models. This

way it becomes possible to highlight a variety of features. Depending on the context, a particular model may be chosen for its ability to emphasise certain basic and important characteristics.

THE PREVENTION MODEL

One of the underlying models used in this book has already been met earlier in this chapter (see p. 2). The three aspects of community health described in the introductory definition are based on Caplan's (1961) model of primary, secondary and tertiary prevention. The format used in this book is presented in Table 1.2.

Table 1.2 Model of health visitor's role: prevention model

Aspect of prevention	Mainly through	Activity
Prevent occurrence of condition	Teaching	a. environmental improvement b. anticipatory guidance (i) child care — physical — behavioural (diet, safety, sleep, immunisation) (ii) adult (young parent, handicap, retirement)
Prevent development of condition	Screening	a. screening (i) clinics— developmental assessment, hearing, vision (ii) parental involvement b. mental health
Prevent deterioration of established condition	Support	a. clients clarify/decide b. tell of helpful agencies c. catalyst: self-help groups

1. Health promotion

Primary prevention is *preventing the occur-*

rence of ill-health and promoting good health. Health visitors achieve this mainly through teaching.

a. Environmental improvement

The same goal may also be achieved by improving the environment, for example, instigating smoke-free zones in public places, ensuring people have adequate social support and helping them attain good housing.

b. Anticipatory guidance

The teaching is usually in the form of anticipatory guidance on safety, nutrition, immunisation, general child care and any aspect of positive health relevant to the people being visited. If people become aware of certain potential health problems, they are then able to take steps to avoid them.

2. Early discovery

Preventing the development of disease or social problems is generally achieved through some aspect of screening, within routine visiting or on a specifically planned occasion. The aim of this secondary aspect of prevention is to discover problems early, enabling them to be dealt with before any irreversible or debilitating damage can be done.

Some models of prevention used in medicine (Williamson, 1981) classify secondary prevention and screening in a different way. They see it as the search only for the precursors of disease in symptom-free people, and not the search for early stages of disease or difficulty. An example of this would be cytology screening, in which the pre-cancerous condition is sought.

a. Screening

Health visitors rarely take part in screening at pre-symptomatic stages. The vast majority are too heavily involved in seeking children's neurological, visual or hearing defects and in keeping an eye open for behavioural, social and other problems. Here, the aim is to bring to light conditions which would benefit from attention. In some schemes, parents are routinely informed of how to look out for signs of physical defects. This sort of parental involvement seems to be on the increase.

b. Mental health

Health visitors are in a good position to keep an educated and informal eye on both the physical and mental health of the adults they visit, in particular the emotional health of the young mother.

3. Supportive care

Tertiary prevention is *preventing the deterioration* of an established condition. The aim is not only to contain the problem but also to achieve rehabilitation, where this is possible.

a. Clients clarify and decide

Listening skills are perhaps health visitors' most useful tool in this aspect of care. Using them in non-directive counselling, health visitors can encourage people to talk through their problems, helping them to gain a better understanding of the difficulties involved and to come to terms with the situation. This sort of approach can also help people clarify their ideas and decide on the sort of solution they would like to seek.

b. Tell of helpful agencies

A good knowledge is needed of people's entitlements and of local voluntary and statutory services to enable people to be informed about agencies that would be able to offer appropriate help. Timely and up-to-date information can help people facing difficulties, such as unemployment or a handicapped baby, start to take positive steps towards coping with and containing their problem.

c. Catalyst: self-help groups

Health visitors sometimes take a background

and/or a catalytic role in the creation of self-help groups. People with major problems, such as those who are bereaved or have a handicapped baby, often find these groups an excellent source of sympathetic under-standing and of basic, practical suggestions for everyday problems. The professional contribution is mainly through bringing people together, helping them to find infor-mation about similar ventures and by offering encouragement and occasional help.

It may help to have an example of the use of the model. A description of a visit to a young mother and her baby will be found in the right hand half of Box 1.1. The column on

Box 1.1 Visit to Mrs Smith: a basis for demonstrating the models

Prevention model	Needs model*	The visit
	1	The house is situated in a suburban estate built in the 1930s. It is a mile from the nearest shops and services. The health visitor arrived on the afternoon arranged by appointment. She was welcomed in and the conversation turned quickly to child care.
Observation, aimed at early diagnosis—to **prevent** (potential) **development** of problems	2	It seems that Mrs Smith had enjoyed using the developmental assessment format, previously suggested by the health visitor. She was delighted to show how Charles was progressing. She said he was now capable of sitting alone for around 15 minutes and holding a cup for drinking. The health visitor heard him say 'dada' and he held two small cubes, one in each hand, in a palmar grasp. He required reassurance before really accepting the visitor but played the game with the cubes quite sociably.
Health education—to **prevent occurrence**	3	The conversation led on to expectations in the future: the emergence of conscience and the effect of mobility in toddlerhood. They talked of the sort of

discipline and play appropriate to that period. Mrs Smith's expectations seemed balanced. She had found one of the recommended child care books especially easy to read and helpful. She remarked on how much her husband enjoyed playing with Charles.

education—to **prevent occurrence** of problems	4	The health visitor gave Mrs Smith a Health Education Council pamphlet on safety, emphasising Charles' needs over the next few months.
test—to **prevent development** of problems	5	The appointment for the hearing test in two weeks' time had arrived and Mrs Smith promised to attend.
listening skills— knowledge of local facilities **preventing deterioration**	6	Just as the health visitor was starting to go, Mrs Smith mentioned a personal problem— extreme loneliness and 'missing work'. She looked rather tired as she described her worries and fears. The health visitor quietly listened and occasionally asked a question which seemed to help Mrs Smith come nearer the core of her concern.
As above	7	A newly set up local mother and toddler group was suggested. A promise was made to introduce Mrs Smith, at the hearing clinic, to another mother who was already attending.
As above	8	Local schemes for minding children of working mothers were discussed. However, Mrs Smith rejected this idea, saying that now she had put it all into words, it did not seem so bad.
As above	9	Her husband, she said, had a good job. She preferred, for the present, to be at home with her baby and would take steps to get adjusted.
	10	The visit ended amicably and with a wave from Charles.

* See Box 1.3

the far left has each of the three aspects of the prevention model set against certain activities—health education, screening and supportive care. The numbers in the central column pertain to the family health needs framework which is explained below.

The model highlights important points, but there can be minor complexities. Things do not always unarbitrarily fall into the pigeonholes chosen. For example, some might argue that the mother in the case described did not have a problem. Therefore, helping her find a group of like-minded mothers would be more likely to prevent its occurrence and so would be regarded as primary, not tertiary, prevention. Others might suggest that the health visitor would be on the look out for early signs of emotional illness and that her response deserves to be classified as secondary prevention!

Borderline delineations, however, are not of great importance. A model is devised only to draw attention to noteworthy features and is successful if it can be used as a tool to clarify thinking and aid learning.

This prevention model is particularly useful in broad explanations of the role and in helping to describe ways health visitors can organise their work.

THE FAMILY HEALTH NEEDS MODEL

Of more practical value to student health visitors preparing their early fieldwork practice

visits is an approach which centres round the health needs of a family. Features pertaining to family preventive health care are brought together under headings of general environment, social, mental/emotional and physical factors. Health is emphasised and facets of daily life and general social needs are included. Box 1.2 gives an outline of this approach. Specific examples will be found in the chapters on visiting antenatally and on the first visit after the birth.

Four areas of health need

1. The section for *general environment* can give an outline of the local area, its facilities and services, the basic social situation of the family, their accommodation and their standard of living.
2. Aspects of the family's *physical health* and daily life, such as nutrition, home safety, hygiene, developmental attainments (in children), medication and other facets of general health, are in one section.
3. Factors such as parental knowledge and attitudes and family members' *mental and emotional health* needs are included in another.
4. The last grouping is for family *social aspect of health*, such as hobbies, child care facilities and support from family, friends or community organisations.

As in the prevention framework, deciding exactly what fits best under any particular

Box 1.2 Some aspects of family health need

General environment	Physical health	Mental/emotional health	Social aspects of health
Community/area	*Parents and children*	*Parents*	*Mother*
Social mix of locality	General health	Knowledge	Support from:
Urban, suburban, rural	Nutrition	Attitudes	— family
Special features	Safety	— expectations	— friends
	Hygiene	Psychological illness	— community
Home	Developmental progress	— postnatal depression	Group activities
Proximity to:	Special screening	Emotional stability	
— transport	— vision		*Family unit*
— shops	— hearing	*Child*	Emotional support
— health services	— chiropody	Play needs	Housing
Availability of:	Medication	— equipment	
— garden/play area		Normal discipline	*Child*
— lift/stairs for flats		Affection	Play—with other children
Standard of living			Stimulation

Box 1.3 Visit to Mrs Smith's home: 'family health needs' analysis

General environment	Physical health	Mental/emotional health	Social aspects of health
Community 1 1930s estate housing, a preponderance of elderly people Relatively remote *Family* 9 Adequate income *Father* In employment	*Mother* 6 seems tired *Child* 2 Developmental assessment: reported and observed characteristics 4 Safety discussed 5 Hearing test arranged 10 Developmental attainment observed	*Mother* 3 Well-read, attitude to discipline relaxed *Father* Involved *Baby* Sociable *Mother* 6 Loneliness discussed	*Mother* 7 ? Mother and toddler club 8 Information: local child-minding facilities

Numbering of the factors corresponds to that in the centre column in the example on page 6, Box 1.1

Features of the *general environment* are important because they make Mrs Smith more vulnerable to loneliness. *Physical* aspects of health covered on this visit were biased towards the baby: observed and reported developmental attainments, safey and Charles' hearing. The *mental/emotional* factors—the mother's knowledge and attitudes, the father's involvement and the baby's social reactions—were all normal and augured well for the future. Mrs Smith's emotional problem of loneliness may be helped by *social* activities with a group of local mothers. Although she misses work, she is not keen to use the child-minding facilities and return to employment at the moment. The family seems to have an adequate income and the father satisfying employment.

category is a matter of personal preference. The way that the visit to the Smith household (Box 1.1) would be viewed from the standpoint of this model is demonstrated in Box 1.3.

THE HEALTH VISITOR CYCLE

A third way of analysing the work of a health visitor is by looking at the behind-the-scenes planning processes. These are not easily detected in an example such as the visit to the Smiths, as this model, outlined in Figure 1.1, is concerned with the way the health visitor works out how best to help the family.

Planning processes

The basic problem is to:
 (i) assess the family's health needs
 (ii) then plan action to be taken (set objectives)
(iii) set about implementing the plan and
(iv) then evaluate the effect of the action.

The information needed to make the assessment and choose priorities for action, comes from several sources:
a. background reading during and after

training and knowledge of the locality
b. prior to the visit, from records and inter-professional communication
c. the client's viewpoint and observations during the visit and
d. the synthesis and outcome of work with the family on previous visits guiding plans for future contact.

The example

The description of the visit to Mrs Smith (p. 6, Box 1.1) does not state how the health visitor was actually thinking. It does seem, however, that (i) the assessment led to (ii) and (iii) high priority being given to child health matters, and that (iv) previous contact with Mrs Smith resulted in her positive involvement in her child's developmental assessment.

Sources of information which help the planning processes, both before and after the visit, are not specified. There is (a) no indication of the health visitor's general background knowledge of relevant research results acquired either during or since her training, or of her understanding of local policies. However, there is an evident awareness of local agencies. It seems likely that (b) the

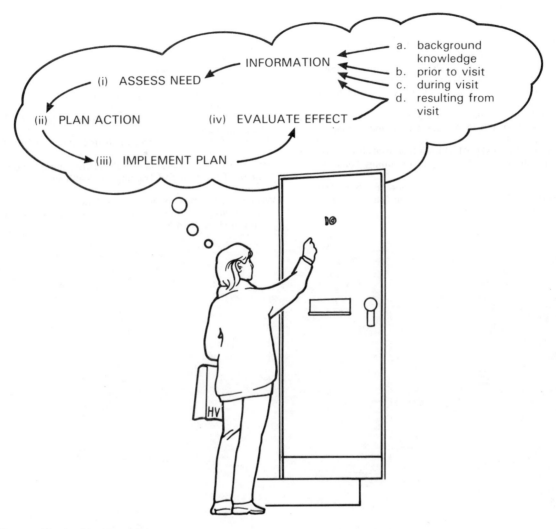

Fig. 1.1 The health visitor cycle

record system triggered the appointment for the hearing test and provided a reminder for the assessment of developmental attainments and safety literature. The description does clearly show, however, that (c) the health visitor's objectives and subsequent actions were modified during the visit, on hearing the mother mention her loneliness. There is (d) no explanation in the case history of how previous visits influenced this one or what is planned beyond the appointment at the hearing assessment clinic.

The health visitor cycle is explained in detail in the next chapter. This model looks at the underlying processes of planning and action: an entirely different perspective from (i), the broad overview which can be provided by the prevention model, and (ii) the more specific and individual approach of the family health needs model. Each scheme makes a useful contribution towards highlighting important aspects of a health visitor's work.

This chapter has been concerned with a brief description of health visiting, a historical perspective and an introduction to the three basic frameworks used in later chapters to help think about and describe the work.

REFERENCES

Baly M B 1980 Nursing and social change, 2nd ed. Heinemann, London. p. 137

Caplan G 1961 An approach to community mental health. Tavistock Publications, London

Clark J 1973 A family visitor. Royal College of Nursing, London. ch. 2

Connolly M P 1980a Health visiting 1850–1900: a review. Midwife, Health Visitor and Community Nurse 16: 282–285

Connolly M P 1980b Health visiting 1900–1910: a review. Midwife, Health Visitor and Community Nurse 16: 375–378

DHSS 1976 Report of the Committee on Child Health Services. Fit for the future. Cmnd 6684 HMSO, London (Court Report)

DHSS 1979 Nurses, Midwives and Health Visitors Act, 1979. HMSO, London

Luker K A 1982 Evaluating health visiting practice. Royal College of Nursing, London

Ministry of Health 1956 An inquiry into health visiting. HMSO, London (Jameson Report)

Orr J 1980 Health visiting in focus. Royal College of Nursing, London

Owen G M (editor) 1977 Health visiting. Bailliere Tindall, London, ch. 1

Robinson J 1982 An evaluation of health visiting. Council for the Education and Training of Health Visitors, London, ch. 1

Williamson J 1981 Screening, surveillance and casefinding. In: Arie T (ed) Health care of the elderly. Croom Helm, London

This chapter looks at some of the sources of information that help health visitors decide whom to visit and how they might best be of help. It introduces three important factors associated with a first visit: establishing a good relationship, explaining the health visitor's role and, where possible, responding to immediate need.

The framework

Examples of first visits

Who . . . and how?
  Background information—for priorities
  Background information—for practical work

Preparing for the visit
  Information—prior to the visit

The visit
  Information—whilst visiting

Plans for subsequent visits
  Short-term objectives
  Long-term objectives

2

Making contact

THE FRAMEWORK

This chapter expands on the health visitor cycle, outlined at the end of the introductory chapter. Making contact with a family is discussed using this framework because it draws attention to important underlying processes that take place. The model highlights health visitors' need to plan their work by gleaning information from various sources and situations, in order to choose whom to visit, to assess their needs and to provide health care.

A particular advantage of the framework is that it concentrates on a range of information sources available at various times to the health visitor. It highlights the everchanging pattern of information on which health visiting decisions are made. It is able, specifically, to draw attention to the family's viewpoint and perspective. This should be a major factor in health visitor planning and care. Success in the work depends upon:
— building up a good relationship
— making it easy for the family to understand how the health visitor is aiming to help
— ensuring that the family feel the appropriateness of that help.

The diagram in Figure 2.1 shows the four sources of information required in the provision of a good health visiting service. The first three sources are:
1. *Background information acquired over time*

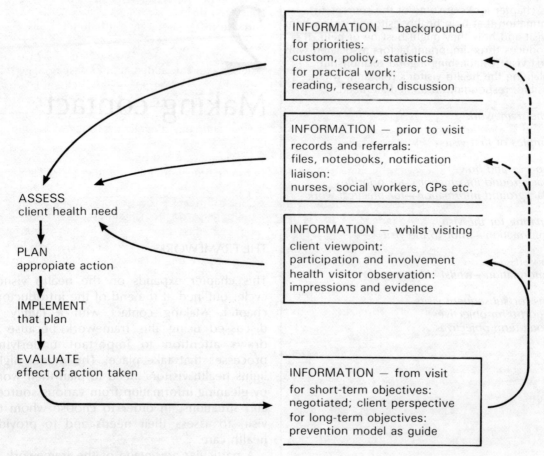

INFORMATION — background
for priorities:
custom, policy, statistics
for practical work:
reading, research, discussion

INFORMATION — prior to visit
records and referrals:
files, notebooks, notification
liaison:
nurses, social workers, GPs etc.

INFORMATION — whilst visiting
client viewpoint:
participation and involvement
health visitor observation:
impressions and evidence

INFORMATION — from visit
for short-term objectives:
negotiated; client perspective
for long-term objectives:
prevention model as guide

ASSESS
client health need

PLAN
appropiate action

IMPLEMENT
that plan

EVALUATE
effect of action taken

Fig. 2.1 The health visitor cycle.

Knowledge of health visiting priorities, and including practical knowledge of how families can be helped
2. *Information acquired before the visit*
Written/verbal communications about each individual family to be visited
3. *Information available when meeting the family*
Information from the family itself, for example any particular wishes, viewpoint, cultural background or situation.

These three together form the basis for assessing health needs and for planning and implementing health care at the first visit.

A fourth source, the last in the diagram in Figure 2.1, is:
4. *Information emerging as a result of the visit*
Closer understanding of the particular

family's circumstances and requirements and, as far as possible, assessment of the effect of the health care given.

This sort of evaluation provides part of the basis on which to plan for care in later encounters, helping to form the health visitor's tentative longer-term and short-term objectives for further work with the family. These objectives are borne in mind and, together with additional information available between visits and at the time of the next visit, they help towards further assessment and provision of care. This is then, in essence, a continuous cycle of drawing together information, planning, action and assessment. The framework is derived from the nursing process.

Use of the health visitor cycle is demonstrated in two examples of a health visitor making contact at a first visit. The matter is then discussed in the rest of the chapter, with this framework providing the format.

EXAMPLES OF FIRST VISITS

The first example is about making contact with a recently bereaved lady in her late 50s. The other is a visit to a young family who have just moved into the area. In each case, the planning processes for the visit and the four sources of information are plotted on health visitor cycle diagrams. Figures 2.2 and 2.3.

EXAMPLE ONE: MISS DENBY

An 'attached' health visitor, Harry Vosper (HV), had experience in bereavement counselling and knew local health policy on visiting recently bereaved people—particularly those with minimal family and social support. The initial visit was usually about two weeks after the death, when family and friends would probably be becoming less involved.

Dr Golding, a GP, referred Miss Denby, aged 58, whose mother had died. The health visitor learned that Miss Denby had given up work four years previously to care for her mother. They had had little contact with the surgery until four weeks before the death. The home was a small Victorian terrace house near the shops. Dr Golding said few people were expected to attend the funeral.

The visit was made on the day suggested on the card the health visitor had posted to Miss Denby. A slim, grey-haired woman with upright posture answered the door. She was very welcoming and offered a cup of tea. This HV accepted, as he wanted Miss Denby to feel there was plenty of time to talk if she wished to. He listened attentively as she spoke, and he concentrated on helping her to express her feelings. He was successful in this and felt the grief and insecurity she showed were normal and typical features of the grieving process.

When Miss Denby hesitated over speaking angrily against her mother and about her guilt feelings, HV responded by saying she need not tell him anything she did not wish to. He went on to explain that such feelings are perfectly normal and that many people find it helpful to talk about them. He reassured her, too, of the confidentiality of their conversation. Miss Denby thanked him and added, a little despairingly, that there was no one else she could tell about such things. In order to help her recontinue, he tried to summarise briefly what she was feeling and saying. Little by little, she explained about her situation, her wishes and how she felt.

Her story was that having taken over care of her increasingly immobile mother, Miss Denby had been left to cope. It seems Mrs Denby had refused all treatment for her Parkinsonism. Her daughter's social life had almost ceased on account of the 24 hour obligations. They did not know about the attendance allowance or what services there might have been available to help. Finally, the old lady had required a very great deal of nursing care. Under great emotional strain, Miss Denby over-rode her mother's wishes and called the doctor. Admission to hospital had been a traumatic experience for them both and the old lady deteriorated fast.

The neighbours had called on hearing of the death. Miss Denby was no longer a church attender, but when HV told her about the local church bereavement visiting service, she said she would like them to call. As he got up to go, HV promised to contact the vicar. He suggested he should come again in six weeks, when, as she had said, she would have had a chance to seek advice on her financial position and entitlements and, perhaps, her chances of finding employment. He drew her attention to the telephone number on his visiting card and told her at what times he could be contacted.

As he reflected on the visit, HV felt a friendly working relationship had been established and she seemed to understand the purpose of his work—at least to the limited extent of his work with her! She had said how much better she felt for having talked about the bereavement. Six weeks would allow the church bereavement visitors time to befriend her and, perhaps, draw her into their circle. He felt the experiences and life-style of the past few years might impede her recovery. She had no close family and had been very isolated. He therefore intended to keep in touch for a while in order to make further assessment until it was obvious she had adequate support or was well on the way to a good recovery.

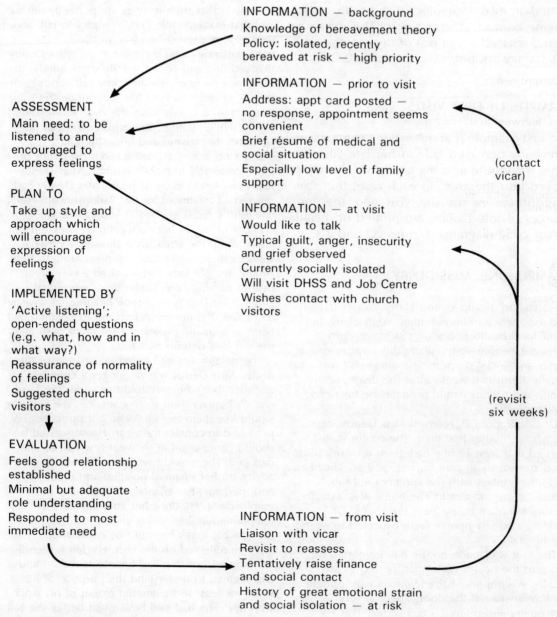

INFORMATION — background
Knowledge of bereavement theory
Policy: isolated, recently
bereaved at risk — high priority

INFORMATION — prior to visit
Address: appt card posted —
no response, appointment seems
convenient
Brief résumé of medical and
social situation
Especially low level of family
support

INFORMATION — at visit
Would like to talk
Typical guilt, anger, insecurity
and grief observed
Currently socially isolated
Will visit DHSS and Job Centre
Wishes contact with church
visitors

ASSESSMENT
Main need: to be
listened to and
encouraged to
express feelings

PLAN TO
Take up style and
approach which
will encourage
expression of
feelings

IMPLEMENTED BY
'Active listening';
open-ended questions
(e.g. what, how and in
what way?)
Reassurance of normality
of feelings
Suggested church
visitors

EVALUATION
Feels good relationship
established
Minimal but adequate
role understanding
Responded to most
immediate need

INFORMATION — from visit
Liaison with vicar
Revisit to reassess
Tentatively raise finance
and social contact
History of great emotional strain
and social isolation — at risk

(contact
vicar)

(revisit
six weeks)

Fig. 2.2 Example one: Miss Denby.

In the event, the church group proved to be very helpful, and after the second visit the health visitor made no further calls until the anniversary of the death.

EXAMPLE TWO: THE TRENT FAMILY

Miss Hazel Vickery (HV) worked in a Health District in which, as is common practice, young families who have newly moved in are visited as soon as possible after notice of their new address is received. The general practice to which she was attached was running an experiment on developmental assessment of young children, using Professor Barber's (Barber et al, 1976) type of visual display charts.

A note in the practice manager's 'transfer in' file informed HV that a young family, parents and

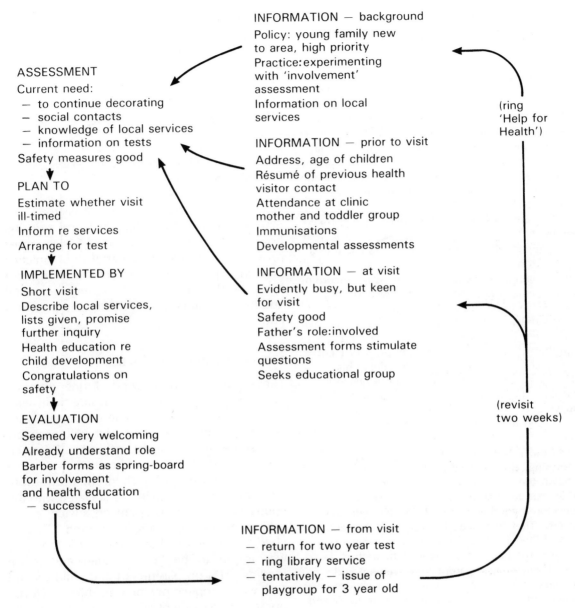

ASSESSMENT
Current need:
— to continue decorating
— social contacts
— knowledge of local services
— information on tests
Safety measures good

PLAN TO
Estimate whether visit
ill-timed
Inform re services
Arrange for test

IMPLEMENTED BY
Short visit
Describe local services,
lists given, promise
further inquiry
Health education re
child development
Congratulations on
safety

EVALUATION
Seemed very welcoming
Already understand role
Barber forms as spring-board
for involvement
and health education
— successful

INFORMATION — background
Policy: young family new
to area, high priority
Practice: experimenting
with 'involvement'
assessment
Information on local
services

INFORMATION — prior to visit
Address, age of children
Résumé of previous health
visitor contact
Attendance at clinic
mother and toddler group
Immunisations
Developmental assessments

INFORMATION — at visit
Evidently busy, but keen
for visit
Safety good
Father's role: involved
Assessment forms stimulate
questions
Seeks educational group

(ring
'Help for
Health')

(revisit
two weeks)

INFORMATION — from visit
— return for two year test
— ring library service
— tentatively — issue of
playgroup for 3 year old

Fig. 2.3 Example two: the Trent family.

children, had just registered with the surgery. Within days, this family's health visitor record cards were received from the previous Health District, noting the change of address.

According to the notes, the mother had been a very regular attender at the clinic with her first baby, now just over three years, and rather less so with her second, now nearly two. The most recent entry pertained to the three year

examination by the clinic doctor. Immunisations for both children were up to date and the mother seemed to have been a staunch supporter of her previous health visitor's mother and toddler group.

Having a 'birth visit' in that area, HV decided to make a brief visit to the Trent household in order to make contact. They were at home. She introduced herself and found the couple in the middle of decorating. She said she would call back at a more convenient time, but they insisted she come in.

The couple had made the room which overlooked where they were working into a huge safe area by using wide, temporarily fitted gates. Here the children were playing and HV was invited to step over the gates to meet them. She congratulated the Trents on their safety precautions. Mr Trent, who was taking a holiday prior to starting his new job, was evidently proud of his children—and his safety measures. It seems the idea had evolved from a discussion at the clinic mother and toddler group.

Not wanting to outstay her welcome, HV asked when she might return to undertake the two year developmental assessment test. In response to a query from the couple, she showed them a copy of the stepladder centile charts used for recording attainments. These led to more questions and discussion on child development.

A date was arranged for HV to return. She gave Mrs Trent a list of child health centres and another of mother and baby groups. Mrs Trent asked about groups with an educational bias. Thinking that the information service, 'Help for Health', might know of some, HV undertook to make enquiries. On parting, the couple were reminded that they could contact HV through the surgery.

As the Trents returned to their wallpaper stripping, HV walked away hoping they had shown their true feelings about her unexpected visit. She felt that it was likely that she would develop a good working relationship with this family. They had made her very welcome and had found their previous health visiting service very useful. The Barber assessment scheme had, as usual, encouraged parental involvement and understanding. Interaction with their children was calm and caring and the children were lively and creative.

Miss Vickery planned, at the next visit, to go through the two year test and to see what views Mrs Trent had about playgroups as preparation for schooling. She made a note in her diary to ring the library 'Help for Health' service the following morning about mothers' health educational groups.

WHO . . . . . AND HOW?

Making contact with families is necessarily preceded by decisions on *who* is to be visited. Reading and discussion can generate useful ideas on *how* these families might be helped and keep up to date the wide range of knowledge needed in the practice of health visiting. They both form an important part of background understanding in health visiting.

BACKGROUND INFORMATION—FOR PRIORITIES

With a remit as broad as a health visitor's, the first question is 'to whom do I give priority, how do I apportion my time?' As in most professions, accustomed patterns of practice play an important role in such decisions, but local health policies and local environmental and health factors also influence the priorities chosen.

Customary patterns of practice

These patterns are learned during training. Students gain experience alongside their fieldwork teachers. They become conversant with current common practice and will probably see some experimental projects. Research suggests that some 70% of health visitors' time is spent on work with children, proportionately more of it in activities associated with the young infant. Time is spent on advice, counselling, reassurance and education. That in child health or well baby clinics, for example, was found to be 26% on diet and infant feeding, 21% on parentcraft and children and 12% with people's personal problems. Developmental assessment accounts for 11% of the time, hearing and vision 5% and immunisation 4%. On average, care for the elderly takes up 6% of the time available (Dunnell & Dobbs, 1982).

The aim is to provide a service at various 'critical periods' (Council for the Education and Training of Health Visitors, 1977), such as ante- and postnatal phases, old age and bereavement. Ann Stanton (1982) has drawn up an outline suggesting one way a new health visitor might arrange her activities, and included some hours set aside for planning, thinking and reading. Ideas are constantly being modified in the light of new research findings, and it is important for health visitors to organise for both keeping up to date and for forward planning in their work.

Jean Orr (1983) has described the influences of recent reports and governmental advisory documents. A lack of money and manpower has stifled many of the developments suggested. Inspired local initiatives, however, have led to improvements in aspects of the work such as antenatal care, child abuse, the elderly, inner city work, 'positive discrimination', out of hours service, 'outreach programmes' and group work. The implementation of newer trends and ideas varies from area to area.

Local health policy

Many factors influence the number of health visitors employed per head of population and an important one is the willingness of the health authority to allocate resources for training and staffing. Metcalfe (1983) points out that, currently, the number of health visitors is regrettably low. It varies quite markedly between some regions (Orr, 1982). Health visitors may find themselves in quite stressful situations, trying to choose how best to spend their time (Schofield, 1982, 1983). Some are obliged to cover two or more caseloads for quite lengthy periods (Thompson, 1983). As Alison Norman (1982) points out, there is a need for more dicussion and investigation of the way caseload size and environmental factors affect health visiting practice.

In most Health Districts, health visitors can decide their own priorities (Fitton, 1983, 1984a, 1984b). Rather than directing the work, many nurse managers use their monitoring role more as that of a consultant advisor and act, to some extent, as a sounding board. In this way, they enable their health visitors 'to come to their own professional decision' (Dingwall et al, 1983). When this works well, it can help them develop new and useful approaches.

There has been some apprehension within the profession because, in some Districts, structured visiting programmes have been drawn up and the health visitors directed to complete them (Health Visitor, 1983). It is feared that some such schemes will result in 'doorstep-hopping, superficial health visiting' (Goodwin, 1982). An obligation to call on a prescribed number of homes each day may increase the number of visits recorded and counted in management terms, but it is unlikely to increase the fruitfulness of the work. The fear is that doorstep visiting will prevent the chance to establish meaningful relationships, the key to useful health visiting, and in the pressure to complete a particular visiting target each day, vital cues to problems may be lost (Health Visitor, 1983).

Local statistics

In order to choose the most important preventive health priorities, it is necessary to know the particular problems prevalent in the locality. Students gain experience enquiring into environmental and health statistics by undertaking a neighbourhood study. Some may have the opportunity to study a caseload profile (Hunt, 1982).

Baroness MacFarlane (1982) suggested that the health visitor should become the primary health care team epidemiologist. Many do become very aware of the environmental, social and health problems of their area and try to tailor their work accordingly. Sheila Jack (1983) has outlined the range of statistics available to the health visitor. Small-scale, local epidemiological information, though, is not a reliable guide (Robinson J, 1983).

Computers can now be used to process the social and environmental data from the 1981 census enumeration district statistics, defining characteristics of small areas with a population size of only a few hundred. From these, quite detailed Health District social profiles can be mapped out. Jarman (1983) and Irving (1983) give examples of how this has been done.

The correlation between levels of health and social circumstances is now well known.

Where local health statistics are post-coded, they could also be mapped and used to overlap the District profile. Such maps, when they are drawn up, are able to provide District Health Authorities with documentary evidence of what health visitors tend already to know: the areas needing special initiatives and, perhaps, proportionately greater investment in primary care services.

There is some debate over the extent to which health visiting should be provided equally to all, or slanted towards those with potentially greater health problems. The Health Visitor Association proposed that there should be a formal inquiry into health visiting, so that the work and the priorities can be properly reviewed (Goodwin, 1982; Health Visitor, 1982). The Cumberlege Report (1986) may help stimulate some solutions.

BACKGROUND INFORMATION—FOR PRACTICAL WORK

Students quickly realise that the health visitors course, although tightly packed with information about, for example, nutrition, psychology and social medicine, and thought-provoking ideas on how to help people, can only be an introduction. Reading, practical experience, advice from colleagues and the search for services and ideas, are all important sources of background information (see Fig. 2.1).

Journal articles

The breadth of the work means health visitors will need to continue to read widely, in order to keep up to date and also to enquire into particular aspects of the work as they are encountered. Professional journals like the *Health Visitor*, the *Nursing Times' Community Outlook*, *Midwife*, *Health Visitor and Community Nurse* and—as will be seen from the lists of references in this book—many others, provide background sources of information.

It is not always easy to maintain a high level of reading alongside the obligations associated with a full caseload. With this in mind, some nurse managers build up and make available a file of useful literature.

Research and library facilities

One of the services some medical libraries provide is access to the Health Visitor Association's *Current Awareness Bulletin*—a very good source for updating work practice. It is important constantly to be seeking the latest and most reliable research results which pertain to practical aspects of the work, in order to provide people with the best possible information.

Hours can be spent by individual health visitors and social workers trying to search out information on, for example, meeting times and places of special interest groups appropriate to invidividuals they are trying to help. If a small team can be specially employed to build up a library of such information and have it available as a telephone, postal or call-in service, it can help provide a much more efficient service.

Robert Gann (1983) has described how the Regional Health Authority set up such a service called 'Help for Health'. It provides patients and all health and welfare workers with accurate and up-to-date information on voluntary organisations. It is especially helpful to health visitors. There is also a wealth of educational material available to both professionals and patients.

Some health visitors accumulate their own small library of favourite reference books which they can lend, for brief periods, to the families they visit (see Ch. 4, Table 4.1 and Ch. 5, Box 5.1).

Discussion and support groups

There are other ways health visitors can share their discovery of useful literature. For example, some meet on a regular basis, perhaps with allied professionals, in order to tell each other of research findings and new ideas that have come to their notice. Working with colleagues on exploratory studies or new projects can also stimulate further thought on how to respond to people's needs. Where they exist, research liaison officers could be invited to help think through ideas for setting up local research into aspects of health visiting.

Clulow (1982, p. 80–99) and Vizard (1983) have described how health visitors meeting together as a support group has helped them cope with, and gain a better insight into, their day-to-day work. Sharing some of their difficult experiences with sympathetic colleagues can lead to new depths of understanding on how to help families. Refresher courses and classes, such as those aimed at improving counselling skills, are also ways of gaining knowledge in order to improve practice.

This section has looked at sources of information for decision-making on priorities and for the knowledge needed for day-to-day work. Both of them are basic to the practice of health visiting and are categorised and shown as 'background information' at the top of Figure 2.1.

PREPARING FOR THE VISIT

INFORMATION—PRIOR TO THE VISIT

Before health visitors can call on any particular family, they need to know where to call and to have, if at all possible, at least an outline of the family size and age structure. Prior warning of any particular needs there might be, means that some forethought can be given to the sort of assistance that might be offered. This information, acquired before the visit and seen in the second grouping in Figure 2.1, shows records, referrals and liaison as important sources of information.

Health visitor records

Record cards give incoming health visitors a picture of the families currently being visited. The cards tend to be filed by one of the following:
— street and neighbourhood
— family surname, in alphabetical order
— age of the youngest child in each family.
Whichever system or combination of systems is chosen, the aim is to facilitate plans to make more frequent visits to families with younger babies and to save time by visiting people living fairly close to each other. Sometimes small sections of the file are set aside for families who for some reason might benefit from more frequent visiting, such as one with a handicapped member.

Annual 'birth books' are used by many health visitors to list, month by month, the births that have occurred within the caseload. These lists make an excellent quick guide to the babies due for hearing tests and other assessments falling at a particular age.

Administrative schemes and referrals

Some Districts use computers for making appointments for developmental assessment and/or for their immunisation programmes. These schemes make it easy to inform health visitors of the families who, for example, have missed three appointments. Follow-up visits can then be arranged.

Notification of the birth enables the District Health Authority to send a health visitor record card for each baby on the GP list of 'attached' health visitors and each one born in the 'geographic patch' of those who are not. There are not such clear-cut arrangements for those who were born outside the area and have 'transferred in'. 'Attached' health visitors may have a special arrangement with the practice manager to have, for example, families newly added to the GPs' practice listed in a notebook. In many cases the newly moved in families may be unknown to the health visitor until the old notes are sent on from the previous area. Getting to know about elderly people is different again and is discussed elsewhere (Robertson, 1984).

Liaison

Where a family is known to the
— midwife
— social worker
— district nurse
— liaison health visitor
— general practitioner
— community psychiatric nurse
— voluntary worker or
— some other agency,
it might be helpful to meet or phone so that, within the rules of confidentiality (see Ch. 8), the situation may be discussed. Contact with other people working with the family lessens the chance of conflicting advice and gives the benefit of the other worker's perspective of the family's needs. However, care needs to be taken that when professionals work in concert like this, they do not become so united in their plan of action that they then take no account of their clients' perspectives and wishes.

In this small section we have had an introduction to the main sources of information acquired before the visit, that is, through records, referral and liaison. These will be touched on again in subsequent chapters.

THE VISIT

A major part of the activity in the health visitor cycle takes place during the visit itself and many interacting factors are at work. For this reason, this section is the longest. Three important elements of success are identified and each is discussed in depth. The two main information sources are, as shown in Figure 2.1, the client's opinion and viewpoint, and the health visitor's own observations.

INFORMATION—WHILST VISITING

The health visitor arrives at a first visit to, for example, a family with young children, a handicapped member or an old person, having given a grading of priority, as explained above, to their potential need for preventive health care. Depending on the depth of information on the family that is available, some ideas will have been formed on the sort of help that might be offered. These are tentative objectives for the visit, but they may be altered radically during the meeting, once the family's own perspective is taken into account and an 'on site' assessment has been possible.

These factors—the client viewpoint and the health visitor's observations—equate, in the health visitor cycle, to the 'subjective' and 'observed' or so called 'objective' elements of the SOAP model of the nursing process (see Ch. 8, p. 140).

The client viewpoint

A great deal is being written now on the importance of client opinion and involvement (Warnock Report, 1978; Department of Health and Social Security and Child Poverty Action Group, 1978; National Children's Bureau, 1981; Dowling, 1983). Health care is no longer seen as something which is 'done *to* people'. Client or parental views and feelings provide what is, basically, the most important information for the health visitor. It is the main springboard from which to begin to plan possible ways of offering help. The Children's Committee (1980) proposed, for example, that parents and professionals should have a partnership in which there is:
— regard for the parents' key position in the life of the child
— sensitivity to the family's social and cultural situation
— parental understanding of the services and
— encouragement for parents helping parents.

In writing about teaching and learning, Elizabeth Perkins (1980) drew attention to the two way processes involved, the need for professional sensitivity to the particular needs of each individual and the central contribution of the parent in preparatory education for childbirth and parenthood.

Health visitor observations

People's beliefs and attitudes are not communicated by the spoken word alone. Betty Raymond (1983) describes how non-verbal signs convey information to the health visitor. The way a door is opened, clothing and general appearance, posture, gesture and mannerisms, facial expression, eye contact and tone of voice, all give an impression of how people are feeling and their approach to life.

It might please some to think of the health visitor as an objective observer of these matters. The fact is, as Betty Raymond points out, there may be several possible interpretations of any given gesture or action. Social science research has shown the inevitability of personal bias. Health visitors as observers are not exempt. The way they view what happens at a visit will be heavily influenced by their background, their training and their various preconceptions. Equally, the behaviour and style of the health visitor also creates an impression, and itself influences the way people feel and act.

Some of the visible information available to health visitors, such as babies' weight and appearance, presents more clear-cut evidence. This type of evidence is likely to be perceived in the same terms by all the parties involved and is not so open to misinterpretation.

There are, of course, enormous limits on the extent to which health visitors may observe the physical surroundings in which they find themselves. They are guests in people's homes and their demeanour needs to be appropriate to the situation. They may not, for example, feel free to allow their gaze to wander around the room, in case this is interpreted as an inspection—and even, perhaps, an intrusion upon privacy. Raymond mentions the need for clients to feel accepted. A non-patronising, non-

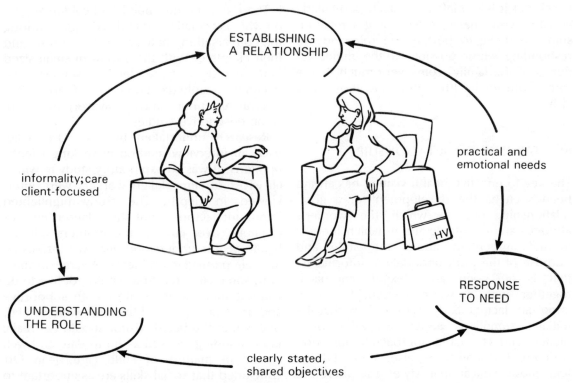

Fig. 2.4 Elements of success in communicating health needs.

judgemental relationship in which the people being visited really feel they are, and are being treated as, equals, is the key to this.

There is sometimes talk of 'seeing people as they really are' as a consequence of the health visitor's calling unexpectedly. However, the Rcn Health Visitors Advisory Group (1983) felt that 'checking up' on people or 'catching them unawares' and other aspects of what might be seen as 'social policing', are no part of the health visitor's role. Appointments systems can help avoid this problem.

There will be an attempt to show, in the rest of this section, that successful communication between the health visitor and the family about health needs and problems, depends mainly on the three interdependent and inter-linked factors depicted in Figure 2.4. These are the quality of the relationship, the extent to which the role is understood and the sort of help that is given. Each is considered in depth.

It could be said that they are, all three, an essential part of all health visiting. However, I feel that it is in making contact, particularly at a first visit, that (i) establishing a relationship, (ii) trying to portray the role and (iii) responding, where possible, to the immediate needs of the family, come very much to the fore—both for health visitors and those they visit.

(i) ESTABLISHING A RELATIONSHIP

The key to effective health visiting has always been seen as the development of a good relationship, one in which the worker's attitudes are acceptable and in which there is mutual agreement about the style and purpose of the work undertaken. Informality, that is an open and flexible approach, together with a warm personality, seem important factors. Early records show that the initial assumptions about the value of a didactic and 'charitable' approach to the work, were rapidly found to be false. A less didactic and more educational style was therefore adopted (Owen, 1983).

More recently, the working party for the Council for the Education and Training of Health Visitors (1977) suggested that establishment of a relationship was central to the discovery of health needs. The working party felt there was a need for adequate time and, in the main, regular contact, in order to achieve this.

Currently, there is a great deal of interest in ways in which the techniques of interpersonal communication and social skills may, or may not, be learned. Discussion is also emerging about the wider implications for health visitor–client relationships.

The evidence

There are two main ways in which to investigate the relationship between health visitors and the members of the families they visit. One way is to observe and/or tape record what actually happens. The other is to ask participants to describe it.

There is very little published evidence, yet, on what is actually said and takes place during the conversations between health visitors and their clientele. With the advent of small sized tape recorders, quite detailed studies have become possible (Dingwall, 1977; Clark, 1984). Several are under way. However, there are some descriptive studies.

Research undertaken by Jean Orr (1980) used an interview method in seeking clients' opinions. It was an exploratory study in which 68 wives of semi-skilled workers were interviewed in depth. The study highlighted important factors about the relationship. For example, over 80% of the mothers felt the health visitor understood and was interested in their particular problems. A large proportion, some 66%, felt they would not like to do without their health visitor. Both supportive and practical aspects of the work were valued, that is that the health visitor should be 'really understanding' as well as up to date and well versed in matters of child care. Jean Orr concluded that social skills are as important to health visitors as is their knowledge base.

Virtually all the women felt that home visits brought no disgrace: association with the health visitor carries no stigma. Many preferred home visiting as it gave more time than was available at the clinic and it was easier to talk openly.

A few mothers were felt to have used appeasing tactics, telling health visitors 'what they wanted to hear'. One explanation suggested was that the mothers might be using this strategy as a way of protecting their personal integrity.

The vast majority would have preferred prior notice of visiting. One of the reasons put forward by the mothers was that they would not feel at a disadvantage if they were able to get ready first. Some saw the value of having the opportunity to prepare questions.

Stereotyping and anxiety

Eighteen mothers in Orr's study felt that an 'ideal health visitor' would be married and have children. Marjory Adams' (1982) personal experience of the helpfulness of a childless, unmarried health visitor, led her to propose that this stereotyped opinion is misplaced. She said that merely having children does not make a person more feeling and thoughtful towards others, and suggested too, that indiscriminate complaining about health visitors often reflects the speaker's own anxieties and inadequacies regarding parenthood. Whatever the basic cause, health visitors should always try to discover their own part in any customer dissatisfaction. The suggestion does remind us, however, as does the example in Clulow's study discussed later in this chapter (p. 27), that the health visitor–client relationship is not always a simple one.

Early motherhood

Field et al (1982) interviewed 78 women. A third were early in their first pregnancy and a third were newly delivered of their first baby. The rest had a first baby of 12–15 months. These researchers also found the same stereotyping about childless health visitors.

Most of the mothers were happy with their health visitor.
Valued attributes were:
— readiness to answer questions
— speedy response to requests for help
— preparedness to listen to problems
— boosting confidence in mothering abilities
— friendliness and
— approachability.
Health visitors who were not liked tended to be seen as:
— interfering
— out of touch
— unsympathetic and
— authoritative.
Again, social skills and relationship play an important part.

Interviewing women from the chosen three stages of early motherhood enabled the researchers to see the value of getting to know the health visitor in the antenatal period, a matter taken up at the beginning of the next chapter.

Observations of style

An American researcher (Mayers, 1973) observed the conversations between public health nurses and some of their patients. It was found that whatever the nurses' style of intervention, whether it was information giving, directive or non-directive (or any mixture of the three), each nurse maintained the same individual interactional style for everyone visited. Whichever the approach, a positive and involved response from the patient was found to relate to the extent to which the nurse paid attention to the patient's point of view.
'Patient-focused nurses'
— demonstrated a sense of concern
— showed personal interest
— engendered a feeling of mutuality in the relationship
— gave the opportunity for their patients to be involved in decisions about solutions to their problems.
'Nurse-focused nurses', on the other hand, reacted to patient initiatives by interpreting

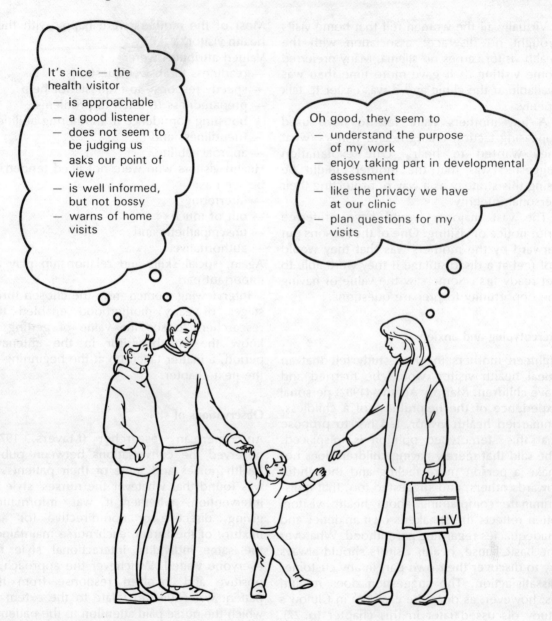

Fig. 2.5 A good relationship.

them according to their own point of view or frame of reference. These nurses relied on their own perspective too, for decisions on solutions to patients' problems.

The sort of relationships that work well have been discussed and listed (see Fig. 2.5), but how do they come about? How can they be achieved?

Some theories

The way people feel and behave towards each other involves deep labyrinths of intricate variation, far too complex for a single, simple explanation. There are, however, a number of useful theories which provide a degree of partial understanding, by piecing together certain observed patterns of behaviour. Many of them are of interest to health visitors. For example, there are the theories on learning and group behaviour and explanations of child abuse.

Eric Berne (1968) likens social transactions between people to games, pastimes, rituals and procedures. This theory provides very interesting and useful perspectives on social custom and practice. Both Berne and Harris (1973) believe that tendencies towards what they classify as the 'Parent', 'Adult' and 'Child' in people, is present in all our behaviour. Harris suggests that by understanding these processes, people can improve their quality of social interaction and attain an 'I'm OK— you're OK' approach to life.

Learning communication skills

Another theory suggests that social skills can be learned through practice, very much as can the motor skills of riding a bicycle or driving a car (Argyle, 1978). This notion has an important role in health visitor social skills training. Enid Lythgoe (1983) has described how communication skills are taught in the Leeds course, using role play and video equipment. With these, the students get feedback on their achievements as well as all the other benefits of experiential learning.

These communication skills are sometimes referred to as counselling skills. Courses aim, not at training professional counsellors, but at helping students develop particular aspects of interpersonal skills. It is hoped that these can be used to help facilitate people's understanding of their own view of their situation and enable them to explore and decide on possible solutions to their problems and needs. Also, all health education and supportive care has to be founded on and tailored to each individual's preconceptions and understanding. The need, therefore, to help people express these thoughts, permeates the whole of a health visitor's work.

Students are given hints on the sort of remarks that can detract from people's ability to give their view or explore their problem. It is generally suggested that untimely advice and opinion giving, and other strategies which draw attention away from the speaker, are best avoided in the early, exploratory stages when the problem or notion is being thought through. A warm, caring and unjudging manner is a basic necessity. Students discuss the sort of non-verbal stance and mannerisms that portray these attitudes.

Learning about these skills and the effect and implications of using them, can be achieved properly only through guided practice and through broadly-based discussion. As a back-up, there are several useful books on counselling and interpersonal skills which give, for example, a good introduction for nurses (Tschudin, 1982), suggest simple exercises to increase self-awareness and to develop particular skills (Munro et al, 1983), and provide a problem management model (Egan, 1981) and a discussion of research into the field alongside a description of the range of social skills needed (Hargie et al, 1981). Listening and questioning are key elements in counselling techniques. Examples of the advice that health visitor students might be given on how to help people to express themselves can be found on p. 26, Boxes 2.1 & 2.2.

It will be interesting to see to what extent these listening and questioning techniques are used in practice—and with what effect. Research is needed in the field because these techniques are so widely advocated. Some recently published, in which tape-recorded health visitor clinic conversation was studied (Warner, 1984), did not report on this specific issue. One of the health visitors in the project was found to be particularly skilled at getting the mothers to ask the 'right' question. However, the researcher was not able to see how she achieved this, despite the availability of the tape recording for analysis. Interpersonal skills do not seem to hinge on any simple and trite formula.

Kate Robinson (1983) is concerned that communication has now become a task to be performed on people. She suggests that treating talk with clients as a professional skill and seeing it as a 'problem', may detract from

Box 2.1 Listening—some points to remember

Environment
If possible, *choose* a situation reasonably
— free from distractions
— comfortable for both
— close to each other

Non-verbal responses
It may help to *show interest* by
— nodding your head in agreement and
  understanding
— using good eye contact
— indicating with 'A-ah' and 'M-mm' sounds that
  the client should continue to talk

Verbal responses
You may be able to *encourage* the client to continue
by
— echoing back last word/words e.g. 'I wish I'd
  called for mother' 'Mother?'
— reflecting back feelings e.g. use of analogy
(as the encounter continues)
— paraphrasing talk so far, perhaps summarising
— appropriate use of questioning
— making sensitive use of silence—to allow client
  thought to develop uninterrupted
You should be aware that you will *detract* from
the client's view or problem by
— stating your opinion
— giving advice—'if I were you . . .'
— over-sympathising—'me too . . .'
These draw attention away from your client and
towards you and your own perceptions and ideas

Box 2.2 Questioning—some points to remember

You may find it helpful to ask:
Open questions
which encourage your client to take the lead in the
dialogue, for example
— How . . . .
— What . . . .
— In what way . . . .
— When . . . .
— How do you feel about . . . .
Your approach should neither be, nor sound,
  inquisitorial
Care should be taken that your questions are
  geared only for the benefit of the client and not,
  for example, to satisfy your curiosity or any other
  matter centred on yourself

You should be aware of the effect of:
Leading questions
indicating particular conclusions, e.g.
— Don't you think that . . . .

Closed questions
able to be answered by 'Yes' or 'No', e.g.
— Would you like to . . . .
— Do you get . . . .
These questions can tend to shut off conversation
and limit client talk

the basic issue of whether or not the conversation and the visit has relevance and value to the participants.

Relationship and clarity about role are linked

The relationship between health visitors and the people they visit necessarily affects the way their role is understood by those families. Both client-focused care and informality are shown in Figure 2.4 as linking factors. Obviously, people who have an involved and participating interaction with their health visitor, will gain direct insight. Working together 'in partnership' means aims and intentions are explained on both sides. As the subsequent health visiting is based on the clients' wishes and perspectives, it is naturally more meaningful, more value to them and better understood.

Similarly, the feeling of informality and

approachability in a good, supportive relationship leads to a closeness in which wider purposes of the visit and the function of a health visitor can be more readily discussed. A brief introduction to the role is, of course, all that can be hoped for on a first visit.

(ii) UNDERSTANDING THE ROLE

'Role' in this context means 'one's function, what (a) person is appointed or expected to do' (Oxford Dictionary). The role in health visiting is a particularly broad one. The Mayston Committee (1969) listed some 60 separate and varied aspects of the work. Just a glance at this formidable description shows it is no easy task to give clients a succinct résumé. More commonly used, shorter descriptions, for example those by the Council for the Education and Training of Health Visitors (1967, 1977), have tended to be broad and non-specific. Alison Norman (1982) says that in her explanations to clients she concentrates on the more practical aspects of the work. These are likely to be much easier for people to understand (see Mayers (1973), later in this chapter on p. 29).

The Health Visitor Association has produced a colourful and practically based pamphlet which can be used on visits to give clients an idea of the health visitor's role. Ann Stanton (1982) suggested that a tailor-made hand-out could be made up by health visitors where no suitable one is available. Not everyone feels such pamphlets are necessary (Schofield, 1982) and many health visitors rely on demonstrating their role through their work.

Research findings

Research on the way health visiting is perceived has looked at three aspects: client opinion, psychological explanations about role, and the way a changing role may be emerging with recent policy and structural changes.

Mothers' opinions

About 80% of the mothers Jean Orr (1980) interviewed knew their health visitor by name. The locally used visiting card may have helped this. The card also stated nursing and midwifery qualifications, but this does not seem to have prevented the health visitors from being perceived as social workers or 'a lady from the welfare', almost as often as a nurse.

All of the mothers in this sample had one pre-school child. The health visitors' work was seen, therefore, in terms of care for children. Over a third seemed unaware of any function pertaining to other members of the family. However, a very wide variety of health and welfare aspects of care were mentioned as having been discussed with the health visitors.

Jean Orr drew attention to the health visitors' use of tact and discretion in advice giving. This and their style of helping people to come to their own conclusions, naturally means that their contribution is not always fully evident to their clients. Health visitors face the dilemma of wanting to make their role understood but, at the same time, finding it necessary to provide a self-effacing and background style which itself makes too many assertive statements about the work impracticable.

Ascribed role

In a study of the effects on marriage of the first baby and preparation for parenthood, Clulow (1982) set up workshops where health visitors could discuss issues arising out of their work with such couples. Clulow said that often families who wanted help had mixed feelings about whether they really did want it. Others who clearly wanted it, were unsure of what help they needed and therefore what role their health visitor should perform. The ambivalence, it seems, could be conveyed in a variety of ways, through both overt and covert communications. Clulow showed how parents might ascribe a role for the health visitor, of which neither she nor the couple were aware.

In an example (pp. 83–5) a health visitor had been chided by a new parent she was visiting over her own abilities as a mother, and was made to feel an inadequate parent. Clulow said these parents had needed the health visitor, not as an expert in child care, but as 'the parent who was found wanting'. He went on to say that they had been comparing themselves against a model of ideal parenthood. He suggested that the 'ascribed health visitor role', by comparison, helped to reduce their anxiety and contributed to building up their confidence.

Many inherent complexities in the role were discussed by Clulow. He felt ideas about the role should not be too rigidly interpreted, in order to give scope for health visitors to be involved with and have better understanding of the people they visit.

Administrative effects on function

The role of the health visitor is to provide a service offering advice and help which families are free to accept or reject as they wish. Dingwall (1982) suggests that the success and continuance of health visiting depend on this non-authoritarian style of dealing with people. Having studied health visiting in depth (Dingwall, 1977; Dingwall et al, 1981), he observed that close supervision and detailed accountability, which tend to be associated with a bureaucratic hierarchy, can undermine this relationship and muzzle professional freedom to react towards clients in the traditional intuitive way. There have been administrative changes in recent years towards a more hierarchical structure for health visiting.

Jane Robinson (1982a) feels that the voluntary relationship that exists between health visitors and those they visit, one in which advice from the so called 'expert' may be accepted or rejected, may be under threat. She is apprehensive about the implications of some recent reports from governmental committees. They urge child health workers to take various initiatives to 'persuade' people to attend clinics and to take other steps towards activities that might be regarded as coercion and as 'social policing'. Structured visiting programmes and 'checking up' on people have both been mentioned earlier in this chapter.

Role and response to need are linked

Clearly stated and shared objectives are shown at the bottom of Figure 2.4 as linking factors. People being visited can understand the role better if the aims and intentions of the health visitor can be made quite clear. Understanding these enables clients to be consulted on and involved in any proposed course of action. Actions mutually decided upon are both more acceptable and meaningful and, themselves, lead to a greater appreciation and understanding of the part played by health visitors.

(iii) RESPONDING TO NEED

Ways that health visitors may be able to help people are discussed in greater detail in most of the later chapters. This section looks at the processes involved in carrying out the work, particularly at the setting of objectives, and draws on some research findings.

The studies

The ways in which health visitors respond to people's health requirements need, of course, to be as effective as possible and to be felt by the people involved to be useful and worth trying. Several research projects have studied health visitors' attempts to respond to people's needs. These have involved short-term, regular visiting, problem and relationship-based responses, and the need for clear explanations about, and agreement on, short-term goals.

Short-term regular visits

In research into the evaluation of health visiting, Karen Luker (1982) looked at the way goals for the work might be measured against results. The study looked at the effect of four consecutive monthly visits on samples of elderly ladies (see Luker, 1982, Ch. 7, pp. 117, 119–120). A significant improvement in their problems was found to have occurred. Much of this was maintained at least six months after visiting ceased.

Two approaches

Looking at young mothers' perceptions of health visiting (see earlier this chapter, page 23), Jean Orr (1980) identified two basic health visiting responses to their needs. These were, firstly, practical aspects such as advice giving and developmental checks and, secondly, relationship-based responses such as willingness to listen to problems and giving support. These were partially mirrored in Jane Robinson's (1982b) study of non-attendance at developmental assessment sessions, as she felt that the health visitors caring for the people in her small sample tended to polarise towards either one or the other of the above approaches to health visiting. To what extent this polarisation is common in the practice of health visiting is not known.

Robinson found failure to attend at clinics tended to be related to the parents' seeing the service as an agency of social control. The case of one mother, 'Mrs Graham', serves very well as an example. She very much resented her first health visitor 'prying' into her private life. Enquiries were made about her husband's income and employment and their food supplies. This discourteous health visitor was asked not to return. Their next health visitor was very friendly–she maintained a low profile and was consulted by 'Mrs Graham' (p. 79). Jane Robinson suggested the first of the health visitors had a 'problem-oriented' approach, whilst the second had a 'relationship-centred' one.

The health visitors in Orr's sample tended to give the mothers satisfaction and seemed to have been functioning from an adequate knowledge base, which gave them the ability to respond to the mothers' requirements. Robinson's 'problem-oriented' health visitor may well have worked from a predetermined list of items, based rather more on bureaucratic notions than on what the family saw as problems. The second was much more sensitive to family feelings and priorities–and was much more effective in being able to provide a preventive health service.

Conversations studied

In her study of health visitor conversations in clinics, Una Warner (1984) showed agreement on goals was associated with success in the work. She found these goals were explained and negotiated in the normal course of conversation.

Marlene Mayers (1973) in her research into public health nurse–patient conversations found that patients who had a better understanding of how the nurse was aiming to help, were those who were cared for by the nurses who thought theoretically mostly in terms of specific, short-range goals–'keep six weeks appointment' or 'get needed medical care'.

Where nurses explained objectives to the researcher in more abstract ideas of personal–social goals—'adjustment to new culture' or 'achieve stable home life'—there was a lower level of understanding by the patients.

Objectives

Aims, goals, plans, intentions and objectives are words commonly used in health visiting to describe what is proposed and what it is hoped to achieve. A time-scale dimension is sometimes used. An example suggesting long- and short-term and immediate objectives is set out in Table 2.1. Intermediate plans for the medium term, many months or a year ahead, become relatively short-term when visiting is infrequent. For this reason, they have not been assigned a special category.

Table 2.1 Time-scale for health visiting objectives

Objectives	Concerned with	Examples
Immediate	Current meeting	Answering queries that arise during the visit Informing family of appropriate services available
Short-term	Present and near future	That the infant receives the full course of immunisations That the mother understands the basic principles of weaning
Long-term	Philosophical aims	That the family attain their full potential for social, mental and physical health Early discovery of family health needs

Long-term objectives in this model include the broad-based, largely unattainable ideals for which to aim. These describe the purpose of health visiting and provide the philosophical framework within which the more tangible and practical objectives are set. It is debatable as to whether these philosophical ideals are better classified as 'aims' or as 'objectives'.

If short-term objectives are made clear and immediate objectives are tailored to what the family feels is important, then client understanding of the aims of health visiting and the extent to which the health visitor can help the family are all likely to be enhanced. This is especially important when making initial contact with the family, such as at a first visit.

The health visitor cycle

Deciding on objectives for a family's care is a complex matter. Three of the sources of information that can help make these decisions—background knowledge and those sources available prior to and during the visit—have already been discussed. The sequences of thought in the health visitor cycle (Fig. 2.1) are, of course, the same as for the nursing process and any other form of management by objectives. These are that an assessment has to be made, based on the information available, so that plans or objectives can be drawn up and put into action. Evaluation and further planning follows. In intuitive, creative activities and in all everyday decision-making, the same processes are gone through but in an unplanned, informal sort of way.

Families are highly individual and present a diversity of environmental and social situations. Also, seemingly routine conversations constantly introduce new notions and perspectives. This brings a need for wide variation in and continually changing objectives. The advantage of the health visitor cycle, as a framework, is that it concentrates on the *sources* of changing ideas—the origins of the subsequent processes of planning and implementation. It has the benefit, too, of being able to highlight the clients' opinions.

Inevitably, objectives have to be founded on inadequate knowledge, but that is a problem common to most spheres of management and decision-making. It is a question of making the best possible use of what is available, and being prepared to vary objectives as new information comes to light.

A checklist

A working party in Northumberland (McClymont, 1983) set out to draw up a standard for measuring health visiting practice (see Ch. 8). They aimed to list criteria for the first visit to a family with a new baby (p. 9–12). It was hoped these items would provide a framework within which help could be given.

They listed statements (p. 7) about the purpose of health visiting and its objectives in general, philosophical terms similar to those Marlene Mayers had found were not satisfactorily explained to, nor understood by the people visited.

Lists of specific items were drawn up. These included:
— factors that should be known prior to the visit
— observations and examinations deemed necessary during the visit and
— matters needing to be clarified.

Some of these 'criteria' would convert quite well into easily understood short-term or immediate objectives for the time-scale model shown in Table 2.1, for example, 'clarification' of the method and routine of feeding and the infant's behaviour, or the suggestions for a physical examination of the baby. The lists had good and poor points and are returned to in Chapter 4.

Health visitor style

Care has to be taken that a predetermined checklist of objectives does not dominate health visitor thought and become counter-productive. A good relationship and sensitivity to the wishes of the family could well prove to be the most important of all objectives.

Figure 2.6 shows a continuum of possible health visitor intention and style. At one end, lack of well thought-out objectives would be likely to result in a confused client, wondering about the purposes of the service.

At the other extreme, where pre-set objectives are rigidly and unthinkingly adhered to, the response would more likely be one of irritation and a strong suspicion of 'social policing'—the experience of 'Mrs Graham'!

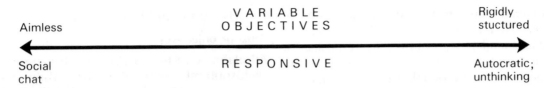

Fig. 2.6 A continuum of possible approaches. A range of health visitor method is shown above the line, whilst below is health visitor style.

In the central range, health visiting is able to respond to clients' wishes, as far as this is possible. Being prepared to vary objectives gives the opportunity for both practical and supportive care, according to what seems to be needed.

Limits on response

Whatever objectives may be drawn up and planned, there are limits on time, and choices have to be made. Jane Schofield (1982) points out that it is *quality* and not quantity that is central to the work. Particularly in places with large numbers of problems, such as inner city areas, some aspects of the work will have to be foregone, in order to provide an adequate depth of service for those with outstanding need.

Karen Luker's study of old people's problems showed focused health visiting, regular and concentrated over a few months, to be productive. Fears about shallow, 'doorstep-hopping health visiting' were mentioned earlier in this chapter (p. 17).

Response to need and relationship are linked

This section has looked at research on approaches to responding to people's health needs. Once again client opinion needs to be central, this time with regard to planning objectives. If health visitors are able to respond to requirements of a practical nature and to the emotional needs of the people they visit (the linking factors shown to the right in Figure 2.4), then this is likely to be appreciated and to further improve the health visitor–client relationship.

In summary, it is the proceedings during the visit itself which should most influence decisions on how best to help the family. The main information source is the people themselves. Encouragement and explanation by the health visitor can play an important part. There needs to be great sensitivity to non-verbal and other signs which express needs and wishes.

Relationship, role and response are all basic and, in many ways, inseparable parts of health visiting. Running through them all is the need for involvement for the client, and for the health visitor, approachability, responsiveness, well thought-out objectives and a flexible and adaptable style. All these are, of course, necessary throughout all aspects of health visiting, but it is obvious that they are urgently required when making contact at a first visit.

PLANS FOR SUBSEQUENT VISITS

Many of the objectives for further visits result from an evaluation of the meeting and discussion with the client. Short-term objectives form an important part in the planning process of the health visitor cycle. Longer-term objectives, more concerned with the underlying philosophical aims of health visiting (see Table 2.1), may rarely be achieved. They can, however, provide useful guidelines and pointers for planning the more day-to-day aspects of the work.

During the visit, several immediate objectives will probably have been achieved. For example, in a first visit it is likely that there would have been explanations about health visiting and how the health visitor can be contacted. There may have been provision of information about local health and welfare services and/or a response to requests for advice and discussion of various issues of importance to the people being visited.

SHORT-TERM OBJECTIVES

As these immediate objectives are identified and, hopefully, satisfied, other objectives come to light in the course of the conversation. Short-term objectives, those concerning matters which will need attention either between this visit and the next, or at some subsequent visit, can be agreed between the parties. For example, the health visitor may promise to return with information on some special topic or problem. There might be plans for a list of queries to be jotted down by the client as they are thought of, so they can be discussed at the next visit.

Another future goal might be assessment of a baby's developmental progress or of an old person's functional ability. These matters might be noted on the record card and/or in the health visitor's diary.

Client perspective

An assessment of the visit will be being made by *all* the participants involved. Both during and after the visit, the health visitors and people they visit will give some thought to how to approach the next encounter in the light of how this one is perceived. These and other assessments of health visiting are very important. However, evaluation is a very complex matter. It is returned to in Chapter 8. The significant point in this discussion about planning objectives for future visits, is that the clients' evaluation and perspectives are clearly important. These need to be understood for the health visitor's work—be it discussions, explanations, assessment or referral—to be either relevant or useful.

It is not easy to assess people's true feelings, but the better the relationship, as already described above, the greater the likelihood of success.

LONG-TERM OBJECTIVES

Aims or objectives

All planning in health visiting is based on the philosophical aim of the work. These have been expressed in different ways. In the time-scale model for health visiting objectives in Table 2.1, these are classified as long-term objectives. This could include, for example, McClymont's (1983, p. 7) list of aims of health visiting

— promoting overall health and preventing disease
— concern with developing and continuing professional help
— assessment of health and ability to cope
— provision of health education

or the Council for the Education and Training of Health Visitors' (1977) four basic principles:

— search for health needs
— stimulation of the awareness of health needs
— influence of policies affecting health
— facilitation of health-enhancing activities.

The prevention model

The health visitor role model in Table 1.2 may provide a particularly useful basis for thinking about overall and long-term objectives. Its three basic aims are described in Chapter 1:

1. *Preventing occurrence* of conditions or problems
2. *Preventing development* of conditions or problems
3. *Preventing deterioration* of established conditions.

This framework can be used to cover the main practical and everyday aspects of the work and can readily convert into more specific longer-term objectives. For example:

1. *Preventing occurrence* of conditions or problems:
   — improvement of the local environment, e.g. smoke-free zones in public places
   — to provide health education, e.g. on safety, nutrition, immunisation and welfare rights
2. *Preventing development* of conditions or problems:

— to seek conditions which will benefit from early attention, e.g. hearing and visual defects, funtional disability in old people, developmental delay in babies, and family emotional problems

3. *Preventing deterioration* of established conditions:
   — to enable clients to express and talk through their problems
   — to help clients know which agency can offer appropriate help
   — to encourage and facilitate emerging self-help groups.

This model also seems capable of providing a guiding framework for some short-term and immediate objectives specific to a particular family. Under '2. *Preventing development* of conditions or problems', for example, can be derived:

— to explain six month developmental assessment to parents
— to involve parents in noting down developmental attainments
— to answer queries raised by these discussions
— to undertake developmental testing, by appointment.

It can be seen that the concepts in this model are pragmatically based. They can tie in with those in the family health needs model, the format used in the following two and some later chapters. They provide a useful basis for planning future encounters in practical terms which could be easily understood by the families involved, as the example in the paragraph above demonstrates.

To conclude, contact has been made and plans are under way for future meetings. By the next visit there may be more information available from the several sources described in this chapter. For example, at the level of background information new pamphlets and other literature may be acquired and, later, used to help a family understand a difficult problem. Liaison with other workers between the visits may give rise to useful guidance.

It is quite likely that by the next visit the clients' circumstances will have changed in some way and some new objectives will need to be drawn up. Mostly, however, the basic and fundamental theme of the objectives tends to remain fairly constant, especially with regard to the underlying long-term philosophical aims and objectives which run throughout this book.

A repeated theme in this chapter has been the need for client involvement and understanding. The importance of a good working relationship, comprehension of role and appropriate response to need, have been demonstrated. The health visitor cycle was proposed as a way of thinking about planning processes. It draws attention to and concentrates on the various sources of information on which health visiting decisions are made—including those when first making contact.

USEFUL ADDRESS

Help for Health
Wessex Regional Library Unit
South Academic Block
Southampton General Hospital
Southampton SO9 4XY
Tel 0703 779091

REFERENCES

Adams M 1982 Health visitors—a tribute from a mother. Health Visitor 55:661
Argyle M 1978 The psychology of interpersonal behaviour, 3rd ed. Penguin Books, London, p. 63
Barber J H, Boothman R, Stanfield J P 1976 A new visual chart for preschool developmental screening. Health Bulletin 34: 80–91
Berne E 1968 Games people play. Penguin Books, London
The Children's Committee 1980 The needs of under fives in the family. The Children's Committee, London

Clark J 1984 Recording health visitor-client interaction in home visits. Health Visitor 57: 5–8
Clulow C F 1982 To have and to hold. Marriage and the first baby and preparing couples for parenthood. Aberdeen University Press, Aberdeen
Council for the Education and Training of Health Visitors 1967 The function of the health visitor. CETHV, London
Council for the Education and Training of Health Visitors 1977 An investigation into the principles of health visiting. CETHV, London, p. 31

Cumberlege Report 1986 Neighbourhood nursing—a focus for care. Report of the Community Nursing Review. Department of Health and Social Security, HMSO, London

Department of Health and Social Security and Child Poverty Action Group 1978 Reaching the consumer in the antenatal and child health services. Report of the conference, April 1978. DHSS CPAG, London

Dingwall R 1977 The social organisation of health visitor training. Croom Helm, London, p. 109

Dingwall R 1982 Community nursing and civil liberty. Journal of Advanced Nursing 7: 337–346

Dingwall R, Eekelaar J, Murray T 1981 Care or control. Decision-making in the care of children thought to have been abused or neglected. A summary of the final report. Social Science Council Centre for Socio-Legal Studies, Wolfson College, Oxford

Dingwall R, Eekelaar J, Murray T 1983 The protection of children: state intervention and family life. Basil Blackwell, Oxford

Dowling S 1983 Health for a change. The provision of preventive health care in pregnancy and early childhood. Child Poverty Action Group in association with National Extension College

Dunnell K, Dobbs J 1982 Nurses working in the community. HMSO, London

Egan G 1982 The skilled helper, 2nd ed. Brooks/Cole Publishing Company, Monterey, California

Field S, Draper J, Kerr M, Hare M J 1982 A consumer view of the health visiting service. Health Visitor 55: 299–301

Fitton J M 1983 Policy constraints on HV practice (letter). Health Visitor 56: 229 Fitton J M 1984a Health visiting the elderly: nurse managers' views. One. Nursing Times Occasional Paper No 10 80, 16: 59–61

Fitton J M 1984b Health visiting the elderly: nurse managers' views. Two. Nursing Times Occasional Paper No 11 80, 17: 67–69

Gann R 1983 It's your line to the health computer. Health and Social Services Journal XCIII: 782–783

Goodwin S 1982 A partnership to promote self help. Nursing Mirror 155, 24: 63–65

Hargie O, Saunders C, Dickson D 1981 Social skills in interpersonal communication. Croom Helm, London

Harris T A 1973 I'm OK—you're OK, Pan Books, London

Health Visitor 1982 The need for a national inquiry into the proper role and functions of health visitors and school nurses (editorial). Health Visitor 55: 445

Health Visitor 1983 Quality visits, not quantity (editorial). Health Visitor 56:225

Hunt M 1982 New approaches in health visiting 3: Caseload profiles: their implications for evaluating health visiting practice. Health Visitor 55: 662–665

Irving D 1983 How statistics can plot areas of need. Health and Social Services Journal XCIII: 1262–1263

Jack S 1983 Research and vital statistics for the health visitor. In: Owen G (ed) Health visiting, 2nd ed. Bailliere Tindall, London

Jarman B 1983 Identification of under-priviledged areas. British Medical Journal 286: 1705–1709

Luker K A 1982 Evaluating health visiting practice. Royal College of Nursing, London

Lythgoe E J 1983 Teaching health visitor students to communicate. Health Visitor 56: 368–369

McClymont A 1983 Setting standards in health visiting practice. National Board for Nursing, Midwifery and Health Visiting for Scotland, Edinburgh

MacFarlane of Llandaff 1982 Responsibility for the future development of health visiting. Health Visitor 55: 273–277

Mayers M 1973 Home visit—ritual or therapy? Nursing Outlook 21. 5: 328–331

Mayston Committee 1969 Report of the Working Party on Management Structure in the Local Authority Nursing Services Department of Health and Social Security, London (Chairman E L Mayston).

Metcalfe D 1983 Trends in the utilisation of the National Health Service. Journal of the Royal College of General Practitioners 33: 615–617

Munro E A, Manthei R J, Small J J 1983 Counselling. A skills approach. Methuen, Auckland, New Zealand

National Children s Bureau 1981 Parents as partners. Intervention schemes and group work with parents of handicapped children. National Children's Bureau, London

Norman A 1982 When sticky plaster is not enough (letter). Nursing Mirror 154, 22: 22–24

Orr J 1980 Health visiting in focus. Royal College of Nursing, London. p 60–64

Orr J 1982 Health visiting in the U.K. In: Hockey L (ed) Primary care nursing. Churchill Livingstone, Edinburgh

Owen G 1983 The development of health visiting as a profession. In: Owen G (ed) Health visiting, 2nd ed. Bailliere Tindall, London, p 5

Perkins E 1980 Education for childbirth and parenthood. Croom Helm, London

Raymond E 1983 The skills of health visiting. In: Owen G (ed) Health visiting, 2nd ed. Bailliere Tindall, London

Robertson C A 1984 Old people in the community. One: Health visitors and preventive care. Nursing Times 80, 34: 29–31

Robinson J 1982a The health visitor—an authority on child rearing or an agent of social control? Health Visitor 55: 113–116

Robinson J 1982b An evaluation of health visiting. Council for the Education and Training of Health Visitors, London

Robinson J 1983 The role dilemma of health visiting. Health Visitor 56: 22–24

Robinson K 1983 Talking with clients. In: Clark J, Henderson J (eds) Community health. Churchill Livingstone, Edinburgh

Rcn Health Visitors Advisory Group 1983 Thinking about health visiting. Royal College of Nursing, London, p 46

Schofield J 1982 Health visiting—quality not quantity (letter). Nursing Mirror 155, 25:37

Schofield J 1983 Visiting can be stressful too. Nursing Mirror 157, 13: 20–21

Stanton A 1982 The listening, liaising, counselling health visitor. Nursing Mirror 155, 22: 57–59

Thompson J 1983 Health visiting: the quality does count (letter) Nursing Mirror 156, 7:18

Tschudin V 1982 Counselling skills for nurses. Bailliere Tindall, London

Vizard E 1983 Twenty months of Fridays — a support group for health visitors. Health Visitor 56: 255–256

Warner U 1984 Asking the right questions. Nursing Times Community Outlook 80, 24: 214–216

Warnock Report 1978 Report of the Committee of Enquiry into Education of Handicapped Children and Young People. Cmnd 7212, HMSO, London

Chapter 3 describes the value of antenatal health visiting and the importance of liaison. It looks at some of the environmental and physical health factors and mental/emotional and social aspects of family health which might receive attention during an antenatal visit.

3

Antenatal visiting

POLICIES AND PRIORITIES

Increasingly health visitors are encouraged to make contact during the antenatal period. These visits have been shown to be a very sound investment, particularly for the post-natal phase (Field et al, 1984), as they provide the opportunity to establish a good working relationship and as part of this, to explain about health visiting and, of course, to offer health education.

The relationship

In a small, in-depth study, an association was found between the extent of the contact with the health visitor in the antenatal period and the degree of support the women felt they had once the baby was born (Field et al, 1982a, 1982b). The researchers pointed out that a brief encounter or two is not enough to establish a good relationship. They found many of the mothers they interviewed had not met their health visitor before the birth of the baby. Two weeks into motherhood, a very vulnerable and emotional time in the adjustment to this new role, these mothers had to face setting up a new relationship with a total stranger.

Competing pressures

However, the ability to visit antenatally is limited for many health visitors by competing caseload priorities and pressures. For example, only 24 of the 40 interviewed in the Cambridgeshire study (Field et al, 1984) undertook antenatal visiting routinely. 14 health visitors did visit, but felt unable to provide this service for everyone.

One health visitor, on the other hand, made a habit of calling three times in pregnancy. It has been suggested that health visitors might aim for this level of antenatal visiting (Stanton, 1982). If, as it seems, the health visitors in Cambridgeshire find this difficult to put into action, then it is hardly surprising that Jane Schofield (1982), working in an inner city area, would find it quite out of the question!

Antenatal visits to first-time mothers were seen as important by the authors of 'Health Visiting in the Eighties' (Health Visitor, 1981). They assigned this aspect of our work even higher priority than the routine visiting of all children to school age. As most women work during their first pregnancy, visits during the earlier part may need to be in the evening, in order to fit in with patterns of work.

Uneven take-up

A review of research into antenatal services intended to prepare people for parenthood, showed them to be inadequate (Pugh, 1980, p. 24–28). The increasing popularity of the National Childbirth Trust and the large number of books on parenting that are now available, give a measure of public demand for, and recognition of, the importance of learning in this phase of life. However, these facilities, both books and antenatal classes, tend to be taken up by the middle classes, people who are likely to face fewer problems overall. Those who may be missing out, such as the very young, the unsupported and couples on low incomes, have a greater need for special initiatives by midwives, health visitors and volunteers.

SPECIAL SCHEMES

Pugh (1980, p. 80) called for professional workers in the field to become more involved

on two fronts: firstly, to provide support and encouragement to enable self-help groups to establish themselves fully and to tell parents about them; secondly, it is suggested help should be provided for particularly deprived families who would not normally join in self-help groups.

Collaboration with parents

One such scheme is currently being undertaken and the experiment assiduously monitored and assessed (Child Development Project, 1984, p. 17–18). It starts with monthly antenatal visiting of primiparae in disadvantaged areas by 'first-parent visitors' and continues for six months after the birth. These health visitors provide a specially designed supportive and collaborative service for which they are given special training.

The aim is to draw out and to develop the dormant potential in parents, rather than to make them dependent on the advice of the health visitor. In the second stage of the project these visitors have been assigned solely to this particular work. The aim is to ensure enough time for preventive and developmental work by removing them from the hurly-burly of responding to urgent calls, pressing clinics and other duties.

Six health authorities are taking part. An earlier phase of the project has shown significant achievements, particularly in raising both the confidence levels of the young parents and their ability to provide a good environment for their children (see also Ch. 5, p. 76).

Creativity and imagination

Sue Dowling (1983) has reported on a very wide range of recent initiatives. She has found that where services are specially modified to have regard for people's particular way of life, contact can be made remarkably easily with most families, even the most socially and economically deprived. Dowling points out that 'creativity' is the basic ingredient needed. She adds, however, that although there are plenty of imaginative workers in health care, apparently 'in the NHS there is some reluctance to recognise, promote and utilise this creativity for change' (p. 167).

Dr Dowling feels that the current emphasis on scientific management, concern with the evaluation and measurement of current practice, the cuts in budgets and the restructuring of the NHS, all tend to lead to a resistance to new ideas. To the managers feeling vulnerable, the old ways are seen as 'safer'. She says that more ideas and experiences of workers in the lower echelons of the NHS hierarchy need to reach their managers and to be included in health care planning. In her book, Dr Dowling describes some health visitors' new initiatives in the community. More are needed.

Even though the importance of preparation is now well recognised (Maternity Services Advisory Committee, 1982; House of Commons Social Services Committee, 1980), health visitors can only take part in antenatal services if they are notified of the pregnancies in their area. Obviously, the earlier these notifications can be received, the better is the opportunity to provide for the needs of the families. Much depends on health authority policy and work practices enabling this contact to be made.

LIAISON

Schemes for informing health visitors about pregnancies vary significantly from place to place. In some cases, the GP or the practice manager will leave messages, or use a notebook to list his pregnant patients. Some hospitals may use a computerised system, a handwritten scheme or send messages through the liaison health visitor. Sometimes local midwives provide the information.

Working together

The health visitor's role during the antenatal period is not always fully understood, interprofessionally, and occasionally rivalries can intervene (Skinner, 1982; Lythgoe, 1982). In order to improve health visitor–midwifery working relationships, the Royal College of Midwives (RCM) and the Health Visitors Association (HVA) produced a joint statement in June, 1982. The document which provided 'a shared vision of ideal arrangements for antenatal preparation', described succinctly the monitoring, supportive and educative responsibilities of the midwife throughout the pregnancy, birth and post-partum period.

The educative role of the health visitor was outlined in the statement, as was the dual responsibility for antenatal education of both professions. Perhaps both should give extra priority to women attending hospital-based, crowded antenatal clinics, as Field et al (1982a) said that in their study these women found it more difficult to discuss their problems than those cared for by domiciliary midwives.

The RCM and HVA suggested that particular attention be given to antenatal education at home for anyone unlikely to attend antenatal classes and that health visitors make extra visits to women whom they would not be meeting at antenatal classes. Sadly, the 'ideal', as set out in the joint statement, rarely balances with current caseloads.

Others' views

Many people may be involved with a woman in her antenatal preparations. For example,
— general practitioner
— community midwife
— hospital consultant
— junior doctors
— hospital midwives
— friends and family
— National Childbirth Trust counsellor
and, perhaps, other organisations such as Foresight and La Leche League.

It can be very helpful if health visitors are able to meet the professionals and volunteers likely to be involved in the care of several of their families. There can then be discussions about the sort of advice commonly given, for example on
— breastfeeding
— smoking

— alcohol
— nutrition
— impact on family relationships
and the sort of literature these people tend to recommend to their patients/clients. Being aware of other advisers' views and working patterns helps to cut down on confusion due to conflicting advice and some repetitiveness of professional questioning.

The best advice

Inevitably, of course, young couples have to face the dilemma of conflicting opinion. Family, friends, voluntary associations, a multitude of books and various professionals each give the advice they feel to be the best. In matters of health, ways of living and child-rearing, cultural variations abound and there is no absolute and indisputable truth. Also, medical views, for example on nutrition or where babies should be born, are vulnerable to change in the light of research findings and further change when these are refined.

Clulow (1982) remarks that health visitors need to be able to live with uncertainty and to cope with it, both in themselves and in the families they visit. An important part of health visiting is to encourage young couples to have the confidence to choose, out of all the views available, those which they themselves feel the most logical and the best suited to their particular circumstances. Books like *Your Body, Your Baby, Your Life* (Philips, 1983)

encourage parents to take an active part in their antenatal care and to make their own choices.

THE VISIT

FAMILY HEALTH NEEDS FRAMEWORK

At an antenatal visit, there are, of course, a very wide range of matters a mother or a couple may wish to discuss with their health visitor. In this chapter and the next, the family health needs framework, the second of the three outlined in the introductory chapter, is used to categorise the topics discussed here.

This model is useful in the context of a specific visit, because it concentrates on the particular requirements of a family, many of which may be considered, and some actually discussed, at such a visit. These matters are categorised in these chapters, occasionally rather arbitrarily, under 'environmental', 'physical', 'mental/emotional' and 'social' factors. Box 3.1 lists some of these issues and expanded in the subsequent text.

It is not proposed to attempt to cover every possible item which might be relevant at antenatal visits. Equally, as in the whole of this book, the range of topics mentioned is not intended to provide an ideal model of what should be discussed. Time at a visit is limited and, anyway, each family will voice a variety of different issues and needs.

Box 3.1 Aspects of family health that might need consideration antenatally

General environment	Physical health	Mental/emotional health	Social aspects of health
The community Social mix Infrastructure Employment	*Mother . . . .* Antenatal checks and education liaison Dental care	*Parental knowledge* Seek information Library: liaison	*Immediate family* Relationships: readjustment
The home Type Surroundings	*. . . and baby* Life-style influences Nutrition Smoking	*Expectations* Difficult to visualise	*Wider family, and friends* Grandmother Others
Standard of living Rights and benefits	*Discussions about* (Immunisation and infant surveillance scheme)	*Adjustment* Mostly for mother Outlook good?	*Community agencies* Antenatal groups and contacts
Working mother		*Discussion points* Breastfeeding Sex in pregnancy Depression	

Use of this model is demonstrated in two examples of a health visitor making an antenatal visit. Many of the issues raised in the examples are discussed in the rest of this section.

EXAMPLES OF ANTENATAL VISITS

The first is to a single parent and the second to a young couple living in the wife's parents' home. Their physical and mental health and some environmental and social aspects of health considered at the visit are described. They are tabulated under these four aspects of family health need in Boxes 3.2 and 3.3.

Some readers may prefer to go straight on to the discussions about family health requirements in the rest of the chapter and then return to these examples.

EXAMPLE ONE: NANCY MANNERS

A 20-year-old student nurse, Miss Nancy Manners, had chosen shared hospital and GP antenatal care. The routine in this surgery was for the community midwife to arrange an appointment for Mrs Hannah Van der Haastrecht (HV) to visit the home at around the 28th week.

Miss Manners lived alone, self-catering, in rented rooms in an Edwardian terrace house close to the Royal Overhampton Hospital where she was in training. The first thing mentioned after

Box 3.2 Example one: Nancy Manners

General environment	Physical health	Mental/emotional health	Social aspects of health
Local community Dominated by hospital and a college	*Mother . . . .* Antenatal checks regular	*Parental knowledge* Keen to learn	*Immediate family* Lives alone
The home Bedsitter: access to bathroom	*. . . and baby* Lifestyle: — Eats at work — Non-smoker — Avoiding alcohol	*Expectations* Non-idealistic Pragmatic	*Wider family, friends* G'mother: mainly telephone contact Landlady supportive
Standard/living Employed, low income Claiming benefits		*Adjustment* Early days good relationship with own mother	*Community agencies* Helpful at work
		Discussed: Breastfeeding, books recommended	*Plans* to tell about useful agencies
		Plans to follow up	

Box 3.3 Example two: the Kirks

General environment	Physical health	Mental/emotional health	Social aspects of health
The community Estate, small houses Poor infrastructure — no public halls — Industrial area	*Mother . . . .* Antenatal checks regular attender	*Parental knowledge* Intend to consult: — G'mother — clinic — library	*Immediate family* Warm relationship between parents Father wishes to help with baby
	. . . and baby Lifestyle: Not discussed	*Expectations* Open-minded	*Wider family, friends* Grandparental support Friends locally
The home Shared with grandparents		*Adjustment* Seems positive	*Community agencies* Invitation to mothers' 'Get Together Group'
Living standard Low wages Saving for own home		*Discussion:* Concerned re coitus in pregnancy	

the normal introductory remarks was how grateful she was that her landlady was prepared to break her own rules in order to let her stay on until a council flat became vacant—promised within a year.

Apparently the *Pregnancy Book* (Health Education Council, 1984) was found especially helpful with regard to its overview of maternity rights and benefits. It seems the hospital personnel department had been very supportive and helpful. Miss Manners had heard there was a hospital creche. The school of nursing had explained with which of the later sets of student nurses she was now likely to qualify. She had been advised to 'eat properly' and to 'keep off baccy and booze'!

When telling people of her intention to breastfeed as long as she could, Miss Manners found she was getting remarkably divergent and confused advice. The health visitor told her that there were in fact quite a number of good ways of setting about it. It was really a question of finding out all one could and then deciding which scheme seemed preferable. The aim then, in health visiting, was to help people achieve their chosen goals. Maire Messenger's (1982) book (probably available from the hospital library) and Garner's (1980) *How to Survive as a Working Mother* were recommended.

Hoping to learn something of Miss Manners' attitudes towards child rearing and her own mother, HV asked 'Now you're to be a mother, how will you bring your baby up? Will it be the same way as your mother did you?' The response was: 'I shall try to. She may not be perfect, but she did her best.' And with a twinkle, 'I don't suppose I shall be perfect either!' In response to a further question asking in what way she would particularly want to be the same, HV was told that her mother had always been moderately firm but had listened to reason and had tried to be just. She added 'You can't ask for more.' Her mother had accepted her pregnancy and had applauded her spirit of independence. She had promised her support in the normal granny role, and was keeping in telephone contact. This all augured well.

It seemed to HV that some of the problems that so frequently beset single parents of employment and housing were not, in the short term, to be a problem to this pleasant, well-organised young woman. She would, however, be on a marginal income and might well have problems over child care and of loneliness.

The health visitor decided to offer to call again in a month. An appointment was made. She planned to discuss organisations such as the National Council for One Parent Families and Gingerbread, and to back up the midwife's invitation to the antenatal classes. The main aim was to provide potential for social links with other parents, if they were desired.

They parted on first name terms. By the following antenatal visit Nancy had realised that she could not possibly afford full-time crèche fees. Her mother had offered to have the baby for the necessary eight months so she could complete her training. After that she planned to cease work until child care arrangements became possible. The birth visit is described in the next chapter.

EXAMPLE TWO: THE KIRKS

Notification of pregnancies from the large maternity hospital where 21-year-old Mrs Kirk was attending for antenatal care tends to come to the health visitors very late. Ms Heather Vaughan (HV) called at the home one evening when Mary Kirk was some eight months pregnant. A mistake in the information she had been given had caused her to deliver the note proposing her visit to the house next door. She had been redirected and was therefore unannounced. HV had generally found a poorer introduction than one that was pre-arranged.

Mr and Mrs Kirk were living with Mrs Kirk's parents, the Grahams. After the introductory conversations, Mrs Graham suggested the young couple take HV into the 'front room' in order to have privacy for their discussions. 'It's their baby' she said. She seemed rather tense and was very apologetic because there was no fire alight in the room. The health visitor apologised again that her visit had been unexpected and explained her normal appointment system.

Fire or no, the conversation flowed very warmly. The young couple were obviously looking forward to having their child. Mr Kirk, a packer at a local factory, said they were hoping to buy a small home within about six months. The Grahams had been trying to help them save for a deposit. There were some difficulties with two families living in so small a house, but they felt the grandparents would encourage them to bring up their baby in their own way.

Mrs Kirk said she would be asking her mother's

advice if she needed it: she trusted her mother's opinion. She hoped also to attend the mobile child health clinic. A group for first-time mothers in the estate (with especial emphasis on trying to draw in mothers receiving hospital antenatal care only) was newly set up and HV invited Mrs Kirk to come to it, both before and after the birth. The health visitor thought how much better an earlier notification would have been.

Mrs Kirk had heard about the mothers' group from one of her school friends who was already attending and she said that meeting the health visitor gave her the courage to come. The group, meeting above the surgery premises, provided the mothers with somewhere to meet regularly and make themselves a cup of tea. Ms Vaughan supplied health education films, tape-slide presentations and other material on topics chosen by the group. It was becoming quite a debating chamber!

When asked whether there was anything they wanted to ask about, the couple said they were concerned as to whether sexual intercourse would be bad for the baby or the pregnancy in any way. They had been abstaining the few weeks previously 'in case'. At the clinic everyone was so busy, there was no one Mrs Kirk dared ask. The matter was discussed. Because the couple agreed that it might be a good idea to follow up the conversation with some relevant reading, HV gave them a photstat of the Savage and Reader (1984) list of books. Several of the books were generally available in their local library. The baby care section there was recommended. The couple had not been in the habit of getting books out of the library, but thought it a good idea to look. Ms Vaughan was glad they had felt able to raise such a sensitive subject. She left, calling her thanks and goodbye to the Grahams, and expecting to see Mary Kirk again at the mothers' group and subsequently at the birth visit.

This young mother became a lively and regular attender at the group meetings. Eighteen months later a full time hospital liaison health visitor was employed by the Health Authority, enabling earlier and more rationally directed antenatal health visiting.

GENERAL ENVIRONMENT

The community

On their way to a home, health visitors naturally make a mental note of the environ-ment and general social circumstances in which the family lives. This helps their general understanding of the sort of problems, or otherwise, faced by the people they visit. Factors such as those in Figure 3.1, considered together, can give an impression of a probable quality and way of life available to the family.

The home

Approaching the dwelling itself, the architec-tural design:
— new or old
— multistorey or single dwelling
— access by lift or steps
— clothes drying facilities
— Safe play areas
— availability of own garden
adds to this impression. For many there is no problem. However, a Child Development Project (1984, p. 9) photograph showing a mother struggling with steps in a modern housing complex, gives a feel for the sort of problems some families face. It is pointed out that there are large numbers of parents living in distinctly disadvantaged circumstances, even in this affluent country.

Problems

People whose basic preconception and concern is a roof over their heads or the avail-ability of accessible employment, may need guidance and support over these basic matters before they can turn their thoughts more fully towards preparation for the baby. Also, there is mounting evidence of the effect of unem-ployment on family health (McLellan, 1985; Maternity Alliance, 1985).

All too often unemployment and poor housing seem insurmountable problems. Port-wood and Steventon (1984) provide some practical suggestions on how health visitors can help unemployed people. Frequently it is they who call before a crisis develops. This provides an advantage. The authors say that help can be given by disseminating infor-mation. Pamphlets and leaflets that explain in simple, straightforward terms, for example how to claim benefits, hunt for a job and keep

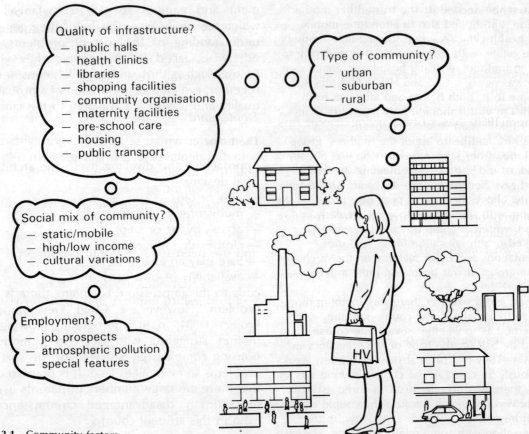

Quality of infrastructure?
— public halls
— health clinics
— libraries
— shopping facilities
— community organisations
— maternity facilities
— pre-school care
— housing
— public transport

Type of community?
— urban
— suburban
— rural

Social mix of community?
— static/mobile
— high/low income
— cultural variations

Employment?
— job prospects
— atmospheric pollution
— special features

HV

Fig. 3.1 Community factors.

mentally active and optimistic, would be of particular value. It is suggested that a local college might be encouraged to produce a booklet that lists agencies of particular help to the unemployed. A sample of the sort of thing that can be produced is available and can be sent for through Dr Portwood.

Some health visitors find that joining an organisation such as their local Radical Health Visitors group means they meet a supportive circle of people concerned with these basic problems and, in addition, find a good source of creative ideas and encouragement as well as useful addresses for people with problems.

Inner city health visiting is considered in the final chapter.

Rights and benefits

Many people will find very helpful the clearly set out and simply stated 'what', 'who', 'when' and 'how' on grants, allowances and other rights and entitlements which can be found in the Health Education Council's (1984, p. 35–39) *Pregnancy Book*. It is a book which is widely available and covers many aspects of pregnancy and early child care. People who wish to know more than this book outlines, may find that specific DHSS leaflets (Department of Health and Social Security, 1984), the trade unionists' *State Benefits* (Labour Research Department, 1984) or *Maternity Rights for Working Women* (Coussins, 1980) give some guidance. Maternity Alliance have some useful leaflets and an informative book (Evans & Durward, 1984).

Working mothers

Coussins provides a table of entitlements

under the Employment Protection Act, 1975, and explains in clear and reassuring terms how to make a complaint to a tribunal, should that be necessary.

Some mothers will want just to talk about the fact that they are choosing to continue in employment after their maternity leave. Leslie Garner (1980) has written giving useful tips, telling of helpful organisations and, perhaps most important of all, putting that niggling sense of guilt that some feel in perspective. On these occasions, the listening role of the health visitor can be particularly useful in helping people think through their feelings, their situation and intentions, and come to their own conclusions.

Confidentiality

Many people talk matters over with their family, neighbours or friends. Others feel they cannot, fearing gossip or interference in their affairs, and, when they need to talk about such things, prefer to discuss these sensitive matters with an objective listener who has a professional obligation to respect their confidence.

PHYSICAL ASPECTS OF HEALTH

Mother. . . . .

Antenatal check-ups

Health visitors may, in some cases, find it necessary to encourage mothers to attend for antenatal care. However, for the most part, health visitors will only come to hear about those who are already attending.

Health visitors who have the opportunity to observe at local antenatal clinics and get to know current local practice, will, when on their visits to people's homes, be more able to work in cooperation with these services. Experience in these clinics could provide useful liaison links and also valuable knowledge for some health visitors, as it is no longer compulsory for a health visitor to have a midwifery qualification.

The mothers may ask advice about a very wide range of issues, though most of the mothers' questions specific to antenatal supervision and the birth of the baby are likely to be asked of their midwives or doctors undertaking this care.

Dental care

One matter which health visitors might raise is that of dental care. Dental treatment is available free for all pregnant women and for the first year of motherhood. Draper et al (1983) found many of their interviewees were visiting their dentists. However, only one of them was aware of the increased possibility of gingivitis and the need for good oral hygiene in pregnancy. Besford (1984) explains about the changes that take place. Some of the Cambridgeshire mothers, having never visited a dentist before, said they were intending to take advantage of the free service.

. . . . . and baby

Life-style influences

Nutrition. There are high levels of professional agreement now on the importance of nutrition in the pre-conceptual period and in early pregnancy (Wynn & Wynn, 1979, 1981; Foresight, 1980; Dening, 1983; Margiotta, 1984). However, by the time notification comes through to the health visitor, the pregnancy is generally well established and it is rather too late for there to be much influence on the growing baby. Even so, if expectant parents seek information about what they should eat, a positive and active response could be a sound investment. This is a long-term matter. There is an obvious need for parents with a new baby to be as well nourished as possible, especially if she mother is breastfeeding. Then later comes the stage of preparing for the possibility of another pregnancy.

What advice should be given? Many hospitals supply diet sheets which parents may wish to discuss. The papers recommended by Pat Margiotta, Jervis's (1983) diet plan and the Community Outlook fact sheet (Pickard, 1983) provide good basic advice on diet, although intended mainly for pre-conceptual care. Discussions about weight gain (Pipe, 1983) and coffee drinking (Shai Linn et al, 1982) can now be guided by some scientifically-based evidence. It is likely that there will be further research into the effects of nutrition (Holt, 1982; Morgan, 1980) and it will be interesting to read about the newer theories as they emerge.

It is not always easy to afford a good diet. Some of those recommended by many hospitals could cost up to a third or a half of some mothers' incomes (Durward, 1984). Lyn Durward gives examples of the sort of diets actually eaten by mothers in the lower socio-economic groups. There is much room for improvement. She provides tables which show the stark differential between the social classes in rates of perinatal death, low birthweight and a specific malformation. For example, in 1981 the perinatal death rate for (legitimate) births was 8.2 for social class I and 15.5 for social class V; birth weight under 2.5 kg was between 5 and 6 per hundred births for social classes I to III, compared with 8.4 for social class V. A malformation ratio calculated for 1977–1979, showed the ratio for anencephalus and/or spina bifida to be four times higher for social class V than for social class I (pp. 3–4).

In general terms, nutritional status tends to improve with income. To what extent are health visitors able to help the poorly nourished? Perhaps the Child Development Project (1984, pp. 41–46,66) will show one of the ways it could be done: a facilitative approach, helping people gain an insight into nutritional alternatives.

Smoking, alcohol and drugs. Tobacco, alcohol and several drugs can cross the placenta by simple diffusion and, on occasions, harm the fetus. Doctors frequently give advice and, through prescription, have control over the use of much unsafe medication (Drury, 1982). It is another matter with social drugs: advice can be given, but, inevitably, it is a personal decision as to whether or not to give them up prior to or during pregnancy.

It seems there is a great deal of variation in the amount that mothers know about harmful effects of drugs, smoking, alcohol and other matters pertaining to their health. Some appear to receive no information, others only cursory advice (Moore, 1984; Draper et al, 1983). The GP is the first point of contact in pregnancy—sometimes as early as six weeks. Health visitors might suggest that the GPs have available and recommend some of the Health Education Council's (1984, p. 78) free leaflets. Their *Pregnancy Book* (Health Education Council, 1984, pp. 15–16,40) provides an excellent base from which to stimulate discussion about these, as well as many other, matters in pregnancy. For topics on which suitable pamphlets are not available from any of the normal sources, a local hand-out might be prepared, for example on alcohol if it is felt that people are likely to find it useful.

In order that people have adequate information early enough, it seems likely that health visitors will need to become increasingly more involved in pre-conceptual counselling—with GPs playing an active part or, perhaps for many, a referral role. The school classroom is, of course, the best place to start this teaching.

Reviews of research findings (Sidle, 1983; Edwards, 1983; Hawkins, 1983; Dowdell, 1981) can help keep health visitors abreast of recent thinking. Literature such as the Health Education Council's 'stop smoking packs' for health visitors (Nursing Times, 1983), and Plant's (1983) clearly stated and brief overview of pregnancy and alcohol, may prove useful for helping people understand the issues involved.

The problem is that it is not easy to give up these addictive drugs. A large proportion of women continue to smoke, even though they know it might have harmful effects, although a few may cut down significantly (Moore, 1984; Black, 1984; Draper et al, 1983). In America, there was a phase when coffee was also thought to be potentially harmful to the fetus. It is now disproved, but it seems it was much easier to give up coffee drinking when it was deemed ill advised, than it was to stop smoking (Shai Linn et al, 1982). For this reason, care has to be taken not to act like an over-zealous missionary and cause feelings of guilt which, instead of leading to the intended positive action, could result in anxiety and perhaps resentment.

It has been suggested that counselling at home may produce the best results (King & Eiser, 1981). There are obvious advantages to home-based work. The subject of alcohol is returned to in Chapter 6.

Discussions about infant health schemes

Frequently, health visitors on an antenatal visit bring the conversation round to matters such as child immunisation or their local infant surveillance scheme. There is an advantage in being able to introduce these notions prior to, and away from, the emotional confusions and the practical preoccupations involved in having a new baby. This is particularly so with a first baby as there are so many new things to think about. Another advantage is that it provides parents with the opportunity to formulate any questions they might like to raise well in advance of any decision they might need to make over aspects of immunisation for their baby or to enquire about postnatal services.

As many health visitors are still unable to provide a full antenatal visiting service, discussion of these matters has been deferred to Chapters 4 and 5.

MENTAL/EMOTIONAL HEALTH

Parental knowledge

Since the advent of smaller families, relatively fewer people expecting their first baby have had much practical experience in child care since their own childhood. Generally, pregnancy is a time when there is a great desire to learn about parentcraft and health. Some seek word-of-mouth information, whilst others prefer to read. If health visitors call into the local library, they can find out what books are readily available. After liaison with the local midwives, they can also discuss with the librarians which books are the most likely to be recommended.

Sometimes at antenatal classes books such as *Family Feelings* (Raynor, 1977) or *New Baby Growing Up* (Scowen, 1981) might be lent to each member of the group for a week of so. Opinions and questions arising out of this reading can then form the basis of a subsequent meeting. However, certain issues can be felt to be too personal, or the parents are too self-conscious, to mention them within the group. At a home visit, they may feel far freer to raise sensitive and delicate matters. Whether they do or not is likely, at least partly, to depend upon their having a good relationship with the health visitor.

Expectations and adjustment

It is very difficult for people to visualise in advance, and therefore to be prepared for, what it feels like to be a parent. The baby's stages and phases may seem, when it comes to it, to present insuperable difficulties. Parenthood can turn out to be very different from that which was anticipated. It is at this stage that someone known and trusted enough to be turned to, can provide part of an important 'safety net' in child care services.

In classes and in home visiting schemes, valuable attempts are made to give parents a chance to think about the emotional implications of parenthood in realistic, non-glamourised and non-idealistic terms. However, there are no glib and simple solutions to this aspect of health education.

Clulow (1982) studied the effect of the first baby upon marriage relationships. Enormous adjustments are needed—especially by the mother. He invited expectant parents to attend discussion groups to see if foreknowledge of the psychological factors associated with having a first baby would reduce the risk of painful problems. In the event, it seems that it is not until problems arise that people can realise to what extent they have been seeing matters in an idealised light. Descriptions by Ann Oakley (1982) and Liz Walton (1983) show just how surprised and emotionally shaken some women can be by the reality of motherhood.

The National Childbirth Trust is one of the organisations which tries to provide a service which will help in these adjustment processes. They give antenatal classes and produce some excellent leaflets and a helpful book: *Pregnancy and Parenthood* (Loader, 1980).

Looking ahead. People vary in the extent to which they are able to make the necessary adjustment. Factors such as
— social circumstances
— family circumstances
— baby's behaviour
— levels of confidence
— mother's personality
— her own childhood experiences
— levels of support from
   — partner
   family
   friends
   professionals
can all have an influence. Health visitors sensitive to these factors may, to some extent, be able to make a reasonable guess at which parents are more likely to be in need of extra support once the baby arrives. Ann Gath (1977) suggested a series of questions which she felt to be friendly rather than personal. These questions were intended to help discover the mothers most at risk of emotional problems. They asked
— how much her partner is able to be with her at this time
— about her relationship with her mother
— what sort of occupation the mother uses for fun and relaxation
There is, of course a need to be sensitive to how much people wish to be questioned, however well intentioned the questioning may be.

Pugh (1980, p. 75) suggests there should be plans to concentrate help upon vulnerable groups such as
— teenagers
— unemployed young people
— those brought up in care
— late attenders at antenatal clinics
— older middle class women

who may have difficulty in adjusting to parenthood. Care has to be taken that people selected in this way should not be considered 'people with problems'. Through their attitudes some professionals can assign such people a lowered status. The problem, if there is one, is in shared misunderstandings. Health visitors, for example, tend to be middle class and, like everyone else, have a limited knowledge of how other people's lives are led. Also they may use jargon terms and have speech mannerisms strange to many of the people they visit (Pugh, 1980, p. 76). These sorts of limitations to good two-way communication and understanding need to be taken into consideration throughout the practice of health visiting.

Discussion points pertaining to emotional well-being

Some of the sensitive issues affecting emotional health which expectant parents may seek to discuss could be sexual activity during pregnancy, postnatal depression and emotional aspects of breastfeeding.

Coitus in pregnancy. It has been suggested that a large proportion of pregnant women would like advice on sexual activity during pregnancy. Savage and Reader (1984) point out that abstention was commonly advised for about two thirds of pregnancy a few decades ago. Extensive research has now shown there is no association between intercourse during pregnancy and adverse outcome of pregnancy (Klebanoff et al, 1984). The advice given now can be far more reassuring. There are, of course, exceptions. For example, abstinence is advised where there has been some bleeding during this pregnancy and may be suggested in the case of a threatened miscarriage or premature labour.

About half the 218 women interviewed by Savage and Reader (1984) received no advice on the subject. Some 40% read books to get the appropriate information. Savage and Reader said that sex in pregnancy should be discussed routinely. They have listed in their article books on the subject and the relevant page numbers, both for professional education and for recommending to pregnant women.

Postnatal depression. It seems that various researchers have associated a multitude of different factors with that of postnatal depression: high anxiety levels, marital tension, earlier doubts about the pregnancy, for example, and problems in relationships with the mother's parents (Ball, 1982). It is a condition which can manifest itself in a variety of ways. Parents who wish to know how they might be able to recognise it and to find out how to help, should it occur in their own family or amongst their friends, may find the National Childbirth Trust's booklet (Waumsley, 1983) a very good starting point. Several mothers' personal experiences are described in it and guidance is given on further reading and agencies that might prove helpful. Postnatal depression is returned to in Chapter 5 (pp. 84 and 93).

Breastfeeding. Three-quarters of the 500 first time mothers interviewed by Hally et al (1984) had already made up their minds about which way they would feed their babies and mostly fed them the way intended.

There are many factors which influence the way people decide whether or not to breast-feed. Solberg (1984) reviewed some of them. Historically, there have been differences between the social classes, and there is a correlation between the experiences of friends and family, for example growing up in an environment where it is commonplace, and breastfeeding.

A positive attitude by the partner means the mother is more likely to breastfeed. Apparently, in a study quoted by Solberg half the mothers who gave up did so due to objections by the father. It seems that the role of the breast in a couple's sexual activities can be influential. For some people, the sexual and the nurturant roles are felt to be incompatible.

Solberg also says that there is conflicting evidence on the benefits or otherwise of physical preparation of the breasts, but that it can be psychologically beneficial if it makes the mother *feel* better prepared.

It seems that the quality of information given to the couple is the key to successful breastfeeding and that the early experiences in breastfeeding are very influential (Hally et al, 1984). *The Breastfeeding Book* (Messenger, 1982) gives detailed and logically presented information and is likely to be popular.

SOCIAL ASPECTS OF HEALTH

Social support systems are of great importance to the young family—those within the immediate family, the broader family network and close friends, and also certain community agencies. They all play some part in ameliorating the loneliness and the strains and tensions which frequently arise from the care of babies and children. Forethought and action in the antenatal period may pave the way for help to be available later, should it be needed. For example, many new mothers can easily become exhausted. Tiredness is the most common symptom in postnatal depression (Hennessy, 1986), and it is worth thinking ahead and planning for its alleviation.

The immediate family

Many mothers give up work for their first baby and therefore become that much more dependent upon their partner economically, for social contact and as 'sharer of problems'. The father, therefore, becomes a key figure.

If antenatal visiting takes place in the evenings, it is more probable that both parents will be met. There is then an opportunity to learn not only the mother's viewpoint and wishes, but her partner's too. An appointment system, where this exists, enables visits to be arranged when both parents are likely to be free.

There is now increasing awareness of the importance of a father's active involvement in the care of his children. Verny and Kelly (1982) described how this can begin even before the birth. The father's voice can be heard by the baby, in utero, and recognised after birth. Bonding and an enhanced relationship can begin this soon, it is suggested, by the father talking to his unborn child and using short soothing words.

To encourage involvement, some mothers may give their partner *The Baby Book for Dads* (Little & Ralston, 1980) or get it from the library. It is well written and shows, in a constructive and humorous way, the important social and emotional role of the father. The advice includes some inaccuracies, but parents have plenty of other opportunities to find more up-to-date advice. Antenatally, for example, there may be classes in the locality where fathers are made welcome.

Wider family, friends and neighbours

Most new mothers enjoy and feel the need for social contact outside their immediate nuclear family. A supportive grandparental link can be much appreciated and very helpful. Friends and neighbours may be able to help fill the gap created by the loss of long-standing social networks associated with going out to work. Mothers who have special circumstances such as a poor marriage, frequent house moving or no support from their own mother, may feel a particular need.

Postnatal groups, where friendships become established antenatally, can be invaluable. Clulow (1982) felt that the 'safety net' factor, the availability of sympathetic support, where people could talk through their problems, was a very important aspect of these groups.

Karin Christiani (Nursing Times, 1982) described Swedish antenatal groups where parents came from the same area and stayed together after the birth of their babies. Similarly, the National Childbirth Trust groups which meet in people's homes can lead on to very valuable friendships and mutual support. Their clientele, however, is predominantly middle class.

Health visitors can help by telling expectant parents about groups and schemes in their area and by encouraging and providing support to new groups and, especially, by concentrating effort on provision for the disadvantaged.

As an alternative to group support, a project based at Lisson Grove Health Centre (Wood, 1985; Hills, 1981) fosters links between established parents and expectant parents in the area. Regular contact is maintained between mothers-to-be and their doctor and health visitor during the pregnancy. An introduction to established parents and attendance at antenatal classes which continue through to postnatal sessions, are offered. When the research on the project is completed, it will be interesting to discover whether this project has been successful and to what extent this sort of approach might be applicable elsewhere. Postnatal groups will be considered in the next chapter.

In this section, we have looked at environmental, physical, mental/emotional and social aspects of health which may be considered or discussed during a health visitor's visit to expectant parents.

AFTER THE VISIT

Record making is increasingly being undertaken during the visit. However, if this was not done, the health visitor will need to make a note of pertinent points immediately afterwards. For example, the date of the next appointment should be noted, assuming one was arranged. It will also be necessary to jot down any particular requests the parent or parents might have made. They might have shown an interest in being put in touch with agencies such as the National Childbirth Trust (NCT) or La Leche League. It might have been agreed that the health visitor should discuss some issue with the midwife. Also, the parents may have expressed an interest in certain health education subjects on which the health visitor has promised to provide further information, or has made a mental note to do so.

It is best if a record of the visit is made as soon as possible. A handbag-sized dictating machine can be invaluable for immediate recording (Robertson, 1982). An audio-typist then transcribes the notes in due course. Such records are generally considered to be much more reliable than hand written records made at the end of the day—or some days later! The problem is overcome, of course, when notes are written up on site.

Recalling and reviewing the visit involves a form of evaluation. As described in the previous chapter, it is part of the process of thinking about how to provide an appropriate service at subsequent encounters. The health visitor would tend to mentally run through:
— how parents seem to feel about the visit and the service provided by the health visitor
— their probable environmental, physical, emotional and social health requirements
— to what extent these were met in terms of:
  1. preventing occurrence: for example, through health education on an aspect such as breastfeeding
  2. preventing development: for example, through assessment of special need, perhaps using social factors as criteria for this assessment
  3. preventing deterioration: perhaps by listening whilst the mother-to-be talks through and sorts out her anxieties

about her intentions to return to work
— which of the family's health requirements seem now to need most attention and to consider these as tentative objectives for the next visit
— immediate objectives for health visitor action, such as liaison with the NCT or midwife, or to find health education information ready for the next visit.

A note of any particular issue needing immediate attention or action at a subsequent visit can then be added to the records. This next encounter might be at another antenatal visit, at antenatal classes or at the birth visit.

This chapter has considered home visiting people preparing for parenthood. It has looked at some schemes currently being tried out and at the need to keep in touch with others caring for these parents-to-be. Some possible health needs have been briefly mentioned. Health visiting at this stage gives an opportunity to provide health education and to explain about the purpose and style of health visiting. This helps the development of a good working relationship, which is particularly important once the baby is born.

USEFUL ADDRESSES

La Leche League (Great Britain)
Breastfeeding Help and Information,
BM 3424 London WCIV 6XX
Tel 01 242 1278

National Childbirth Trust,
9 Queensborough Terrace,
London W2 3TB
Tel 01 221 3833

REFERENCES

Ball J 1982 Stress and the postnatal care of women. Nursing Times 78: 1904–1907

Besford J 1984 Good mouthkeeping or how to save your children's teeth and your own, too, while you're about it. Oxford University Press, Oxford, p 40–41; 122–124

Black P 1984 Who stops smoking in pregnancy? Nursing Times 80, 19: 59–61

Child Development Project 1984 Child development programme. Early Childhood Development Unit, Senate House, University of Bristol, Bristol BS8 1TH

Clulow C F 1982 To have and to hold. Marriage, the first baby and preparing couples for parenthood. Aberdeen University Press, Aberdeen, p 105

Coussins J 1980 Maternity rights for working women. National Council for Civil Liberties, London, p 24–25

Dening F 1983 Infant morbidity and preconceptual care. Nursing Times Supplement 79, 29: 3–6

Department of Health and Social Security 1984 Which

benefit? Leaflet FB.2/ Nov 84. Department of Health and Social Security, London

Dowdell P M 1981 Alcohol and pregnancy. A review of the literature 1968–1980. Nursing Times 77, 43: 1825–1831

Dowling S 1983 Health for a change. The provision of preventive health care in pregnancy and early childhood. Child Poverty Action Group, London

Draper J, Field S, Kerr M, Hare M J 1983 Women's knowledge of health care during pregnancy. Health Visitor 56: 86–88

Drury V W M 1982 Prescribing in pregnancy. Maternal and Child Health 7: 351–352

Durward L 1984 Poverty in pregnancy: the cost of an adequate diet for expectant mothers. Maternity Alliance, London

Edwards G 1983 Alcohol and advice to the pregnant woman. British Medical Journal 286: 247–248

Evans R, Durward L 1984 Maternity rights handbook.

Know your rights: the questions and answers. Penguin Books, London

Field S, Draper J, Kerr M, Hare M J 1982a Interaction with health care personnel Part 1 The antenatal period. Midwife, Health Visitor and Community Nurse 18, 5: 197–198

Field S, Draper J, Kerr M, Hare M J 1982b Interaction with health care personnel Part 3 The postnatal period. Midwife, Health Visitor and Community Nurse 18, 7:279; 287

Field S, Draper J, Thomas H, Farmer S, Hare M J 1984 The health visitor's view of consumer criticisms. Health Visitor 57: 273–275

Foresight 1980 Guidelines for future parents. The Association for the Promotion of Pre-conceptual Care, Woodhurst, Hydestile, Godalming, Surrey GU8 4AY

Gath A 1977 Emotional needs in a new family. Nursing Mirror 143, 28: 52–54

Garner L 1980 How to survive as a working mother. Jill Norman, p 25–37

Hally M R, Bond J, Crawley J, Gregson B, Philips P, Russell I 1984 What influences a mother's choice of infant feeding method? Nursing Times Occasional Paper No 4 80, 4: 65–68

Hawkins D F 1983 Drugs and pregnancy. Human teratogenesis and related problems. Churchill Livingstone, Edinburgh

Health Education Council 1984 Pregnancy book. A guide to becoming pregnant, being pregnant and caring for your newborn baby. Available through District Health Authority Health Education Units (in telephone directory under name of Health Authority: eg Winchester Health Authority)

Health Visitor 1981 Health visiting in the eighties. Health Visitor 54, 2: centre pages supplement

Hennessy D A 1986 Should health visitors also care for mothers? Proceedings of the Rcn Research Society, 1985 conference. Royal College of Nursing, London (in press)

Hills A 1981 Getting it right first time. Health and Social Services Journal XCI:892

Holt K S 1982 Diets and development. Child: care, health and development 8: 183–201

House of Commons Social Services Committee 1980 Second Report, Session 1979–80 Perinatal and Neonatal Mortality. HMSO, London (Chairman Renee Short)

Jervis R 1983 Planning a balanced diet. In: Foresight Supplementary Chapters to Guidelines for Future Parents. The Association for the Promotion of Preconceptual Care Godalming, Surrey

King J and Eiser J R 1981 A strategy for counselling pregnant smokers. Health Education Journal 40: 66–68

Klebanoff M A, Nugent R P, Rhoads G G 1984 Coitus during pregnancy: is it safe? The Lancet II: 914–917

Labour Research Department 1984 State benefits. A guide for trade unionists. LRD Publications Ltd, London

Little P and Ralston D 1980 The baby book for dads. New English Library

Loader A (editor) 1980 Pregnancy and parenthood. Oxford University Press, Oxford

Lythgoe E J 1982 HVs and antenatal care (letter). Nursing Times 78:1475

McLellan J 1985 The effect of unemployment on the family. Health Visitor 58: 157–161

Margiotta P 1984 The importance of pre-conceptual nutrition. Nursing Times Health Visitors' Supplement 80, 42: 11–12

Maternity Alliance 1985 Born unequal: perspectives on pregnancy and childbearing in unemployed families. Maternity Alliance, 59–61 Camden High Street, London NW1 7JL

Maternity Services Advisory Committee 1982 Maternity care in action Part 1: antenatal care. DHSS (Leaflets) PO Box 21, Stanmore, Middlesex HA7 1AY. p 17, 19

Messenger M 1982 The breastfeeding book. Century Publishing Co Ltd, London

Moore J 1984 Antenatal ignorance. Nursing Times Community Outlook 80, 19: 147–148

Morgan J B 1980 Nutrition during pregnancy. Nutrition Bulletin 5, 6: 300–308

Nursing Times 1982 Parent groups help in pregnancy. Nursing Times: 78, 37:1532

Nursing Times 1983 Helping people to stop smoking. Nursing Times 79, 23: 62–65

Oakley A 1982 From here to maternity. Becoming a mother. Penguin Books Ltd, London

Philips A 1983 Your body, your baby, your life. Pandora Press, London

Pickard B 1983 Fact sheet on pre-pregnancy care. Nursing Times Community Outlook 79, 23: 255–258

Pipe N G J 1983 Weight gain in pregnancy. Maternal and Child Health 8: 370–375

Plant M 1983 Alcohol in pregnancy: is it safe? Nursing Mirror Midwifery Forum 157, 14: ii–iv

Portwood D, Steventon B 1984 Health visitors and the unemployed. Health Visitor 57: 17–18

Pugh G (ed) 1980 Preparation for parenthood. Some current initiatives and thinking. National Childrens' Bureau, London

Raynor C 1977 Family feelings, Understanding your child from 0–5. Arrow Books Ltd, London

Roberston C A 1982 Becoming a health visitor—an obstacle course? Nursing Times 78, 36: 1508–1512

Royal College of Midwives and Health Visitors Association 1982 Joint statement on ante natal preparation. Health Visitors Association, 36 Eccleston Square, London SWIV 1PF

Savage W, Reader F 1984 Sexual activity during pregnancy. Midwife, Health Visitor and Community Nurse 20: 398–402

Schofield J 1982 Health visiting—quality not quantity (letter). Nursing Mirror 155, 25:37

Scowen P (editor) 1981 New baby growing up. B Edsall and Co Ltd, London

Shai Linn P H, Schoenbaum S C, Monson R R, Rosner B, Stubblefield P G, Ryan K J 1982 No association between coffee consumption and adverse outcomes of pregnancy. The New England Journal of Medicine 306, 3: 141–145

Sidle N 1983 Smoking in pregnancy—A review. Hera Unit, The Spastics Society, 12 Park Crescent, London W1N 4EQ

Skinner V 1982 HVs, midwives and pregnant women (letter). Nursing Times 78:1236

Solberg S M 1984 Indicators of successful breast feeding. In: Houston M J (ed) Maternal and infant health care. Churchill Livingstone, Edinburgh

Stanton A 1982 The listening, liaising, counselling HV. Nursing Mirror 155, 22: 57–59

Verny T, Kelly J 1982 The secret life of the unborn child. Sphere Books Ltd, London. p 17–18

Walton L 1983 Thoughts of a new mother. Health Visitor 56: 208–209

Waumsley L 1983 Mothers talking about postnatal depression. National Childbirth Trust, London

Wood T 1985 Formal and informal support systems for mothers with newborn. Midwife, Health Visitor and Community Nurse 21: 42–49

Wynn M, Wynn A 1979 Prevention of handicap and the health of women. Routledge and Kegan Paul, London

Wynn M, Wynn A 1981 The prevention of handicap of early pregnancy origin. Some evidence for the value of good health before conception. Foundation for Education and Research in Childbearing, 27 Walpole Street, London SW3 4QS

Chapter 4 looks at activities in preparation for and associated with the birth visit. It provides another example of how the family health needs framework can be used to systematize matters that pertain to or may be considered or discussed during the call. The classification this time is under physical, emotional and social aspects of health.

Behind the scenes
  Information gathering

The visit
  Meeting the family
  The framework in action

Examples of birth visits
  Physical health
  Mental and emotional health
  Social aspects of health

Arranging further visits

4

Birth visit

BEHIND THE SCENES

By tradition and law

The first home visit after the birth usually takes place between the tenth and fourteenth day postnatally. In many places, the day chosen depends on traditional arrangements made between the midwives and the health visitors. In some instances, the 'hand-over' date is decided on an individual basis. If there is a clinical problem, the midwife may maintain contact with the mother up to the 28th day.

Some health visitors have been known to refer to this first visit as their 'statutory visit', but this is a misnomer. The statutory obligation is on the Health Authorities, under the National Health Services Act, Part II, Section 24

to make provision in their area for the visiting of persons in their homes by . . . . . . health visitors for the purpose of giving advice as to the care of young children, persons suffering from illness and expectant or nursing mothers . . . .

There is no compulsion in the visiting. Although the service must be provided, it does not have to be received. The system depends entirely upon these nurses being seen as acceptable and helpful visitors as was discussed in Chapter 2.

INFORMATION GATHERING

The law requiring notification of the birth by

the midwife enables this information to be passed on to the health visitor. Parents have six weeks in which to notify the Registrar of Births.

The record card

Normally, with each new birth a health visitor record card is sent through the administrative system to the health visitor's desk. Besides the child's
— surname
— home address
— and date of birth
there may be an indication of its
— sex
— weight
— length
— 'at risk' factors, if any
— congenital malformation, if any
— phenylketonuria test date
— hearing test date
— and other tests.
Regarding the mother, it may show her
—age
— number of previous births
— general practitioner
— midwife
— and where the birth took place.
The amount of information actually recorded on the card varies according to local custom and practice. In some places, for example, the phenylketonuria test may be considered so commonplace as not to be worth recording—unless a problem has been detected.

Liaison

The health visitor may be informed of much of the information mentioned above or alerted to relevant medical or social factors through an obstetric discharge computer print-out or a form filled in by the midwife. These papers may be sent to the health visitor through the administrative system, given to the liaison health visitor or left with the mother to hand on at the visit.

The McClymont (1983, p. 10) working party suggested that useful information might include: type of delivery; apgar score; the condition of both mother and infant, and several factors that would give an indication of social background. Some of the factors useful in helping to identify the families for whom health visitors should give extra consideration and support, were mentioned in Chapter 3 (page 46). There is also a need to know the discharge address if it differs from the mother's normal place of residence.

Both early notification of important information and personal liaison between the midwife and the health visitor, mean a better service can be given. The same applies, of course, to liaison with the general practitioner.

It seems that around three-quarters of the health visitors interviewed by Dunnell and Dobbs (1982) and Draper et al (1984) felt they had a very good or good working relationship with the GP. However, it follows that a significant number found communication inadequate.

Ann Bowling (1983) studied primary health care teamwork and reviewed some of the pertinent literature. She mentioned Bruces' report that, like GPs, health visitors could also find it difficult to share information, unless it was especially requested.

Health visitors' and GPs' hesitancy about sharing information could be for the same reasons. In both cases, their work is of an independent nature and, for many, a special effort has to be made to make contact. Many from both professions may feel worried when confronted by seemingly contradictory ideals: on one hand, the ideal of information sharing and on the other, the individual's right to privacy and confidentiality. In some cases there may be a fear that clients would not be helped so much as become 'labelled'—branded as having a problem—and denigrated or patronised. This recedes as an issue when the health visitor and the GP (or any other member of the primary health care team) have witnessed improved care through teamwork and have learned, over time, to trust each other's ability to help the families involved.

However, people's basic right to confidentiality and their assumption that medical and personal details will go no further than the professional person in whom they confide, still remains. The matter is returned to in the last section of Chapter 8.

Frequent and flexible meetings on practical issues as they arise, provide a forum for feedback and discussion. These can help to build up this understanding and trust and to overcome common difficulties in teamwork, such as

— problems of role definition
— friction and stereotyping
— concerns over status and leadership.

Telephoned and written messages can ensure speedy communication in between meetings.

Pamphlets

Several books and papers are available which may be felt to be worth having to hand on this visit (see Table 4.1). The choice of matters introduced during the call and, therefore, the supportive literature which would be needed, will be influenced by what topics have been discussed antenatally and, also, whether other opportunities for early contact with the family are anticipated.

If, for example, the health visitor is carrying a double caseload, a great deal will have to be fitted into this first visit after the birth. On the other hand, weekly visiting may be the norm, perhaps until the baby is six weeks or so. In this case, certain papers such as pamphlets on immunisation or information about developmental or hearing tests, might be introduced later, at one of those weekly visits, and be organised to suit the parents' wishes.

Preparing to call

The mother may well appreciate advanced warning of when the health visitor expects to visit, either through a telephone call or through a standard arrangement with the midwife.

It is likely that the agreed visit would be written into the health visitor's diary, the date

Table 4.1 Examples of literature the health visitor might have available at a birth visit

Items		Source
Cards, lists and forms to leave with the family	Health visitor visiting card—where can be contacted and tel no Immunisation request and consent form—to be completed and returned	Health Authority admin
	Lists of: — child health clinics and out of hours health visitor service — family planning clinics — local mothers' groups — local crying baby telephone and other support services	Health visitor office (need frequent updating)
	Green card: infant care guide	Foundation for Sudden Infant Death Syndrome
Leaflets and booklets to lend or leave	Safety: HS2 Keeping pets: ID5 Feeding: NT4; NT5 Childminding: CW30; CW31 'Now You're a Family' CW2 'You Know More Than You Think You Do' CW7 Local specially designed leaflets	District Health Authority Health Education Dept
	'The Book of the Child' Child Health Record Booklet	Scottish Health Education Group Edsall, publishers
Books as visual aid or to lend for a week or so	Leach P 1977 Baby and Child. Penguin Books Jolly H 1981 Book of Child Care. Sphere Books Messenger M 1982 The Breastfeedng Book. Century Pub. Scowen P, editor 1981 New Baby Growing Up. Edsall Richards M 1980 Infancy. Harper and Row Rayner C 1977 Family Feelings. Arrow Books	Usually health visitor's own property

of birth, name and address put into the appropriate section of that year's birth book, and the record card filed away in the compartment for current visiting, probably with the record cards for other members of that family, should there be any.

THE VISIT

MEETING THE FAMILY

This call may be on a family already known to the health visitor, perhaps through previous children or through antenatal contact. Where there is a high turnover of staff or it is a first baby, and particularly in inner city areas, it is not unusual for this to be the introductory visit.

Making contact with a family was considered in Chapter 2. We looked at some of the elements of success such as establishing a good relationship, helping people understand the purpose of health visiting and making an appropriate response to family health requirements. The 'fact gathering' associated with this visit make it worth mentioning two further points.

Knowledge kept in the background

Health visitors arrive at these households with a fair amount of information about the circumstances of the birth and the baby. However, it is probable that for reasons of diplomacy, they will not wish to *appear* too knowledgeable. There are several reasons. For one thing, they would prefer to encourage the parent or parents to describe various things, in order to gain an understanding of their perspective.

In some cases, parents may be too hesitant to explain, if they feel they may be repeating something already known to their listener. A second reason is that a 'know-all' health visitor may be resented and (perhaps properly) be labelled as a potential autocrat. Thirdly, some issues can be very delicate and people may be better choosing their own time to mention them, should they wish to.

It may help to give an example of this third reason—a delicate topic. Let us say a record card shows

previous births: 1 + 0

indicating one previous birth and no miscarriages. The case is one where there is no earlier record card in the files and so the health visitor is not aware of a previous child. Liaison may have enabled forewarning of a previous still birth or adoption. Whether they know the whole story or not, many health visitors would not themselves raise the subject, unless it seemed absolutely necessary.

It is the experience of the author that often a small remark, perhaps when the baby is being looked at, a remark such as, 'You must be very proud of your little girl', will cause people to refer back to an earlier, hurtful experience, as part of an explanation as to why they are so happy now. They can then explain in their own way and at their own pace.

This 'background approach' when visiting has the advantage of enabling positive client participation, but it has the disadvantage that health visitors may appear to 'know nothing'. There are, however, many ways in which they can make suggestions and show themselves to be knowledgeable and useful. Some are described in later sections of this chapter under physical, emotional and social aspects of family health need.

Avoiding implied criticism

Health visitor attitude and visible usefulness seem to be the key to success in the work. It is, therefore, somewhat dismaying to read the McClymont (1983, p. 11) working party's list of factors suggested as needing 'to be observed' by the health visitor during this primary visit. The general tenor might easily be interpreted as critical and health visitor centred. Phrases like
— 'ability of mother to cope'
— 'organisation of household, cleanliness'
— 'maturity of parents'
— 'attitude of mother . . . (and) . . . other
  relatives to HV'

are used. All these are matters on which the health visitor's observations must have a strongly subjective bias. Household standards, just as one example, are a distinctly questionable means of measuring either the quality of a family's loving relationships or a person's skills in parenting (Goodwin, 1982).

However, the working party did not claim to have all the answers—in fact the reverse (p. (i)). They published the outcome of their activities because they could *not* provide clear answers to the questions posed and they hoped to encourage further study.

Their list of matters suggested as needing 'to be clarified' during the visit is much more helpful (p. 11–12). This list includes factors about the baby and the family situation such as

— feeding method and routine
— sterilisation of equipment
— whether benefits have been claimed
— family planning services
— mother's return to work
— sibling relationships.

Its value lies in its drawing together a range of possible discussion points which the family may wish to raise, or perhaps develop, if they were introduced by the health visitor.

However, as shown in the previous chapter and in the list of factors in Box 4.1 and discussed in the following sections of this chapter, the McClymont list should *not* be taken as providing an ideal model of what should be achieved in the visit. There are limitations on time and every family has differing priorities on what they would like discussed during the visit. Added to this, there will be other matters which might be raised and need to be considered. There is not room in a review of this kind, to mention every possible relevant item.

THE FRAMEWORK IN ACTION

As in the previous chapter, a family health needs framework has been chosen to demonstrate one way of organising a mental checklist of the sort of matters that might be

Box 4.1 Some aspects of family health considered at the first visit after the birth

Physical health	Mental/emotional health	Social aspects of health
Mother General health Postnatal factors: — physical condition — postnatal check — medication	*Parental knowledge* Many possible queries	*Mother and father: family network* Important source of help and support Isolated?
Baby Examination e.g. — general appearance — vision — hearing — weight — CDH — record card Boys: foreskin Hygiene and safety Immunisation Artificial feeding	*Expectations, adjustment and emotional well-being*	*Mother* Lonely? Advice on local support services for young mothers Child health clinic
	Mother: baby Baby's behaviour Bonding Breastfeeding: support needed	
	Siblings Rivalry Special attention	*Siblings* Playgroup Toddler and mother group.
	Father: mother Attention to baby means less time for each other Sexuality Contraception	

considered during a visit. The model, seen in Box 4.1, emphasises some of the physical, mental/emotional and social aspects of health requirement family members may have at this stage of their life.

A section on environmental factors has not been included in this chapter. This is in order to allow more space for matters specific to the health visitor's first visit to a family with a new baby. Environmental factors were introduced in Chapter 3 (page 41). Naturally, these become increasingly significant with the arrival of young children in a family and their exclusion is in no way intended to minimise their importance or to belittle their influence on family health.

EXAMPLES OF BIRTH VISITS

Once again, two examples are given in order to show the framework in action. The first is the birth visit to Nancy Manners, who featured in the previous chapter as an example of an antenatal visit. The second is to the Clarks, who already have a three-year-old child. Outlines will be found in Boxes 4.2 and 4.3.

EXAMPLE ONE: NANCY MANNERS

The information on the health visitor birth card delivered to Mrs Hannah Van der Haastrecht's (HV) desk, showed that Nancy Manners had had a girl by caesarian section three days previously. The Apgar score (10 after 10 minutes) and other indicators were satisfactory.

The primary health care team weekly meeting was held six days later, when the baby was 10 days old. The GP reported that Miss Manners had been very disappointed not to have a normal delivery but had adjusted to the circumstances well. He had visited the home that day and had examined the baby fully. Glancing down the list of items on the notes, HV saw no abnormality recorded. The community midwife (CMW) said

that breastfeeding, on demand and currently around two hourly, was successful so far. Nancy's mother was staying for a week or so to help. HV and CMW arranged to visit together for the handover.

On the morning of the fourteenth day, as pre-arranged, they called. Mrs Manners answered the door and HV was pleased to have a chance to meet her. The baby had just finished being fed. Breastfeeding was progressing very satisfactorily, now generally at three or four hourly intervals. Nancy, who was still taking 'no baccy or booze' very seriously, had told the midwife how much she had appreciated her motherliness and support, especially over breastfeeding. She seemed pleased when HV said she would be able to call weekly for a few weeks.

Baby Pauline was tending to be wakeful in the evenings, but, it seems, Nancy and her mother were making it an opportunity to cuddle and to play with her. Whilst the nappy was being changed, they enjoyed showing HV and CMW the baby's ability to make eye contact and to respond to facial expressions. Pauline startled and blinked in response to a loud hand clap, she looked well, her eyes were clear and HV noted that her umbilicus was dry. The baby was weighed by CMW. She had regained her birthweight of 3 kg and it was recorded on the 50th centile. The doctor had checked her hips four days previously.

When HV asked how the delivery had been, Nancy explained about the breech presentation and the subsequent decisions. She said that in her training, she had heard a good deal about 'bonding'. She was worried in case her relationship with her baby should be inadequate on account of not seeing her immediately after the birth. They discussed current ideas on bonding theory.

When CMW asked if there was anything in her feelings for her baby that made her worry, Nancy said they were a little mixed. As they talked on, particularly about her behaviour with her baby, Nancy realised that she had no real problem. Some pages from a booklet HV had in her bag, 'Now You're a Family', proved useful.

The health visitor described the facilities at the clinic, including those for getting to know other mothers. Nancy said she had met a few mothers at the NCT antenatal classes but felt a closer bond with the people she had met at the Gingerbread meetings. They had made her very welcome and she was grateful to HV for telling

Box 4.2 Example one: Nancy Manners

Physical health	Mental/emotional health	Social aspects of health
Mother Caesarian stitches Breasts comfortable Not smoking No alcohol Postnatal exam at hospital nearby	*Parental knowledge* Given booklet CW2 Messenger book still useful *Adjustment* and *emotional well-being*	*Mother* Grandmother supporting Gingerbread contacts NCT discontinued Contact with nursing friends Invited to clinic
Baby Examined by GP including CDH Vision: eye contact Hearing: startles Skin: good colour Fontanelle: normal Passing urine; faeces normal Weight: 3 kg	*Mother: baby* Breastfeeding: seeks support Baby wakefulness: acceptable 'Bonding' discussed	

her about the local group. Some of the members were babysitting for each other and Nancy planned to join this scheme.

Hannah Van der Haastrecht was glad her caseload was small enough to allow her to keep closely in touch with Nancy. They arranged a date for a morning the following week. As some time was likely to be spent at the mother's home, HV made a note of the telephone numbers, both of this house and of the mother's home.

EXAMPLE TWO: THE CLARK FAMILY

Henrietta Varley (HV), a health visitor in an inner city area, heard of the Clarks, recently moved in, through one of her monthly meetings with the community midwife. The midwife said that Mrs Clark (36 weeks pregnant) did not wish to breastfeed and that they had a three-year-old daughter. A grossly handicapped boy, born five years previously, had lived only four days. An antenatal visit was not possible due to workload pressures: HV was covering the caseload of a colleague on maternity leave.

The baby was born about a fortnight after that meeting and the birth card came through to HV. Mr Clark answered the door when she called. He had taken two weeks' leave to look after his wife and daughter. Three-year-old Tracey hung around the living room doorway and HV engaged her in conversation about playschool and about 'her' baby.

Mrs Clark said the discomfort in her breasts had gone; however, an episiotomy wound was proving uncomfortable. She was tired by evening but felt reasonably energetic earlier in the day.

Baby Ian was presenting 'problems'. Mr Clark seemed particularly distressed by the baby's crying each evening. They had 'tried everything'. The baby was possetting and they were considering changing the milk formula. Having explained how to do this in a gradual way, HV went on to describe the minimal differences between the milks. She asked how the feeds were currently being made up.

The baby was asleep, but the couple wanted HV to examine him. She enquired about vision, hearing, whether they had seen the hip test done, remarked on the normality of the fontanelle and mentioned foreskin care. The couple explained that their deepest fear had been that he might be handicapped. In a way, they

Box 4.3 Example two: the Clark family

Physical health	Mental/emotional health	Social aspects of health
Mother Breasts comfortable Painful perineum No medication	*Parental knowledge* *Discussion about:* — *milk formulae* — *possetting* — *foreskin care* — *sexual activity* — *Pamphlets on immunisation*	*Mother* Husband supportive Grandparental homes 200 miles away Newly moved in One friend locally
Father Appears well·		
Toddler Alert child	*Adjustment and emotional well-being*	Intends to: — join mothers group — attend clinic
Baby 3–4 hourly feeds = SMA Possetting Sleeping prone Hearing: startles Vision: eye contact CDH test Fontanelles: not depressed	*Parents: baby* Anxious re handicap *Mother: father* Cooperating *Toddler* Involved with care Receiving parental attention	*Toddler* Plans for playgroup

found it difficult to believe their luck. It sounded as if they would be very active in monitoring his developmental progress in the record booklet which HV gave them.

Ian had regained his birthweight and, for most of the day, was reported as sleeping between three and a half to four hourly feeds. The couple said they would talk later about what had been said about the milk formulae and might wait a while before deciding whether to change it. Having Hugh Jolly's child care book in her bag, HV showed them his reassuring remarks about possetting and they all joked about his (very practical) ideas on placing towels everywhere to protect clothing and floors against the 'overflow'.

The Clarks had involved their daughter in the baby's examination. Later she went to the other side of the room and played quietly.

The forms requesting immunisation were discussed and as the couple wished to 'think about it', HV gave them up-to-date pamphlets and promised to answer their questions next time they met.

Mrs Clark had made a friend through the antenatal clinic. She was very pleased to have the list of local mothers' groups and organisations and also to find it provided addresses of playgroups. The health visitor explained that two retired ladies help entertain the toddlers at her baby clinic so that the mothers would have a chance to talk and get to know each other.

Towards the end of the visit, HV followed up the earlier remark about the painful episiotomy wound. It transpired that it had been very painful during attempted intercourse. The matter was discussed and HV recommended it should be mentioned at the six week postnatal check, if it was still painful. She made a mental note to mention it at her next visit.

As she left, the health visitor gave the couple her telephone number. Mrs Clark said she had been a regular attender at the clinic with Tracey and she intended to be with Ian.

PHYSICAL HEALTH

Mother

Liaison with other members of the primary health care team may have alerted the health visitor to a particular problem of general health which the mother may find relevant and wish to discuss. At this visit, matters such as the condition of the breasts, perineum or lochia, dental care and postnatal exercises may be of concern.

Arrangements for the six week postnatal examination and any difficulties likely to arise over attending it, may be discussed. Georgina Ray (1984) discussed and described this visit for parents and reminded mothers to take with them, as appropriate:
—a sample of urine
—their maternal cooperation card
and if attending their GP, their baby's National Health Service registration card, so, presuming they wish it, the baby can be registered there.

Dr Gunn (1983) describes the physical examination and encourages mothers to ask questions about their labour, their current condition and what they might expect in a subsequent pregnancy. He provides a useful checklist of 20 possible questions about such things as:
— vaginal discharge
— when the next period would be expected

— use of tampons
— discomfort of stitches
— painful intercourse
— lumpy breasts
— how long to breastfeed
— caesarian scar
— likelihood of another caesarian/forceps/ episiotomy
— the reason for needing to be induced
— method of contraception
— how to help get figure back.

Medication and lactation

Some drugs are best avoided by breastfeeding mothers. Lewis and Hurden (1983) provide an overview of the subject. They include a list of drugs where deleterious effects have been reported, another of drugs about which there is some doubt and a third list showing those which are probably safe for nursing mothers.

Grant and Golightly (1984) describe how new information from research can mean that reviews can soon be out of date. They outline the Drugs and Breast Milk Information Service (DIBMIS) which is available both to the professions and the public. It has already been made use of by health visitors and breastfeeding counsellors as well as many others.

Canadian researchers looking into postpartum consumption of alcohol (Davidson et al, 1981), were concerned to find that a significant proportion of the 260 women taking part in their study, *started* to drink at this time—on *professional advice*, suggesting that it would aid lactation and relaxation. Only two women had been warned to avoid alcohol both in pregnancy and for the breastfeeding period. The question arises as to whether this hazardous sort of 'medication' is being advised here too—and encouraging the lone drinking discovered in the Canadian study.

Father and siblings

The general health of the father and the baby's siblings is, naturally, also of importance in the family equation. Basic health matters such as safety, nutrition and sleeping patterns might receive consideration. In the current economic climate, the relationship between health and unemployment becomes a significant factor (Fagin & Little, 1984).

Baby

It may not always be convenient to the family for the baby to be disturbed for an examination. A separate appointment may have to be made. Even so, the family are generally very pleased for their visitor to admire their baby in its cot. If there are felt to be any problems, it is not unusual for the parents to be anxious for the health visitor to make a thorough check, even if this means disturbing a peaceful sleep.

The extent to which the baby should be examined will vary according to the local service provided. Awareness of local GP and hospital routines will increase the chance of being able to guess which babies could possibly have fallen through the normal infant screening safety net, and therefore, need greater attention.

A paper by the Department of Health and Social Security (DHSS, 1980a) suggested 6–10 days as one of the key ages for the baby to be examined, and proposed that this examination should be carried out by a doctor trained for this purpose. Health visitors curious to know about likely procedures, will find outlines by Illingworth (1982) and Curtis Jenkins and Newton (1981).

Curtis Jenkins emphasises the effect of the examination on the mother—for better or for worse. He says that appropriate demonstrations and explanations, and a well-performed examination, may make the examining doctor 'a friend for life'. Particularly important is showing the baby's ability to see, hear and, usually, to smile. The author provides pictures which show the doctor demonstrating patterns of infant behaviour. Witnessing these can significantly increase the mother's understanding of her baby's skills and abilities and the baby's need for talk and interaction.

Health visitor examination

What form then, should the health visitor's examination take? The phraseology and listing in the McClymont (1983, p. 12) criteria for the 'examination to be made during the visit' imply that the health visitor *must* undertake an investigation in which every part of the baby should be seen. This would mean stripping the baby—possibly risking irritating parents who feel the baby is currently all right and have, anyway, witnessed a recent and thorough inspection by a doctor.

If the health visitor examination is to be a brief one with the baby dressed, then the health visitor's basic nursing habit of observing general appearance is likely to take note, perhaps without comment, of the baby's
— range of facial expression
— skin colour and condition
— apparent temperature
— fontanelle: depressed?
and certainly, to investigate or enquire after
— eyes discharging?
— mouth: thrush?
— umbilicus: still moist?
— vision (making eye contact)
— hearing (startled by sudden loud noise).
In some locations, a record is made of
— naked weight
— head circumference
— length
— certain reflexes
giving the health visitor a better baseline from which to observe and compare with possible later changes.

Foreskin care

This examination provides an appropriate cue for telling parents of boys about correct foreskin care. Griffiths (1984) found people tended to be poorly advised and says initial 'masterly inaction' followed by routine penile hygiene from the age of three or four, will prevent many childhood circumcisions for phimosis, which is the reason for 80 per cent of the circumcisions currently performed.

Congenital dislocation of the hip

The tests for congenital dislocation of the hip (CDH), ably described by Monk and Dowd (1981), are neither simple nor easy. Fixen (1983) feels that health visitors should be properly trained on how to do it and what to be on the lookout for. Perhaps the best way to become more proficient, is to ask to attend the clinic of a local orthopaedic surgeon, who would probably be delighted to help.

It seems that many CDHs have been missed. The reasons were found, in a study by David et al 1983, to be due to failure
— to examine the baby's hip
— to follow up abnormalities
— to follow parental observation of problem
— of parents to understand the significance of abnormality

Clearly the current system has room for improvement.

There has been some debate about the significance of clicking or grating hip (Cunningham et al, 1984a, 1984b). It is now generally felt that hip examinations should continue after the first month or two of a baby's life. The matter is, therefore, returned to in Chapter 5 (p. 91).

The modern tendency to advise parents to lay their babies in the prone position, thought also to help prevent development of infantile ideopathic scoliosis (McMaster, 1983), could be particularly beneficial to those babies with an undiscovered tendency towards hip dislocation (Wilkinson, 1983). McMaster remarks, however, that only a quarter of the 568 normal infants in an Edinburgh study were, in fact, nursed prone. It would be interesting to know in what position people elsewhere place their babies and how this correlates with these orthopaedic problems.

Parents' own record

In some places, child health record cards for the parents' own record, are made available (Green & Macfarlane, 1985). These are likely to be explained to the parent or parents either during or after the health visitor examination.

General baby care

There are many practical matters which parents may like to discuss. 'Wind', possetting, stools, 'colic' and sleep patterns, for example, are neatly covered in books such as Penelope Leach's (1979) *Baby and Child* and Hugh Jolly's (1981) *Book of Child Care*.

Some health visitors keep a spare copy of their favourite child care book for lending, short term, to parents. They can then take time to think things over and compare the ideas in the book with other views available to them. The book can be picked up at the next visit or when the baby is brought to the clinic.

Hygiene and safety

There is a Community Outlook 'checklist' (Swaffield, 1983) which usefully sets out the major points on how to avoid nappy rash and diarrhoea. The Health Education Council's (198(1)) *Play It Safe* covers the major potential hazards for small babies, through suffocation or choking (p. 7), falls (p. 11) and car travel (p. 29). Cat nets and pram brakes (Scowen, 1984) are also topical at this stage.

A green card outlining infant care guidance on feeding care, crying and the baby's temperature is available to all parents from the Foundation for the Study of Infant Deaths. Situations in which a doctor should be called are described and emergency procedures are listed. It can be hung up in the kitchen for quick and easy reference and for reassurance.

Immunisation

Jenkinson (1982, p. 94) describes the organisation involved in immunisation and provides a table showing the basic programme for children.

Immunisation, since its beginnings, has been a controversial subject and it is still under debate (Jenkinson, 1982; Robertson, 1984; Wells, 1984). It can often be very confusing for parents. It is they who have the responsibility for deciding the relative risks involved—from the disease or from the immunisation—and for deciding what action should be taken for their baby.

Parents need to be fully informed and to have time to consider and raise questions about the matter. Where at all possible, there is much to be said for introducing the subject either antenatally or at a follow-up visit, if one is planned shortly.

Pertussis immunisation has been, in recent years, the main one to suffer from a media scare. The ensuing debate stimulated research, the earlier findings of which have been reported on elsewhere (Robertson, 1984). Some of the important points raised were: the influence of professional opinion, uncertainty about interpretation of contra-indications and inadequacy of records systems. These are outlined below.

Professional advice was found to be such a significant factor in parents' decision-making that, in Calderdale, a special training scheme was offered to professional staff involved in immunisations. It improved professional advice and immunisation procedures and brought good results.

Increasing public awareness of contra-indications for immunisation was made part of the Calderdale programme. Valman (1982) suggested that an appropriate questionnaire, given to parents in the doctors' waiting room, would allow them time to think about possible contra-indications. However, there was another problem. Governmental recommendations on contra-indications were found to be liable to wide variation in interpretation—both within and between the various professional groups whose opinion might be sought. Health visitors may need to seek clarification on local policy and the reasons for the approach adopted.

The National Childhood Encephalopathy Study (NCES) unit which was set up to research the effects of pertussis vaccines found, like some other researchers, that central recording methods could be poor, particularly regarding the details of the vaccine and the date it was given. Some parents were found to have no personal record. Some did not know what immunis-ations their children had been given. A record in the personal record booklets (Green & Macfarlane, 1985) mentioned above, would provide parents with a useful reference—and a reminder for boosters as the child grows up.

In the event, the results of the NCES and other studies have been reassuring (Bellman et al, 1983; Pollock et al, 1984; Waight et al, 1983) especially for adsorbed preparation of the vaccine.

Current advice is that an interrupted course of immunisation should not be started again. It is now thought the effect of the earlier dose lasts a few years. Also, the frequency of side-effects is liable to increase with the number of injections (Smith, 1983; Waight et al, 1983). A suggested target for pertussis uptake in the community has been put at 80% (Jelley & Nicoll, 1984).

Keeping abreast of current thinking and research in this important aspect of health visiting, will need wide reading and support from the health authority, nurse manager, peer group and professional organisation (see Ch. 2, p. 18).

Feeding: artificial

A significant proportion of women are still choosing to bottle feed their babies. There are some clear step-by-step descriptions available for those who need reassurance or instruction on preparing the feed or sterilising equipment (Health Education Council, 1984; Leach, 1979, p. 64–71). The government has provided guidelines on good feeding practice (DHSS, 1980b; Health Visitor, 1981).

There are several important aspects of artificial feeding in which health visitors may be able to be particularly helpful. For example, they need to to explain, in simple terms, the very small differences between milks (Jeffs, 1983). Downing and Howkins (1984) have described the tendency for some people to blame the milk when there are small difficulties for the baby such as skin rashes or wakefulness. They also described common mistakes in making up feeds and parental concern over constipation. All these may need advice and guidance.

In this section we have looked at some of the physical aspects of a family's health that might be considered during a health visitor's first visit after the birth. Breastfeeding, which might have been included in this part, has been held over until the next, in order to highlight, once again, some of its emotional aspects.

MENTAL AND EMOTIONAL HEALTH

Care has to be taken that physical aspects of infant health do not completely overshadow aspects of a family's emotional welfare. Reasons why this might happen could be, for example, that limitations of time at a visit may lure health visitors in giving total priority to, and concentrating on infant care. Also, if this visit is the first time they have met, both sides may hesitate to step into sensitive areas of discussion.

A. Parental knowledge

The sort of issues that parents may wish to raise will depend, primarily, upon the worries currently uppermost in their minds, the extent to which they are encouraged to express them and, of course, just how well they feel they know and trust the health visitor. It will, of course, also depend on what topics have already been covered at previous meetings. Some of the things that might be discussed can be found in this and the previous section, matters such as immunisation, hygiene and safety, infant feeding and developmental progress.

The problem of conflicting advice was mentioned in Chapter 3 (p. 37). Breastfeeding is such an important issue at this stage, that it would seem well worth making special efforts to find out the the sort of advice generally given by the GP and midwives and to keep in touch with changes of policy. In many places, now, there is a locally devised booklet given out at clinics and the hospital.

B. Expectations, adjustment and emotional well-being

Mother

It is fairly common for the mother to feel a degree of fatigue and tension. She, the main carer for the family, needs, herself, to feel cared for. The health visitor, in showing a particular interest in the mother and the way she is feeling can, for many women, provide some part of that support. There is a need for the health visitor to provide opportunities in the conversation for the mother to express her anxieties and how she feels in herself (Fig. 4.1).

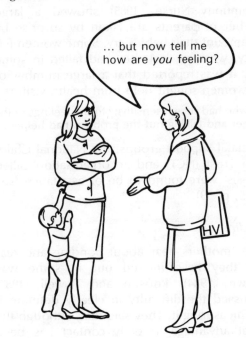

Fig. 4.1 Care for the carer.

Common problems are confused feelings over an unexpected pattern of behaviour in the baby, anxieties about 'bonding' and worries about family and, perhaps, sexual relationships. Breastfeeding mothers are especially in need of support.

Mother: baby

Unexpected behaviour

Mothers, especially of first babies, can feel particularly worried on coming home to what amounts to sole responsibility for the new baby. This is lessened if the baby is readily comforted, sleeps a good deal and feeds well. If the baby does not behave as expected, it can cause great concern and feelings of guilt about ability to care for the baby. Common worries are:

— amount of crying
— amount of sleeping
— bowel movement
— spitting up/possetting
— feeding
— lack of pattern in sleeping and feeding.

A recent study (Midwife Health Visitor & Community Nurse, 1985) showed a large number of parents are taken by surprise by the amount their babies cry. Some women felt guilty, worrying lest they had failed in some way. It was reported that a large number of the women sought help from health visitors:

. . . who had shown sensitivity to the feelings of the mother and talking out the problem had helped.

Postnatal support groups, the National Childbirth Trust (NCT) and an organisation called 'Cry-sis' were found to be of assistance (see Ch. 5, p. 59).

Bonding

Some mothers hear about bonding and fear that they have missed out in some way (Brown, 1984). Robson and Powell (1982) discussed the difficulty in clearly defining it and measuring it. They said that, although the initial advantage in early contact has been demonstrated, it is not currently possible to show what the more important long-term effects are.

What seems to be more important is an ongoing sympathetic interaction between mother and baby which is synchronised to suit them both. Enabling a mother to become aware, early, of her baby's skills in communication and perception, can enhance the interactive potential between herself and her baby (see p. 60)—and the baby and the father (Robertson & Robertson, 1982).

Many mothers will find it reassuring to hear that several studies have shown that some 40% of first time mothers feel some indifference towards their newborn babies. Robson and Kumar were reported by Robson and Powell to have found that initial feelings of maternal indifference soon wore off for most mothers.

Breastfeeding

For women who wish to breastfeed, an important key to success seems to lie in the mother's confidence in her ability to do so. It is well known that milk flow is very sensitive to psychological inhibition. Some mothers who originally wished to feed but 'fail' and change to artificial feeding, feel guilty (Houston, 1984a). Women need support in these early days. Pre-arranged, regular visiting seems to help significantly.

Mary Houston (1984a, 1984b) has researched and written on professional support at home for breastfeeding mothers. She found mothers liked to have the same person giving advice and to have appointments made for further visits. This enabled mothers to cope with problems that arose, knowing that help would be coming.

In her small study groups, Dr Houston found Social Class I mothers coped well with or without special support. Social Classes II, III and IV tended to benefit from the extra visiting. This raises the question as to whether health visitors' traditional creed of equal visiting to everyone, should be changed. She suggested it might be better for there to be a bias towards more visits to the social classes less likely to turn to the NCT or La Leche League and towards devoting more time to the encouragement of local self-help groups.

A health visitor, Marion Kelly (1983), compared the duration of breasfeeding of 19 mothers she visited weekly until six weeks and fortnightly to twelve weeks, providing structured practical and emotional support, and a control group who were visited at 11 days, three, six and twelve weeks. A greater number in the study group breastfed for three months, apparently benefiting from the morale boosting and encouragement. The results of a small sample can, of course, provide no more than an indicator.

Books and organisations. The wide range of books available on breastfeeding reflects a large demand by parents feeling the need of support and guidance. Penelope Leach (1979, p. 48–63) has provided some very practical advice and clear explanatory drawings, which mothers might find helpful. Maire Messenger's (1982) *The Breastfeeding Book* was mentioned in the previous chapter and a recently published book by Celia Worth (1984) may prove to be popular.

Another response to this need can be seen in the emergence of La Leche League and the National Childbirth Trust and their work in support and counselling in breastfeeding. Health visitors can refer mothers to them. Alison Spiro (1984) describes how NCT counsellors can work together with midwives and health visitors to help give women emotional and practical support. These organisations do tend, however, to have a bias towards catering for the more articulate and middle class mothers.

Enabling, and avoiding discouragement. Caroline Flint (1984) highlights the fact that breastfeeding is an intimate experience between two very individual people and, to a certain extent, one which they will naturally have to work out for themselves. She sees the role of the professional as an 'enabler'— offering a great deal of encouragement—and avoiding the symbols of impending failure: bottles of water or test weighing.

In the community, the 'symbol of failure' might easily be a sample packet of infant milk food. Bergamin et al (1983) studied the effect of giving mothers samples of formula feed. They found this tended to shorten the duration of breastfeeding, especially for first time mothers, the less well educated and mothers who had suffered some small illness postnatally. Complementary 'topping up'

feeds at night have been found to tend to undermine breastfeeding and mothers' confidence (Houston & Howie, 1981).

Siblings

The arrival of a new baby necessitates adjustment for everyone within the family circle. There is a need for each family member to be involved with and supportive of the others and this is no less true for the children. Claire Rayner (1977, p. 44–46) describes how they can feel. She stresses the normality of sibling jealousy and makes practical suggestions for ways in which problems might be prevented or, at least, minimised.

It is interesting to note that in Dunn and Kendrick's (1982) small in-depth study of the relationship between siblings, breastfeeding a second baby did not create jealousy in the first born. For whatever reason, the siblings in this sample were less likely to interfere and irritate when their mothers were breastfeeding the baby than were those whose mothers were bottle feeding.

During visits to a family with a new baby, health visitors tend to give special attention to older brothers or sisters, so that they also feel important and included.

Father: mother

Research on the way fathers can be affected is mentioned by Maureen Laryea (1984). The arrival of a baby, particularly the first, means a significant change in their way of life—changing routines, greater responsibilities and, alongside this, less of their wives' attention devoted entirely to themselves.

The father's active involvement with the children can be an important factor in the support of his wife, as well as in the benefit both he and the children have from it. It is good if the father is at home during the health visitor's call, as he can then be involved in the discussions and explanations.

Parenthood and sexuality

Loss of sexual interest is not at all uncommon

amongst women during the first year after the baby is born. Claire Rayner (1977, pp. 14–17) suggests several possible reasons for a woman losing libido at this time:
— current satisfaction
— hormonal changes
— tiredness
— damage creating pain
— fear of pregnancy
— fear of failure
— other psychological problems.

She describes the Masters and Johnson 'sensate focus' exercises, which many couples may find very helpful to know about.

Some practical advice on sexuality and breastfeeding is provided by Maire Messenger (1982)—discussions about feelings whilst feeding, the possibility of breasts leaking whilst love-making and a caution about contraception.

The various methods of family planning have been brought together in *The Which? Guide to Birth Control* (Kane, 1983). Rose Shapiro (1984) provides a brief overview. She reminds nurses of how they need to be as aware as possible of the influence in discussions of their own bias and prejudices, and how they need to be sensitive not only to what people know, but also how they feel about various methods of contraception.

These, then, are just some of the mental and emotional factors which a family may wish to discuss with the health visitor. Also, at this stage a health visitor might be thinking of the possibility of a future postnatal depression. It tends to affect a larger number of women some twelve weeks after the birth and is therefore included in Chapter 5 (pp. 84; 93).

SOCIAL ASPECTS OF HEALTH

Families' social needs tie in closely, of course, with their emotional needs for communication and support. Health visitors, as the professional people most closely involved with young families, are in a good position to be able to offer help where it is needed.

Mother and father: family network

Immediate and close family are usually the main sources of help for babysitting, shopping, advice, acting as confidant and all the other aspects of support that are needed when the children are small. Many young parents, however, move a significant distance away from their parents' home. To supplement the help they can give each other, they need assistance from a circle of friends and/or from community organisations.

Mother

Loneliness and isolation can be major problems for young mothers. Some women have no difficulty in finding supportive neighbours and joining friendship groups, whereas others can be more shy and need help to find friends. People with young children and with no one to turn to for support, should be considered an important priority.

Gillian Pugh (1980) suggested that health visitors, on their first call, should take a list of all the locally available schemes and services offering help and support to young families. It is not known how many already do so. She also suggested that lists of services should be clearly displayed in such places as clinics and doctors' waiting rooms.

Mothers may wish to know about organisations and services such as:
— local church groups
— National Childbirth Trust
— National Housewives Register
— mother and baby groups
— keep fit classes
— community centres
— mother and toddler groups
— babysitting services
— out of hours services from health visitors
— telephone contact for worried and stressed parents.

First time mothers and those newly moved in, need to know about the health care facilities at local child health clinics. At this visit, the health visitor can tell them about times, days, alternatives available, whether they are organised with a crèche to entertain the toddlers and if they provide facilities where mothers can meet for a cup of tea and a chat. Many health visitors are involved in setting up mothers' groups in order to help provide both for social and health educational requirements, a matter returned to in the following chapter.

Siblings

If their parents know where to find
— mother and toddler groups
— playgroups
— nurseries
toddlers' social needs, as well as the mothers', can be helped to be satisfied. These facilities should also be included on the listing described above. Keeping the list of mother and toddler groups up to date can sometimes be difficult, but is obviously well worthwhile.

Many pregnant mothers like to see their older children settled into this sort of group well before the arrival of the baby. Others wait until the newness of the baby's arrival has worn off to avoid possible feelings of exclusion.

We have been looking at some of the physical, mental/emotional and social health needs of the members of a family with a new baby and at some of the ways in which a health visitor might be able to help during a first visit after the birth.

ARRANGING FURTHER VISITS

If parents know in advance when the health visitor is likely to call again and at which clinics they will probably be able to talk with 'their' health visitor, they can then prepare questions, knowing when and where help is available, and can plan to use the service in the way that suits them best.

In some areas, a day-time health visiting telephone contact service is provided and, in a few, a seven day health visiting service has been set up. Parents need to have their attention drawn to such services, where they exist, and to be given the telephone numbers involved. Generally, health visitors have a visiting card with their office telephone number and address on it and, before they leave, inform the parents of the times they can be contacted personally.

Priorities

Where health visitors are unable to visit every family equally, they have to decide who should take precedence in their visiting schedule. Some of the families who would be considered an important priority will be met in subsequent chapters, for example, families with a handicapped baby or who have recently immigrated. Some people who would have priority, such as those who have extra difficulty in adjusting to parenthood or who are socially isolated, have already received a mention, though rather briefly, in this and the previous chapter.

Guidance for health visitor priority also comes from the evidence of the Black (1980) Report and other studies which have demonstrated the problem of higher levels of ill-health amongst people from the lower socio-economic groups and yet their lower use of the health services.

It can sometimes be very difficult to respond to this need. The problem is most common in inner city areas and this is where health visitors are more likely to be coping with double caseloads on account of staff shortages and an above average turnover of staff. The problem presents a special challenge. Inner city health visiting is considered in the final chapter.

Sometimes particular circumstances regarding the baby lead the health visitor to give an above average priority to visiting a family. For example, parents of babies recently discharged from the special care baby unit will need extra support. Added to this, the health visitor will need to have assigned time to getting up to date on and becoming familiar with the care of low birth weight babies (Amick, 1984). This becomes less necessary when a specialist community nurse from the unit undertakes home visiting.

Another example of such a priority for more frequent follow-up visiting, would be that of multiple births. Twins occur in about one in eighty pregnancies. They take a great deal of time and ingenuity, particularly in the early days, and there are special problems involved in their care. Parents, especially the mother, need extra help and support (Bryan, 1983; Linney, 1980; Stables, 1980). Recently published books on the care of twins may prove helpful to the parents (Leigh, 1983; Friedrich & Rowland, 1983) The opportunity to be told about such books antenatally, would be preferable, of course.

Choosing priorities for visiting is a complex matter as there are so many factors involved. It is helpful to parents to know to what extent the service is available to them and, for many, to know when to expect the next visit.

In this chapter we have looked at the health visitor's first visit to a family after the birth of their baby. Some behind-the-scenes preparations and considerations were described and some of the matters that may be discussed at a birth visit were classified under physical, mental/emotional and social aspects of family health need.

USEFUL ADDRESSES

Cry-sis, British Monomark Cry-sis,
London WC1N 3XX
Tel 01 404 5011

Foundation for the Study of Infant Deaths,
5th Floor 4/5 Grosvenor Place,
London SWIX 7HD

La Leche League (Great Britain)
Breastfeeding Help and Information,
BM 3424 London WCIV 6XX
Tel 01 242 1278

National Childbirth Trust,
9 Queensborough Terrace,
London W2 3TB
Tel 01 221 3833

National Housewives Register,
National Office,
245 Warwick Road, Solihull,
West Midlands B92 7AH
Tel 021 706 1101

Scottish Health Education Group,
Woodburn House,
Canaan Lane,
Edinburgh EH10 4SQ

Twins Club Association
Mrs D Hoseason (sec) 'Pooh Corner',
54 Broad Lane, Hampton,
Middlesex

REFERENCES

Amick J H 1984 Support for parents of babies in special care units. Midwives Chronicle and Nursing Notes 97: 170–175

Bellman M H, Ross E M, Miller D L 1983 Infantile spasms and pertussis immunisation. The Lancet I: 1031–1034

Bergamin Y, Dougherty C, Kramer M S 1983 Do infant formula samples shorten the duration of feeding? The Lancet I:1148–1151

Black D 1980 Inequalities in health. Report of a research working party. Department of Health and Social Security, London (chairman Sir Douglas Black)

Bowling A 1983 Teamwork in primary health care. Nursing Times 79, 48: 56–59

Brown J 1984 I can't love my child. Parents 100, 7: 80–81

Bryan E 1983 Twins in the family. Nursing Times 79, 28: 50–52

Cunningham K T, Beningfield S A, Moulton A, Maddock C R 1984a A clicking hip should never be ignored. The Lancet I: 668–670

Cunningham K T, Beningfield S A, Moulton A, Maddock C R 1984b A clicking hip should never be ignored (letter). The Lancet I: 1184–1185

Curtis Jenkins G, Newton R C F 1981 The first year of life. Churchill Livingstone, Edinburgh, pp 36–38; 71–77

David T J, Poynor M U, Simm S A, Parris M R, Hawnaur J M, Rigg E A, McCrae F C 1983 Reasons for late detection of hip dislocation in childhood. The Lancet II: 147–148

Davidson S, Alden L, Davidson P 1981 Changes in alcohol consumption after childbirth. Journal of Advanced Nursing 6: 195–198

DHSS 1980a Prevention in the child health services. Department of Health and Social Security, London

DHSS 1980b Present day practice in infant feeding. HMSO, London

Downing L J and Howkins E J 1984 Infant feeding in practice. Nursing Times 80, 6: 57–60

Draper J, Farmer S, Field S, Thoms H, Hare M J 1984 The working relationship between the general practitioner and the health visitor. Journal of the Royal College of General Practitioners 34: 264–268

Dunn J, Kendrick C 1982 Siblings. Love, envy and understanding. Grant McIntyre, London, p 49–51

Dunnell K, Dobbs J 1982 Nurses working in the community. HMSO, London

Fagin L, Little M 1984 The forsaken families. The effects of unemployment on family life. Penguin Books, Harmondsworth

Fixen J 1983 Congenital dislocation of the hip and club foot in the young child. Health Visitor 56: 281–283

Flint C 1984 Midwives and breastfeeding. Nursing Times 80, 15: 30–31

Friedrich E, Rowland C 1983 The twins handbook. From prebirth to first school days—a parents' guide. Robson Books, London

Goodwin S 1982 HV—by appointment only. Nursing Mirror 155, 2:19

Grant E, Golightly P W 1984 Providing an information service on drugs and breast milk. Journal of the Royal Society of Health 104: 99–101

Green A, Macfarlane A 1985 Parent-held child health records—a comparison of types. Health Visitor 58: 14–15

Griffiths D M 1984 The health visitor and the foreskin. Health Visitor 57:275

Gunn A 1983 Why you need a post-natal check. Mother and Baby March: 38–39

Health Education Council 198(1) Play it safe! A guide to preventing children's accidents. Health Education Council and Scottish Health Education Group in association with BBC

Health Education Council 1984 Pregnancy book. A guide to becoming pregnant, being pregnant and caring for your newborn baby. Health Education Council, London. p 70–72

Health Visitor 1981 Present day practice in infant feeding: 1980 New revised version of 1974 Oppé Report. Health Visitor 54:179

Houston M J 1984a Home support for the breast feeding mother. In: Houston M J (ed) Maternal and infant health care. Churchill Livingstone, Edinburgh

Houston M J 1984b Supporting breast feeding at home. Midwives Chronicle and Nursing Notes 97: 42–44

Houston M J, Howie P W 1981 The importance of support for the breast feeding mother at home. Health Visitor 54: 243–244

Illingworth R S 1982 Basic developmental screening: 0–4 years, 3rd ed. Blackwell Scientific Publications, Oxford, p 38–40

Jeffs J 1983 Happy bottle-feeding. Mother and Baby March: 40–42

Jelley D M, Nicoll A G 1984 Pertussis: what percentage of children can we immunise? British Medical Journal 288: 1582–1584

Jenkinson D 1982 Immunisation. In: Hart C (ed) Child care in general practice. Churchill Livingstone, Edinburgh

Jolly H 1981 Baby and Child Care. The complete guide for today's parents, 3rd ed. Allen and Unwin, London

Kane P 1983 The Which? guide to birth control. Consumers Association and Hodder & Stoughton, London

Kelly M 1983 Will mothers breast feed longer if health visitors give more support? Health Visitor 56: 407–409

Laryea M G G 1984 Postnatal care. The midwife's role. Churchill Livingstone, Edinburgh, pp 64–66, 69–71

Leach P 1979 Baby and child. From birth to age five. Penguin Books, Harmondsworth

Leigh G 1983 All about twins. A handbook for parents. Routledge and Kegan Paul, London

Lewis P J and Hurden E L 1983 Drugs and breastfeeding

In: Hawkins D F (ed) Drugs and pregnancy. Human teratogenisis and related problems. Churchill Livingstone, Edinburgh. p 217–218

Linney J 1980 The emotional and social aspects of having twins. Nursing Times 76: 276–279

McClymont A 1983 Setting standards in health visiting practice. National Board for Nursing, Midwifery and Health Visiting for Scotland, Edinburgh

McMaster M J 1983 Infantile ideopathic scoliosis: can it be prevented? Journal of Bone and Joint Surgery 65-B: 612–617

Messenger M 1982 The breastfeeding book. Century Publishing Co Ltd, London. p 94–100

Midwife Health Visitor & Community Nurse 1985 Jottings by Janus. Midwife Health Visitor & Community Nurse 21:149

Monk C J E, Dowd G S E 1981 The problems of early diagnosis and prevention of congenital dislocation of the hip. Journal of Maternal and Child Health 6: 76–85

Pollock T M, Mortimer J Y, Miller E, Smith G 1984 Symptoms after primary immunisation with DPT and with DT vaccine. The Lancet II: 146–149

Pugh G (ed) 1980 Preparation for parenthood. Some current initiatives and thinking. National Children's Bureau, London. p 37

Ray G 1984 Probing postnatal check-ups. Mother April: 42–43

Rayner C 1977 Family feelings. Arrow Books Ltd, London

Robertson C A 1984 Preventive health care for infants. In: Houston M J (ed) Maternal and infant health care. Churchill Livingstone, Edinburgh

Robertson J, Robertson J 1982 A baby in the family. Loved and being loved. Penguin Books, Harmondsworth

Robson K M, Powell E 1982 Early maternal attachment. In: Brockington I F, Kumar R (eds) Motherhood and mental illness. Academic Press, London

Scowen P (ed) 1984 New baby. A health visitor's handbook for parents. B Edsall and Co Ltd, London, p 63

Shapiro R 1984 Putting the sex back into contraception. Nursing Times Community Outlook 80, 15: 123–131

Smith J W G 1983 Interrupted immunisation. Archives of Disease in Childhood 58:167

Spiro A 1984 Counsellors can help. Nursing Times Community Outlook 80, 38: 314–316

Stables J 1980 Breastfeeding twins. Nursing Times 76: 1493–1494

Swaffield L 1983 Clean babies. Nursing Times Community Outlook 79, 51: 369–371

Valman H B 1982 Whooping cough. British Medical Journal 284: 886–887

Waight P A, Pollock T M, Miller E, Coleman E M 1983 Pyrexia after diphtheria/tetanus vaccines. Archives of Disease in Childhood 58: 921–933

Wells N 1984 Childhood vaccination, current controversies. Office of Health Economics, London

Wilkinson J A 1983 Your child's congenital dislocation of the hip: a guide to parents. The author, Southampton General Hospital, Southampton

Worth C 1984 Breastfeeding basics. Unwin Paperback, London

Chapter 5 looks at the part played by a health visitor in preventive health care for a family with very young children. The work is considered through the perspective of the prevention model. Ways in which help may be given are classified in three groupings: strategies aiming to prevent the occurrence of health problems, those to prevent their development and, thirdly, those to prevent deterioration of established conditions.

Using the prevention model

Examples of work with families with very young children

Anticipatory guidance

Screening and surveillance
Behind the scenes
The programmes

Giving support

5

Families with young children

USING THE PREVENTION MODEL

In these next two chapters, we look at the sort of contribution that the prevention model can make to planning and describing health visiting. This is demonstrated by taking the phase which follows the birth visit, that is, work with families who have children under school age. In this chapter, we look at anticipatory guidance, screening procedures and supportive care for families with babies and children up to about the age of three. Looking at such a wide section of a health visitor's work in only a chapter, means a great deal must be left out. However, it does give an indication of the sort of work entailed and a chance to look briefly at some of the important factors involved.

The prevention framework was the model most fully introduced in Chapter 1 (see pp. 4–7). It will be recalled that facets of the health visitor's role were pigeon-holed into three aspects of prevention:

—*preventing the occurrence* of potential future problems, such as by immunising babies against whooping cough in order to avoid the possibility of unfortunate side-effects of the disease, or, as another example, by promoting good health through health education.

— *preventing the development* of difficulties or handicapping conditions through early discovery and appropriate action. For example, finding deafness in a baby early enables timely use of hearing aids and special teaching and leads to the best possible development of speech.

— *preventing deterioration* of established conditions or circumstances by helping people cope with and/or overcome, for example, babies' sleep and feeding problems. The aim is that a greater dysfunction does not develop out of the current situation and that, so far as is possible, it is improved.

Table 5.1 Families with very young children: the health visitor's work

Aspect of prevention	Examples of activities	Important considerations
Preventing occurrence of condition (Anticipatory guidance)	*Discussion of*: family diet, smoking safety, breast cancer, immunisation, sleeping, play 'discipline', tooth care, illness, recognition	Parental involvement Promotes self-confidence 'Family visiting' Reach those in need Querying own advice Querying own practice
Preventing development of condition (Surveillance of family health)	*Screening re*: postnatal depression, developmental progress, hearing, vision and speech, weight, length and head circumference, hip dislocation, special schemes	Accessible treatment Early discovery Physical and general welfare Search *and* teach Parental involvement Reach those in need Review monitoring
Preventing deterioration of established conditon (Supportive work)	*Sympathetic listening; Information about services; Encouraging self-help groups;* re: common baby and childhood problems, isolation and lack of confidence, postnatal depression, bereavement	Support and teach Availability of service Individual initiative Congeniality of clinic Strategies for problems: — wide-ranging — more rare

This approach, which in essence describes the reasons why the work is undertaken, is particularly useful for looking at our work, both over a range of time and from a case-load-wide perspective. The family health needs framework of the previous two chapters, is rather more useful for looking at what factors need to be considered at a single or at a particular type of visit.

The presentation of the prevention framework in this chapter, shown in Table 5.1, has been modified a little from that in Table 1.2. This is to make space for listing important considerations pertaining to the work, such as availability of the service or parental involvement, whilst still leaving room in the table for lists of the basic health visitor activities.

It may be found helpful if we can start by giving a couple of examples of a health visitor's work with a family and show how this framework can highlight important factors.

EXAMPLES OF WORK WITH FAMILIES WITH VERY YOUNG CHILDREN

The first example outlines some of the work of a health visitor with a couple in their first two years as parents. The other example is of a health visitor in an inner city area, and gives a brief overview of her work with a disadvantaged young family. The factors mentioned are listed in the prevention format, in Tables 5.2 and 5.3.

EXAMPLE ONE: THE FORESTS

Mrs Honor Vincent (HV) had very vivid memories of her early visits to the Forest family. She had just completed her health visitor course and their first baby, Sarah, was the first birth visit on her new caseload. They had had no antenatal visit. In order to give them something of a quick overview of her work with young families, she had shown them the Nelms and Mullens list, photostatted for her studies. The Forests had encouraged her to keep it in her bag. It proved, at several of the visits, to be a useful trigger to some pertinent questioning, for example on stimulation and

Table 5.2 Example one: the Forests

Aspect of prevention	Examples of activities	Important considerations
Preventing occurrence of condition (Anticipatory guidance)	*Discussion of*: immunisation, safety, stimulation family diet	Promote self-confidence Parental involvement 'Family visiting
Preventing development of condition (Surveillance of family health	*Screening re*: **mother**: postnatal depression **daughter**: hearing, vision, weight developmental progress and head circumference **son**: special scheme	Accessible care Early discovery Search *and* teach Parental involvement Service reviewed
Preventing deterioration of established condition (Supportive work)	*Sympathetic listening; Information about vol. groups re*: Sleep problem—book lent Postnatal depression— ref. NCT Crying baby service	Support *and* teach strategy for support service available

Table 5.3 Example two: the Lambournes

Aspect of prevention:	Examples of activities	Important considerations
Preventing occurrence of condition (Anticipatory guidance)	*Discussion of*: Safety, stimulation (Deferential mother) New scheme set up	Promote confidence Parental involvement Querying own practice Reach those in need
Preventing development of condition (Surveillance of family health)	*Screening re*: weight and head circumference, developmental progress, hearing and speech Vision—re amblyopia: orthoptist seen	Search *and* teach Parental involvement Early discovery Accessible treatment
Preventing deterioration of established condition (Supportive work)	Sympathetic listening; Encouraging self-help groups; re: Loneliness— local women's group Clinic	Strategy for problem Individual initiative Attempt to improve

family diet, by the parents and particularly over safety at each phase of development. They enjoyed being able to look, with her, at a phase or two ahead and they said it made them search things out in the baby manuals they had been given.

The father was usually at home for the visits. He was a night worker, and they chose appointments in the morning so he could join in. Both parents were amused by the lists of hints on whether or not the baby could hear and see, and found them fun to try out. They did not wish to attend the baby clinic and weighed their baby at the chemist, taking a spare set of clothes to weigh in order to be able to deduce the naked weight. They filled in a centile chart themselves and had promised to call into the clinic or ring

HV if they were worried. In the event, they did not need to. Also, they did not use the 'crying baby' service, run on a rota basis by some of the health visitors.

There had been a rather worrying patch when, eight weeks postnatally, Mrs Forest's self-assessment questionnaire had shown her, as she had felt, to be depressed. However, both a fortnight and four weeks later, she was seen to be gradually returning to normal, as she became less restless at night and less despondent and less irritable. She had, however, followed up HV's suggestion and contacted the National Childbirth Trust (NCT) and had said she intended to remain with the group. Mrs Forest was evidently grateful to be able to pour out her feelings, both with the NCT counsellor and with HV. Follow-up assessments showed no problems. The scheme had done what it was intended to do and had alerted the parents and the health visitor to the possibility of postnatal depression. The health visitor was glad that, in this small town environment, her caseload pressures were light enough to enable more frequent visiting, eight times in the first year.

The eighteen month visit had been the most recent one. They had checked Sarah's developmental progress, talked over measles vaccination and the Forests had proudly shown HV their latest safety devices and schemes. They had reported that Sarah's sleeping habits had become unacceptable, and HV had lent them her copy of 'My Child Won't Sleep' which they returned to her through the surgery two weeks later. Mrs Forest had said she was two months pregnant.

Today the practice midwife had told HV that Mrs Forest had had a premature birth and a small baby boy. This baby was likely to qualify as 'high risk' in the newly set up infant surveillance scheme and would be scheduled for weekly weighing until he reached 3 kg or the expected date of delivery, whichever were the later. Mrs Vincent was grateful she now had her own portable baby weighing scales to take with her to the home. She had planned anyway to make extra visits as Mrs Forest had been determined to breastfeed this baby and had previously had postnatal depression. In the event, baby Mark progressed well and Mrs Forest showed no indication of a repeat of the depression.

EXAMPLE TWO: THE LAMBOURNES

The Lambournes were moving to another part of the city and, as Hazel Vickery (HV) glanced through their records before sending them on to the next health visitor, she was reminded of the change of attitude in her client.

At both the antenatal and the birth visit, Mrs Lambourne had been rather deferential and seemed unconfident. The health visitor found herself wishing that she had been trained in the skills employed in the Child Development Projects and knew a few more tips on how to help parents take the initiative in their discussions.

During the next visit HV had shown and discussed the leaflet 'You Know More Than You Think You Do', following up an interest expressed by the mother. She was beginning to suspect the mother could not read, and when at six weeks

HV had shown Mrs Lambourne the four aspects of development listed in the stepladder centile charts, she felt pretty sure. She always took care after that, casually, to read aloud things like the phases of development and the lists of 'hints for parents' or any papers they were studying.

Looking together at the developmental centile charts, led on to discussions, particularly about stimulation and safety, and gradually Mrs Lambourne gained the confidence to state and expand on her own view. When they went through the nine month assessment tests together and chatted about the next phase of developments, Mrs Lambourne mentioned how much fun her husband was having 'romping' in the evenings with their baby son. They had bought second-hand gates and a fireguard.

Mrs Lambourne had attended the clinic which was very formally set up, just once. Around that time HV had tried, unsuccessfully, to get the rest of the staff involved in their draughty church hall clinic to agree to a rearrangement to try to make it more welcoming and 'social', and had finally decided she needed to find another solution. She had talked with the GPs in the practice about the isolation and loneliness of women, particularly those such as Mrs Lambourne, on a marginal income and living some distance from their families.

One of the GPs was very sympathetic and persuaded the others to allow the use of an upstairs room once a fortnight for a self-help group, provided HV was prepared to act as background support for it. It was decided it should have a three months trial period. Now, it had been going for a year: the group showed no signs of lack of support and the slow beginnings had been well worth weathering.

The members of the group had picked up issues that caused them concern, and, as they had gained in confidence, had determined together to do something about them. Their latest campaign had been for safety around their blocks of flats, particularly aiming at limiting motor access and in setting up play areas for the young children. They had invited two of their local councillors to come and join them and had shown them a health education film that helped make their point about local safety needs. They had found the road safety officer from the environmental health department very helpful. Mrs Lambourne said she had not realised just how much can be achieved by contacting and talking with such people, and that it was fun working with the other members of the group.

The most recent incident on her card referred to the fact that the Lambournes had been playing with their son and they found he reacted against one of his eyes being covered over. They had been trying out 'helpful hints on vision' and felt he might have a squint. It was in the family. A secondary screening service was available at the orthoptists clinic which meant they would not have to wait on a long waiting list to see the ophthalmologist. Reduced vision in one eye was confirmed, an early case of amblyopia which would need attention. Fortunately the house to which the Lambournes were moving would be within walking distance of the hospital and so trips to visit the orthoptist's clinic would not prove as expensive as they would have in bus fares from their current flat.

ANTICIPATORY GUIDANCE

The greater amount of most health visitors' time is taken up with trying to help parents of babies and very young children avoid future potential problems. Health education is undertaken in various ways and is included in work in clinics, in the home and in group work; it is interwoven into screening sessions and supportive care, and provided in special projects.

Many of the topics discussed with parents can be found in well-known manuals and are not repeated here because they could only be covered in a very shallow way. Some of these books are listed on this page, Box 5.1. They are the sort that might be recommended to parents and that some health visitors keep available in their car to help in giving anticipatory guidance.

In this section we shall look at some of the issues that health visitors need to think about when planning and undertaking this aspect of their work, such as helping people to know some of the details about aims and intentions, so the service can be used better; the need to boost morale; discriminatory provision of the service in favour of those with greatest need; and questioning one's day to day advice and practice.

Parental involvement

If parents can have a fair understanding of the way in which the health visitor is aiming to help, then it is much easier for them to make good use of the service. There are some lists available that give an outline of the sort of matters that are of concern in health visiting. Examples are will be found on page 75, Box 5.2. Some health visitors find that one or two of these make useful visual aids when they are telling parents about the wide range of topics discussed in the course of their work. The main disadvantage of these papers is that, in

---

Box 5.1 Books which might be recommended to parents of very young children

Green C *Toddler Taming* A parent's guide to the first four years Century Publishing, 1984	**Leach P** *Baby and Child* Penguin Books, 1979
Scottish Health Education Group *The Book of the Child* Pregnancy to 4 years old 2nd edn Scottish Health Education Unit, 1980	**Jolly H** *Book of Child Care* The complete guide for today's parents Sphere Books, 1981
Rayner C *Family Feelings* Understanding your child from 0 to 5 Arrow Books, 1977	**Douglas J & Richman N** *My Child Won't Sleep* Penguin Books, 1984
Scowen P (ed) *New baby Growing Up* Edsall & Co Ltd, 1981	**Koch J** *Superbaby* Over 300 exercises and games to stimulate your baby's intellectual, physical and emotional development Orbis Publishing Ltd, 1982

Box 5.2 Lists showing areas of concern in preventive health care for children under three years

Book	Lists	Indicates
Nelms B C & Mullins R G *Growth and Development* A Primary Health Care Approach Prentice Hall Inc, 1982	pp. 70–73	The sort of background information sought; a range of possible tests; interest in feeding, safety and development; possible anticipatory guidance
Ingalls A J & Salerno M C *Maternal and Child Health Nursing* C V Mosby Company, 1983	pp. 328–341	Physical, motor and language development, listed along with photographs; a range of possible anticipatory guidance; some psychosocial factors
Sheridan M D *The Developmental Progress of Infants and Young Children* HMSO, 1975	Most of booklet	Wide range of developmental stepping-stones listed under: posture and large movements; vision and fine movements; hearing and speech; social behaviour and play
Sheridan M D *Children's Developmental Progress*. From Birth to Five Years: the Stycar Sequences NFER Publishing, 1975	Most of book	Similar information to booklet above with clear line drawings demonstrating attainments and hearing and vision tests
Lee C *The Growth and Development of Children* 3rd edn Longman, 1984	pp. 170–183	Child's physical development; his feelings; social behaviour and his needs
	pp. 190–191	Some suggested play materials
Pringle M K *The Needs of Children* Hutchinson, 1974	p. 159	'Ten child care commandments'—aspects of children's needs

them, concern is centred entirely upon the child. Also, by looking at child care so intensely, they may give the impression that health visitors have a vision of and hope for 'ideal parenthood' in the people they visit.

A morale boosting, family visitor!

Excellent antidotes to misconceptions about perfect motherhood or parenting, can be found by referring parents to the booklets 'Now you're a family' and 'You know more than you think you do' (see Table 4.1) and the book by Claire Rayner (1977). Perhaps, even better, is another book for parents called *Toddler Taming* by Dr Christopher Green (1984). It is well presented and amusing, as well as giving very practical advice, and looks fairly and squarely at *parental* needs when confronted with the vagaries of a robust and energetic toddler.

This book covers many matters of importance to health visitors. For example, Dr Green points out that there are no 'right answers' and aims to boost parents' confidence. He tells his readers to beware of books and advisers that set unattainably high goals—and consequently generate feelings of parental inadequacy. A brief history tells how deviant behaviour in the last century was felt to be caused by 'bad breeding', and was later explained, eventually in an extreme form in the 1950s, by 'poor environment'. The doctor explains how, at that time, blame was put on the mothers, consequently giving them enormous feelings of guilt and unhappiness. He warns that some 'helping professionals', still guided by the 'archaic ideas of the 50s', cannot give practical advice without psychoanalysing the parents (Green, 1984, pp. 9, 23–30)! The advice given by Dr Green, in contrast, recognises that some children are more difficult than others and gives parents many useful ideas on how to encourage 'good' and cope with 'bad' behaviour.

Naturally, most health education for families

with very young children centres around child care. It tends, therefore, to detract from the image of the health visitor as one concerned with the health of the whole family. The balance is restored a little when subjects are discussed which directly concern other members of the family. An example of this could be asking a mother if she wishes to know about self-examination of the breast (Laurence, 1983; Dening, 1983; Rowden, 1983; Nichols, 1983).

Greatest need

An important aspect to be considered is the extent to which the service is provided for those who need it most. Initiatives are necessary to make provision for the people who do not tend to use the standard services. This matter was touched on in Chapter 3 (page 36). The Child Development Project (1984) was mentioned with regard to antenatal care. In the postnatal period, the specially assigned health visitor calls on each family monthly for six months or so and stays for about an hour at each visit. An assessment is made of recent nutrition, and pamphlets and recipes are available for the parents. The child's health and development are noted. The service is provided in this first, most critical period of parenthood, and is being given to first time parents to get maximum benefit for the family. Good use is made of humour, through cartoons, and the parents are encouraged to contribute to the pool of ideas.

There are 600 'intervention' and 400 control families taking part in this stage of the research project. The work has, of course, been more successful with some families than with others. However, a general pattern is emerging of a greater awareness by 'intervention' mothers of development and good nutrition and of an alertness in their children (Child Development Project, 1984). Health visitors are very appreciative of these encouraging developments (Cranshaw, 1984; Fairs, 1984; Percy, 1984).

The Black (1980, p. 108) Report found evidence that went against the commonly held view that health visitors visit everyone equally without regard to positive discrimination in favour of people in particular need. It seems that looking at 'class' or 'father's occupation' alone gives a distorted view. They describe a study in Glamorgan and in South West England, which found that, when factors such as local social amenities, overcrowding and parental education were taken into consideration, the 'disadvantaged' tended to receive more health visits right through the first three years.

This same Report noted that accidents account for one third of deaths in children, and show a strong class differential (Black, 1980). It is obviously an important matter for preventive health care. The Report suggests that there is much that can be done without great cost to the public to improve the safety of children. Health visitors might try, locally, to 'influence policies affecting health' (CETHV, 1977), perhaps with the help of the Child Accident Prevention Trust, an organisation which undertakes research and is concerned with influencing decision-makers and their policy. Health visitors may know, for example, of low standards of safety in rented accommodation and unsafe areas for children to play, and liaison with environmental health officers, local councillors and voluntary organisations might help instigate improvements.

Safety should be, of course, an important subject of discussion during health visits (Health Education Council, 1981; Moore, 1982; Ray, 1982; Community Outlook, 1982; 1984; Ahamed, 1982), and the effect of poverty on the ability of disadvantaged families to provide a safe environment needs special consideration. Colver and Pearson (1985) showed the value of knowing exactly what grants families on supplementary benefits were entitled to for stair-gates, cookers and fire guards, and also where and at what cost safety items could be purchased. Their study showed a small amount of well-informed, relevant guidance could be very effective.

Questioning common practice and advice

A great deal of the sort of advice that health visitors give on child care has not been, and in some cases cannot be, tested properly. Much of that found in the well-known child care manuals varies significantly. For example, there is little agreement between them on views about the use of dummies (Darbyshire, 1985). More 'scientifically'-based advice, such as that founded on 'evidence' about salt in the diet, is still open to controversy (The Economist, 1984; Johnson & Silman, 1985; Stretch, 1983). It seems best for health visitors to try to provide, in their discussions, information about the range of current ideas and to attempt to be as aware as possible of the extent to which these theories have been validated.

In many ways this lack of certainty helps to make it easier to develop a partnership between parent and professional. It also tends to put in perspective what some professionals see as 'non-compliance', where people continue to carry out their own ideas—despite the wonderful advice they have been given! The aim, of course, in health visiting is not to order people's behaviour, but to help them make informed decisions and then to support them in whatever choice they make. Health visitors can learn a great deal from the varied perspectives and the practical experiences of parents. Also, it pays to listen. Offering dogmatic advice which takes no account of the family's views is liable to generate antagonism. Even worse, it can lead to feelings of guilt and inadequacy on account of failure to comply with the instructions. These are very counter-productive and create an atmosphere in which it is most unlikely there could be open discussion with the health visitor about the true situation.

All common practices need to be examined for their value and for their potential for counter-productivity. Questions are being raised, for example, about the propriety and the effect of health visitors' giving out samples on behalf of the infant food manufacturers (Rowe, 1985; Stretch, 1983). The correlation between mothers' being given milk samples and lowered rates of breastfeeding, was noted in Chapter 4 (p. 65).

Rajan's (1985) small study of the result of giving away samples of babies' weaning foods at clinics, found it correlated with early weaning, again, the reverse of what is being advised as the best policy. There is a clear need for further research. Either way, health visitors do need to be fully aware of the extent to which they are being 'wooed' by baby product firms as a route through to persuading mothers to buy their goods. They need to think carefully, too, about the use of their professional position with regard to their giving that 'preferential consideration' (UKCC, 1984).

These, then, are just some of the issues that health visitors need to consider when planning and thinking about how to prevent the occurrence of problems and conditions, be it through liaison or through anticipatory guidance on matters such as nutrition, safety, and immunisation, for the families they visit.

SCREENING AND SURVEILLANCE

Trying to prevent the development of problems by discovering them early, comes into most aspects of a health visitor's work, both at the clinic and out on home visits. Weighing and measuring babies, searching out vision and hearing defects and surveillance of developmental progress and mothers' emotional health, provide some examples of this sort of work with families with very young children. It involves behind-the-scenes planning and evaluation as well as the more visible practical aspects of screening and surveillance.

BEHIND THE SCENES

There are many questions the primary health care team need to think about when planning and evaluating screening and surveillance

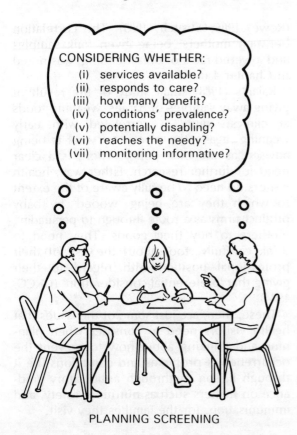

CONSIDERING WHETHER:

   (i)   services available?
   (ii) responds to care?
  (iii) how many benefit?
  (iv) conditions' prevalence?
   (v) potentially disabling?
  (vi) reaches the needy?
 (vii) monitoring informative?

PLANNING SCREENING

Fig. 5.1 Some factors considered in planning screening.

programmes (see Fig. 5.1). Time should be set aside for this, to try to ensure that the service provided is the one most appropriate to local circumstances and needs. Some of the questions which may be considered are:

Are services available and accessible?

There is no point in discovering conditions that cannot be improved in any way, once they have been identified. Services may be provided, but there may be problems of geographic inaccessibility or of a long wait for treatment to be made available. Distance from the clinic is, of course, particularly important to the people least able to afford the bus fares and who do not own a car, especially if they have more than one young child. Health visitor managers and administrators should be informed about clinics affected by travelling

difficulties, so that some attempt can be made to provide clinics in the localities where this is known to be a common problem.

If the way cases are referred on to clinics is inadequate or the service is poorly organised, there may be delays in receiving treatment and its effectiveness may be diminished. Health visitors should know about alternative methods of referral and have some idea of the length of the waiting lists. For example, if a squint is discovered, the quickest form of referral is necessary, be it via the GP or straight through to the local eye department/specialist or the local optician. The length of time spent on the waiting list for the orthoptist or/and the consultant, is very important, as very lengthy delays may affect the way the condition responds to treatment. A year between first suspicions of a squint and seeing the specialist, does not seem to be unusual (Johnson, 1984). Where significant delays between discovery and treatment are found, liaison is needed to draw attention to extent of the problem and to find appropriate solutions.

Will conditions improve with attention?

Consideration needs to be given as to whether problems are likely to be discovered early enough and also whether the degree of improvement is likely to justify the efforts involved. A hearing defect at nine months, for example, can affect the development of speech. The earlier the discovery, the more successful will be the outcome. Encouraging parental involvement in monitoring their children's ability to hear can maximise the chance of discovery (Latham & Haggard, 1980) and takes only a little time to explain (see Fig. 5.6).

Are there problems to justify the service?

Efforts to estimate what the service is likely to bring to light, help to clarify the objectives of the programmes being provided. If research on the epidemiological spread, for example, of vision or hearing defects is available, then this might provide benchmarks against which to plan these aspects of the programme and to compare results (Robertson, 1981). However, looking for medical defects is only one aspect of child surveillance programmes. Health visitors tend to consider a very wide range of features, such as a child's apparent nutritional state and any signs of illness, social aspects of development and indicators of emotional development. They note, for example, a baby's expression and eyes, its apparent relationship with its mother and whether it is alert, withdrawn or subdued (Connolly, 1983).

Are the problems potentially disabling?

It is only worth seeking to discover and treat problems that are potentially harmful in some way. Many screening programmes aim mainly to discover conditions which threaten life. This is not so in child health surveillance programmes, though such cases have been reported (Powell, 1985). The aim is, rather, to make an early discovery of factors that affect the quality of life, such as hearing and vision defects, developmental delay and social and emotional problems for the various members of the family.

The surveillance programme should also act as a teaching aid and promote parental awareness of the pre-requisites for good health. In this way, it should help avoid the occurrence of potentially harmful situations at a later date. For example, assessment of a toddler's developmental progress may bring to light behavioural problems. Discussions at the screening session, and later parents' involvement in monitoring their child's developmental progress, may increase their understanding of the needs and limitations of their child. This, in turn, can help them think of better ways they might handle and give attention to their child. Thus the programme should help them avoid 'behavioural difficulties at a later stage, as well as helping them cope with the current minor problems.

Does the programme reach those who need it?

It can be very time consuming to follow up people who either do not wish to, or who are unable to attend clinics. However, it is a very important aspect of surveillance and screening programmes. What is needed is to be able to make contact with these families, in order to explain the purpose of the programmes, offer the tests at home, and/or explain what the parents should be on the look-out for, so that serious problems will be found early. For example, missed vision or hearing defects in babyhood and childhood, can have very serious consequences for a child's ability to learn or to communicate later on. If long-standing problems are not being discovered until the children get to school, then the system is obviously failing.

It has been reported that children can remain unscreened due to shortages of staff, or due to triple duty nursing (health visiting combined with district nursing and midwifery) in which other work is given higher priority (Morris & Hird, 1981). Managers should, of course, be kept up to date on the extent to which inadequate staffing affects the service. However, methods of working out staffing levels such as those in Cheltenham are becoming available (Bell & Moules, 1985). It is important that any such scheme is able to provide indicators of the sort of social problems and the level of 'at risk' factors in a community and that have been assigned to each health visitor. The Portsmouth surveillance scheme (Powell, 1985), for example, can provide such indicators. This sort of information can also help managers be fully aware of the sort of pressures their staff are under, and would, of course, provide some measure of the adequacy of service available to those who most need it.

Not everyone finds the currently provided services to their taste. Where people do not respond to invitations to clinics, it can be a very useful exercise to try to find out what it is that they find difficult or dislike about them. Jane Robinson's (1982) small study of non-attendance found that those who did not come, cared just as much about their children's welfare as those who did. Her study raised some very important questions about, for example, the provision of services, and further research of this sort is needed.

There is the question, too, as to whether health visitors are aware of the whereabouts of all the children in their area. For example, does the Housing Department notify the health visitors of homeless families placed in hostels? Are the children in long-stay hospitals, residential and foster care, receiving the service? Parliament's Social Services Committee (1984) recommended that social services departments should be statutorily obliged to notify the appropriate health authorities of movements of children in their care. In the meantime, it is a matter over which cooperation should be sought between the local services.

Communications can be another barrier. Where lack of a common language leads to a poor service for some families, then efforts should be made to employ staff of the same culture and language. This aspect is returned to in Chapter 10.

Is monitoring informative?

This question is important from several points of view. One is with regard to information on the overall outcome of the programme and how much feedback this information gives to health visitors on what they are achieving. We return to this in Chapter 8. Another is to do with the validity of any screening tests used, that is, the extent to which they bring to light relevant problems. This is a matter which needs urgent attention (HVA, 1985, p. 24). A third aspect concerns to what degree the chosen screening test is informative for parents and is useful in helping to improve their understanding of their children's needs and development. Some valuable attributes of screening tests are listed in Table 5.4.

These then are just a few of the matters that may be raised in appraisals of potential or current screening and surveillance schemes. The Health Visitors' Association's policy statement on the health visitor's role in child health surveillance covers several more. For example, it considers health visitor training for screening, the role of the doctor in child health surveillance, the requirements of chil-

Table 5.4 Factors which can help make a test for surveillance of children particularly useful

Factor	Special value	Comment
A minimum of equipment needed	Easier to use in the homes of families not attending clinics or surgery, making service available to all babies whose parents wish it	E.g. Prof Barber's test needs a bell, a rattle, small cubes and brick— and the records
Scheme includes most important and indicative test items only	Leaves time for parental queries and to explain value and purpose of surveillance and screening, so that parents can take an active part in the scheme	Properly researched validation of tests needed
Has spread of test items to accommodate the wide range of variation within normality	Can demonstrate to parents a general picture of development and the individuality of each baby's progress	E.g. Sheridan (1975a), very wide range—very time consuming for health visitor, but can be explained to parents
Simple system of recording, preferably in diagrammatic form	Makes it easier for both examiner and parent to monitor child's progress at a glance, and to compare current attainments with previous and normal performances	E.g. Prof Barber's centile charts (Barber et al, 1976); Bar charts (Bryant, 1980)
Standardised scheme for local use	Enables systematic research and validation of the tests, making it possible to compare different wards and areas	Professor Barber's scheme allows for computerisation of results

dren with special educational needs and the conditions for satisfactory testing of vision and hearing (HVA, 1985). Several other documents also make a useful contribution to the debate (Royal College of Nursing Health Visitors Advisory Group, 1983; 1984; Royal College of General Practioners, 1982; General Medical Services Committee of the British Medical Association, 1984).

HAD Scale

Name: Date:

Doctors are aware that emotions play an important part in most illnesses. If your doctor knows about these feelings he will be able to help you more.

This questionnaire is designed to help your doctor to know how you feel. Read each item and place a firm tick in the box opposite the reply which comes closest to how you have been feeling in the past week.

Don't take too long over your replies: your immediate reaction to each item will probably be more accurate than a long thought-out response.

Tick only one box in each section

I feel tense or 'wound up':
Most of the time ....
A lot of the time ....
Time to time, Occasionally ....
Not at all ....

I still enjoy the things I used to enjoy:
Definitely as much ....
Not quite so much ....
Only a little ....
Hardly at all ....

I get a sort of frightened feeling as if something awful is about to happen:
Very definitely and quite badly ....
Yes, but not too badly ....
A little, but it doesn't worry me ....
Not at all ....

I can laugh and see the funny side of things:
As much as I always could ....
Not quite so much now ....
Definitely not so much now ....
Not at all ....

Worrying thoughts go through my mind:
A great deal of the time ....
A lot of the time ....
From time to time but not too often ..
Only occasionally ....

I feel cheerful:
Not at all ....
Not often ....
Sometimes ....
Most of the time ....

I can sit at ease and feel relaxed:
Definitely ....
Usually ....
Not often ....
Not at all ....

I feel as if I am slowed down:
Nearly all the time ....
Very often ....
Sometimes ....
Not at all ....

I get a sort of frightened feeling like 'butterflies' in the stomach:
Not at all ....
Occasionally ....
Quite often ....
Very often ....

I have lost interest in my appearance:
Definitely ....
I don't take so much care as I should.....
I may not take quite as much care ....
I take just as much care as ever ....

I feel restless as if I have to be on the move:
Very much indeed ....
Quite a lot ....
Not very much ....
Not at all ....

I look forward with enjoyment to things:
As much as ever I did ....
Rather less than I used to ....
Definitely less than I used to ....
Hardly at all ....

I get sudden feelings of panic:
Very often indeed ....
Quite often ....
Not very often ....
Not at all ....

I can enjoy a good book or radio or TV programme:
Often ....
Sometimes ....
Not often ....
Very seldom ....

Do not write below this line

Printed as a service to medicine by 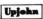 **Upjohn**

Fig. 5.2 Example of self-assessment questionnaire: Hospital Anxiety and Depression (HAD) scale. Reproduced by kind permission of Dr R P Snaith, Department of Psychiatry, St James University Hospital, Leeds.

IDA Scale

[Ref: R. P. Snaith et al. Brit J Psychiat (1978), 132, 164–71]

Name: Date:

FOLD HERE

Instructions for Use

First write your name and date in the space above. This form has been designed so that you can show how you have been feeling in the past few days.

Read each item in turn and then UNDERLINE the response which best shows how you are feeling or have been feeling in the past few days.

Ignore the letters and numbers at the left-hand side and at the end of the questionnaire.

Make sure to complete both sides.

D				I feel cheerful:
0				Yes, definitely
1				Yes, sometimes
2				No, not much
3				No, not at all
	A			I can sit down and relax quite easily:
	0			Yes, definitely
	1			Yes, sometimes
	2			No, not much
	3			No, not at all
D				My appetite is:
3				Very poor
2				Fairly poor
1				Quite good
0				Very good
		O		I lose my temper and shout or snap at others:
		3		Yes, definitely
		2		Yes, sometimes
		1		No, not much
		0		No, not at all
D				I can laugh and feel amused:
0				Yes, definitely
1				Yes, sometimes
2				No, not much
3				No, not at all
		O		I feel I might lose control and hit or hurt someone:
		3		Sometimes
		2		Occasionally
		1		Rarely
		0		Never
	A			I have an uncomfortable feeling like butterflies in the stomach:
	3			Yes, definitely
	2			Yes, sometimes
	1			Not very often
	0			Not at all
			I	The thought of hurting myself occurs to me:
			3	Sometimes
			2	Not very often
			1	Hardly ever
			0	Not at all

PTO

Fig. 5.3a Example of self-assessment questionnaire: Irritability-Depression-Anxiety (IDA) scale. Reproduced by kind permission of Dr R P Snaith, Department of Psychiatry, St James University Hospital, Leeds.

D					I'm awake before I need to get up:
3					For 2 hours or more
2					For about 1 hour
1					For less than an hour
0					Not at all, I sleep until it is time to get up
	A				I feel tense or 'wound up':
	3				Yes, definitely
	2				Yes, sometimes
	1				No, not much
	0				No, not at all
		I			I feel like harming myself:
		3			Yes, definitely
		2			Yes, sometimes
		1			No, not much
		0			No, not at all
D					I have kept up my old interests:
0					Yes, most of them
1					Yes, some of them
2					No, not many of them
3					No, none of them
		O			I am patient with other people:
		0			All the time
		1			Most of the time
		2			Some of the time
		3			Hardly ever
	A				I get scared or panicky for no very good reason:
	3				Yes, definitely
	2				Yes, sometimes
	1				No, not much
	0				No, not at all
		I			I get angry with myself or call myself names:
		3			Yes, definitely
		2			Yes, sometimes
		1			Not often
		0			No, not at all
		O			People upset me so that I feel like slamming doors or banging about:
		3			Yes, often
		2			Yes, sometimes
		1			Only occasionally
		0			Not at all
	A				I can go out on my own without feeling anxious:
	0				Yes, always
	1				Yes, sometimes
	2				No, not often
	3				No, I never can
		I			Lately I have been getting annoyed with myself:
		3			Very much so
		2			Rather a lot
		1			Not much
		0			Not at all

FOR OFFICE USE ONLY	
D (4–6)	A (6–8) ....
IN. IRR (4–6)	OUT. IRR (5–7) ....
Figures in parentheses denote borderline ranges	

Fig. 5.3b Example of self-assessment questionnaire: Irritability-Depression-Anxiety (IDA) scale–overleaf. Reproduced by kind permission of Dr R P Snaith, Department of Psychiatry, St James University Hospital, Leeds.

THE PROGRAMMES

For the mothers

Postnatal depression

It is logical, when seeking early signs of family ill health, to start with the mother. Her health, particularly her emotional health, is a cornerstone of family welfare. As the main carer, the mother's mental state is likely to be reflected in the way she copes with her responsibilities. Jacqueline Habgood (1985) a former health visitor, has described how postnatal depression affected her and her relationship with her child. She felt and looked ill and drained of strength over a six-year period. Mrs Habgood had shouted at and smacked her little girl, who had needed a great deal of good mothering to compensate, once the depression was overcome.

Some 20–30% of mothers are affected by postnatal depression and it is important to recognise it early. Mrs Habgood says health visitors in Edinburgh use a self-report screening test designed by Dr Cox (1986; Holden, 1985) to detect postnatal depression. There is an obvious advantage if parents can learn something about it antenatally as was discussed in Chapter 3.

Self-assessment tests from Leeds University have been available for a while. These are the hospital anxiety and depression (HAD) scale (Zigmond & Snaith, 1983) and the irritability-depression-anxiety (IDA) scale (Snaith et al, 1978), shown in Figures 5.2, 5.3a and 5.3b. The IDA scale, perhaps the more appropriate for the postnatal period (Snaith, 1984), and its scoring system are very clearly explained by Snaith et al. The HAD scale, which is managed in the same way, may, however, be more acceptable to mothers. Some may be rather sensitive about the questioning on irritability. Both of the scales could be completed, perhaps whilst waiting in a clinic, and, certainly, in the privacy of the mother's own home. They are both readily available (information included with references), the IDA scale with a small charge, the HAD scale free.

Recognition of the condition is the first important step, and there is an obvious advantage to parents who have had forewarning that it might occur and have learned something about it in the antenatal period. It cannot come as such a shock. There are, however, very many views about postnatal depression and what should be done about it (Kumar, 1982; Atkinson, 1983). The National Childbirth Trust booklet (Waumsley, 1983) points out that merely knowing there is someone who cares and will listen, is of great importance, a subject returned to in the next section (p. 93).

For babies and very young children

Suggested pattern

In 1976, the Court Report (1976) made proposals for child health services. By 1980, the Department of Health and Social Security (DHSS) had issued guidelines for practice. The DHSS (1980) proposed that health visitors should undertake health surveillance on babies and toddlers at six weeks for general welfare and development, and again at seven to eight months but with special attention to sensory problems and to vision and hearing. In a further test at eighteen months, the Department advised that health visitors should undertake a review of development to include vision, hearing and early language, mobility, manipulative skills, social relationships and also to discuss the range of normal growth and behaviour.

In a policy statement, the Health Visitors' Association (HVA) suggested that the six week test could be undertaken, either by a health visitor alone, or jointly by a doctor and a health visitor. Whether it was alone or together would depend on the sort of information received about the previous examinations at or soon after birth and any particular concerns the parents or professionals might have (HVA, 1985, p. 11). The HVA suggested that thereafter babies should be screened at seven to nine months, at eighteen months and at two-and-a-half to three years of age. It proposed that these three tests should be undertaken by the health visitor alone, with doctors providing further assessment as a support service.

Many schemes inadequate

An inquiry in the late '70s and early '80s found a wide variety of tests in use in the, then, Area Health Authorities (Connolly, 1983). Thirteen of the 88 Authorities provided guidelines involving Sheridan, Denver, Griffiths and locally devised tests. In 54, set schemes were issued and for these specially designed record forms were provided. It was found that none of these forms incorporated scales or grading schemes. It was not possible, therefore, to accommodate individual differences in children's progress.

Stepladder, centile charts

A very good scheme has been devised in Glasgow by Professor Barber et al (1976a; Barber, 1982). The test is designed for use by health visitors, employing the sort of timing proposed by the DHSS and HVA. When reviewing recent literature on developmental screening, I felt this scheme was the best of all those reported (Robertson, 1984). Stepladder, centile charts have been devised, using specially selected and graded test items for each of the main four aspects of development: gross motor development; speech and language; vision and fine movement; and lastly, social aspects of development. There are four tests for hearing under nine months, and vision is given special attention early on. There is a booklet which describes exactly how the tests should be conducted (Barber et al, 1976b).

As can be seen from a glance at Figures 5.4 and 5.5, these charts provide immediate visual comparison with previous attainments and allow for continuous comparisons over time, similar to that of weight and height charts. In this scheme, children who are seen outside the standard time, either because they need extra attention or because they were missed at the scheduled time, are able to have a relevant and valid test, recorded appropriately on the graph. An important plus point is that it would take little explanation to enable parents to understand the scheme and, therefore, to be more involved.

A bar chart

The Denver developmental screening test is another test which uses a visual record, this time a bar chart. It is a system based on the percentages of population able to achieve various activities by a given age and is explained very clearly by Ingalls and Salerno (1983) and Bryant (1980). The latter described how Cardiff health visitors had tested babies aged nine months with a modification of this test, one adjusted to match the local population. The scheme was limited as it was undertaken only at nine months.

The Denver test was tried out on 198 preterm children (Elliman et al, 1985). It was found that, when using the test at their actual age, about 40% would be rated as possibly having abnormal development, a significant rate of over referral for the assessment clinic. The problem was that using an age corrected for the preterm birth, the test was unable to pick up several who did, in fact, have abnormal progress. It seems some 7% of babies born are preterm and, therefore, need special consideration. It was concluded that the over-referral rate for more detailed assessment would be small enough to be outweighed, easily, by the advantage of being able to provide early identification and treatment for those who needed it. The advice given was that tests should be undertaken at the true age in order to find need for further assessment, and also at the adjusted age in order to prevent undue anxiety.

Listed attainments

Surrey's (Owen, 1982) structured system of health surveillance provides an example of a scheme without pictorial or graphic feedback.

SOCIAL

1. Able to dress — except laces and back buttons (H).
2. Dry at night (H).

3. Washes hands (H).
4. Pulls pants up and down (H).

5. Drinks and replaces cup (H).
6. Dry by day (H).

7. Drinks from cup without spilling (H).
8. Indicates toilet needs (H).

9. Puts cubes into box after being shown.
10. Finds toy under cup.

11. Rings bell.
12. Chews and swallows biscuit (observed).
    Copes with solid food.

13. Puts objects into mouth (cubes).
14. Reaches for and shakes rattle.

15. Aware of and responsive to bath (H).
16. Enjoys being handled by mother (H).

17. Smiles when spoken to (H).
18. Some vocal sounds (H).

(H) = History of achievement sufficient

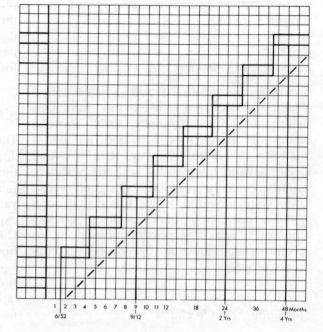

A

HEARING AND LANGUAGE

1. Hears whispers at 0.9 m (3 ft) — R&L (Reed test).
2. Grammatical speech articulated correctly.

3. Says first name.
4. Knows own sex.

5. Simple sentences (H).
6. Plays with miniature cup and saucer.

7. Points to parts of body.
8. Says five or more words (H).

9. Obeys simple commands e.g. clap hands.
10. Says less than 5 words excluding
    "Mama" "Dada" "Baba" (H).

11. "Mama" "Dada" "Baba".
12. Hearing tests above ear level.

13. Unintelligible babble.
14. Hearing tests at ear level.

15. Turns eyes to sound.
16. Looks round meaningfully when spoken to.

17. Stills to bell.
18. Stills to mother's voice.

(H) = History of achievement sufficient.

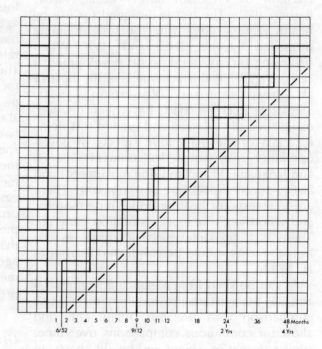

B

Fig. 5.4 Step-ladder charts for recording pre-school developmental progress: social and hearing and language. Reproduced by kind permission of Professor J H Barber, University of Glasgow Department of General Practice. (Note change in scale after 12 months.)

GROSS MOTOR

1. Descends stairs one foot per step.
2. Hops.

3. Climbs stairs in adult fashion.
4. Walks on tiptoe (H).

5. Up and down stairs holding on, 2 feet per step (H).
6. Kicks ball.

7. Climbs stairs, hand held, 2 feet on each step (H).
8. Kneels without support. (H).

9. Pulls to standing on furniture.
10. 'Cruises' round furniture.

11. Sits steadily on floor without support for few mins. (H).
12. Stands holding on to furniture.

13. Sits against wall or hand — no lateral support — 2/3 secs.
14. Hold round waist, lower abruptly exclude scissoring.

15. Pull from lying. Little or no head lag.
16. Ventral suspension. Holds head above plane of body.

17. Ventral suspension. Head in plane of body.

(H) = History of achievement sufficient.

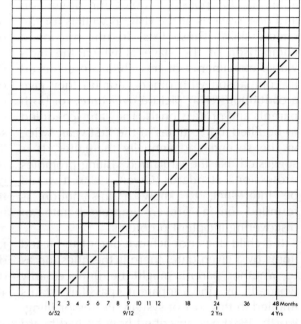

A

VISION AND FINE MOTOR

1. Picks up and replaces very small objects, e.g. pins, with each eye covered separately.
2. Copies a square.

3. Copies a circle.
4. Builds a bridge of three bricks when shown.

5. Makes a vertical line when shown.
6. Makes a tower of six bricks when shown.

7. Makes a scribble on paper.
8. Makes a tower of three bricks when shown.

9. Pincer grasp using a small object e.g. Smartie.
10. Bangs bricks together when shown.

11. Side of finger grasp using a small object e.g. Smartie.
12. Matches cubes.

13. Picks up cube from table or hand.
14. Transfers cube from one hand to another.

15. Holds a pencil briefly.
16. Follows a moving person with eyes.

17. Follows a moving face with eyes.

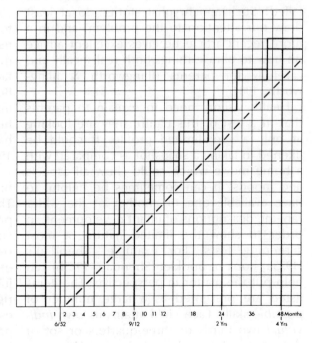

B

Fig. 5.5 Step-ladder charts for recording pre-school developmental gross motor and vision and fine movements. Reproduced by kind permission of Professor J H Barber, University of Glasgow Department of General Practice. (Note change in scale after 12 months.)

Lists are used with 'yes/ no' and 'remarks' columns, for possible topics for discussion and observations at the visit, as well as for the child's skills. These lists do not provide a comparison of the stage at which the individual attainments of this child are achieved in comparison with others, nor do they give a continuous clear picture over time, for both parents and professionals. They are scheduled to be filled in five times in the first year, twice in the second and annually thereafter. It is suggested that the structured visiting promotes professional standards (Owen, 1982). It would be interesting to know if this notion is founded on a proven improved rate of discovering incipient problems.

If a child does not achieve one of the listed items by a given date, there is the question as to whether parents might be unnecessarily worried by the apparent pass/fail status implied in this sort of system. Professor Illingworth (1981) has described how he had heard of health visitors 'failing' 40% in a 6 month test and telling the mothers their babies had failed! Such apochryphal stories do at least draw our attention to the problem, and in a more recent article he gives excellent advice on how to phrase things both realistically and carefully for parents (Illingworth & Illingworth, 1984).

Health visitors need to explain to parents that in a test of this nature they are looking at only a very limited profile. It could be likened to taking a snapshot as compared with a home movie which could show all aspects and moods! It can sometimes be helpful to have available one or another of the wider ranging descriptions of infant development, in order to show the limited nature of most screening tests. For example, Sheridan's (1975a) book or booklet (Sheridan, 1975b) can help put the matter in perspective. The items listed are presented as a large number of *possible* skills. Each child attains its *own individual* two thirds or three-quarters or so, of the range, by each stated age. Where a mother is suspicious about her child's development, health visitors should not be too reassuring (Sheridan, 1975a).

Special programmes

Sudden infant death is receiving more and more attention (Knight, 1983; Golding et al, 1985). Various schemes have been set up. In these, infants thought to be at increased risk of dying unexpectedly from preventable causes, are identified. This is done by comparing all babies against a researched scoring system, at birth and again a month later. Studies have been undertaken in Sheffield and Portsmouth. Increased visiting by health visitors, paying particular attention to the babies' weight gain, feeding, developmental attainments and general health, and allied health education, is given to these families. These areas have seen a significant decrease in the number of unexpected infant deaths (Carpenter et al, 1983; Powell, 1984; 1985).

Jean Powell described how the Portsmouth study was set up. She explains how in her scheme selection factors differ from those in Sheffield. She also describes a pattern of visiting undertaken by health visitors, according to estimated risk for the baby. A computer is used to help sort out the 46 variables from the midwives' birth information and the scoring factors arising out of a visit at four weeks. Both the GP and the health visitor are informed of whether each baby is low risk, high risk or very high risk. So far, 10% of the babies have been classified as high risk and 1% as very high risk.

The schedule arranges for 19 visits in the first year of life for very high risk babies. Those deemed to be at high risk are programmed to receive 11 visits, which can be compared with the 5 visits planned for low risk babies. The health visitors in one sector of the District have chosen to follow their own judgement about visiting, rather than to stick rigidly to the guidelines. It would be interesting to know to what extent their actual pattern of visiting varies from the guidelines, in what ways they choose to tackle the problem using another approach, for example through group work, and what effect this has on the infant mortality and morbidity rate.

Weight, length and head circumference

Early discovery of failure to thrive or abnormal weight gain, can be achieved only with accurate methods and adequate recording. Abnormalities of growth can also be found—with the same provisos. Describing weighing in clinics, Davies and Williams (1983) remark on the lack of guidance given on this widely practised procedure. They feel that abnormal weight gain often goes undetected and that, all too often, normal weight gain is misinterpreted as abnormal. The problems are:

— unreliable techniques in weighing
— insufficient use of centile charts
— inadequate understanding of normal patterns in weight gain
— insufficient understanding of nutritional influences on weight.

They describe how centile charts are now widely available and are becoming increasingly used in clinics, and they have provided very good diagrams to show the difference between normal and abnormal patterns on a centile chart. It is interesting to note that in the Portsmouth surveillance scheme, each health visitor has her own portable weighing machine in order to enable adequate and accurate weighing in the home. Hopefully, this idea will spread to become the norm.

Professor Tanner (1985), who has devised height and weight charts for child health clinics (Tanner & Whitehouse, 1973), describes the diagnosis and treatment of various growth disorders which are best treated as early as possible. Harvey and Wallis (1978a, 1978b) have given some very helpful hints, with photographs, on how to measure a baby's length (up to two years of age) and, later, height. They say that the commonest cause of low stature in a Newcastle-upon-Tyne study was social deprivation, and that it accounted for a third of the cases.

The value of head circumference as a measure is explained by Wood and Walker-Smith (1981). Its size relative to length and weight can be a useful measure for indicating stunted growth. Its size relative to chest size can also be an indicator.

Vision, hearing and speech

There seems little doubt that the more parents are involved with monitoring the vision and hearing of their babies, the greater will be the chance of early diagnosis and treatment (Robertson, 1984; Robinson, 1983). A checklist of general signs of ability to hear in the first year of life, and another suggesting some simple tests for vision that parents should know about, will be found in Figure 5.6 and Table 5.5. McCormick (1983) has described the successful outcome, in Nottingham, of improvements in training health visitors to test babies' hearing, and gives good advice for District Health Authorities who may wish to check their policies and procedures on this issue.

Speech and language are said to be the most common developmental problem in young children and Professor R J Robinson (1982) suggests that it should receive attention because it

— may be a sign of deafness or an other underlying condition
— commonly leads to emotional and behavioural problems

Table 5.5 Indicators of a baby's ability to see

	Does the baby:	Comments
Early weeks	Have eye-to-eye contact with the mother	Seek mother's opinion, but may be observed
	Fixate on the mother's face?	May be observed or reported
	Follow a moving object?	Early test: follows a dangling object 3 cm (12 in) away, through a quarter of a circle
Early months	Recognise familiar sights?	Seek mother's opinion
	Follow a moving person with his eyes?	May be observed during screening
Later months	Object to having one of his eyes covered when playing games?	Parental opinion should be sought, as this could indicate quite a marked loss of vision in the uncovered eye

Nottingham Health Authority ——**Hints for Parents**——

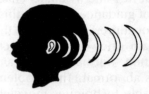

"Can your baby hear you?"

Here is a checklist of some of the general signs you can look for in your baby's first year:-

YES/NO

Shortly after birth
Your baby should be startled by a sudden loud noise such as a hand clap or a door slamming and should blink or open his eyes widely to such sounds.

By 1 Month
Your baby should be beginning to notice sudden prolonged sounds like the noise of a vacuum cleaner and he should pause and listen to them when they begin.

By 4 Months
He should quieten or smile to the sound of your voice even when he cannot see you. He may also turn his head or eyes toward you if you come up from behind and speak to him from the side.

By 7 Months
He should turn immediately to your voice across the room or to very quiet noises made on each side if he is not too occupied with other things.

By 9 Months
He should listen attentively to familiar everyday sounds and search for very quiet sounds made out of sight. He should also show pleasure in babbling loudly and tunefully.

By 12 Months
He should show some response to his own name and to other familiar words. He may also respond when you say 'no' and 'bye bye' even when he cannot see any accompanying gesture.

> Your health visitor will perform a routine hearing screening test on your baby between seven and nine months of age. She will be able to help and advise you at any time before or after this test if you are concerned about your baby and his development. If you suspect that your baby is not hearing normally, either because you cannot answer yes to the items above or for some other reason, then seek advice from your health visitor.

Fig. 5.6 Hints for parents on testing their children's hearing. Reproduced by kind permission of Dr Barry McCormick, Children's Hearing Assessment Centre, Nottingham Health Authority.

— has a strong association with later difficulties in reading, writing and spelling

— is likely to improve with skilled intervention.

The professor says there should be concern about a child not using words with meaning by 21 months or constructing simple sentences by 3 years, but cautions us against the unthinking use of arbitrary cut-off points of this nature. Understanding statements is particularly important, and it is suggested that a child who does not understand simple commands at eighteen months should also be referred for assessment.

Congenital dislocation of the hip

Some cases of hip dislocation (see Ch. 4, page 61) cannot be detected at birth. In half the 'missed' cases looked at by David et al (1983) there had been no routine hip checks after three months. They advised follow-up of babies with transient instability or clicking hips at birth, at six weeks, three months, six months and twelve months, and at six monthly intervals until they walk normally. Babies at high risk, such as breech deliveries or where there is a family tendency, should receive special attention. In a quarter of the cases studied, there was no record of the test having been undertaken at birth. Health visitors should check on this to see if it was, in fact, undertaken, and to find out the result.

Again, it helps if parents are aware of the need for vigilance. Stephen Ware (1984) describes how he gives parents an outline of the mechanics of the disease and suggests they gently abduct their babies' hips each time the nappy is changed and report any asymmetry immediately to the health visitor or the GP. He tells the parents, too, that abduction normally becomes more limited as the baby gets older.

In this section on screening and surveillance, we have looked at planning and monitoring screening programmes, at assessment of mothers' emotional health and at a variety of tests available for use with babies and very young children.

GIVING SUPPORT

Supportive aspects of the work can range from helping couples who are experiencing the day-to-day anxieties associated with early parenthood, through to helping young families who have come up against a major problem, or even a tragedy. The aim in either case is to ameliorate the position, in order to prevent greater dysfunction growing out of the current difficulties.

Common problems

Although sympathetic listening is an important therapeutic aspect of the service they can give, health visitors would wish to provide other practical help too, where this is possible. Some will not only keep available books they can lend people (see Table 5.4), but also their copy of well-written, reassuring and helpful articles on common problems. These might be, for example, infantile colic (Jones, 1984), unacceptable sleeping habits (Richman, 1983; Kitzinger, 1985) and 'hyperactivity' (Delvin, 1984). Such articles can be found through the HVA Current Awareness Bulletin.

It seems probable that discussions on how to cope are more successful, particularly in the longer term, if they are backed up by background information which helps the parents understand more about the mechanics of what is happening. Health education is intertwined with supportive aspects of health visiting, just as it is in screening and surveillance. Being able to give information about relevant voluntary and statutory agencies is also very important (Webb, 1985), a matter discussed in earlier chapters.

It is important to plan how to help people facing these common problems. They can be very distressing. Crying babies can serve as an example. In a study reported by Sheila Kitzinger (1985), a quarter of the mothers who had responded to the questionnaire had felt like smacking their crying baby, one in ten had actually done so. This was a self-selective, non-random sample, but it does give an indication of how distraught people can become.

Sheila Kitzinger's advice to mothers was:
— find a 'support network' before baby's birth
— there is no need to fear asking for help
— arrange for a break away from the baby
— the excessive crying generally stops by six months of age
— get partner to help
— talk to someone about the crying
— note some useful addresses of relevant organisations.

Four out of five of the mothers in the study had talked with their health visitor and this was found to be very helpful.

Availability

Access to our service is important. Field et al (1983) said that parents facing decisions as to whether or not their child is ill, particularly those living alone, can feel very confused and delay seeking help. Besides needing to know and be confident about normal behaviour and common illnesses, Field et al said that parents need also to have both GP and health visitor services available at unsocial hours when they require it.

Health visitors in Richmond (Beech, 1981) and Plymouth (Bogie, 1981) have written about how they have organised out-of-hours service for parents with crying babies. More recently, a seven day health visiting service has been set up in Peterborough (Rawdon Smith, 1984). The telephone number of the service is given routinely to new mothers. The service has been particularly helpful to parents with very young babies. It has been found to be very well used and inexpensive to run.

Mothers can also routinely be told of voluntary organisations in the locality interested in supporting mothers. There may be nearby groups from, for example, the National Childbirth Trust, Meet-a-Mum Association or Parents Anonymous. Laura Swaffield (1984) has described how Cry-sis, a voluntary group which aims to help distraught mothers, is seeking to make itself known to, and to work in cooperation with, people like health visitors.

Work with groups

The importance of mothers' need for each other's company, mutual support and guidance they can give one another, is well recognised by many health visitors who have set up groups (Wood, 1985; Moulds et al, 1983; Hennessy et al, 1978). Deborah Hennessy (1983) has provided practical advice on planning and setting up support groups, making suggestions for matters such as:
— leadership arrangements
— length of meetings
— number of meetings
— size of group
— supervision of children
— drawing meetings to a close.

Two health visitors have described their work with self-help groups. Diana Balter (1985) was approached by a group of women who organised themselves a course on health topics. She ordered films and acted generally as a background resource. It is interesting to note that the group were able to obtain grant aid to pay for their accommodation through a special social services fund. Nina Trick (1985) discussed the problem of first time mothers' loneliness with the doctors in the rural practice to which she was attached. They offered a room in the surgery for a weekly meeting. This team venture has been successful and has resulted in increased confidence for the mothers.

Child health clinics which are appropriately geared for it can make an excellent place for mothers to meet and give each other sympathetic support and encouragement. Formal clinics where mothers have to queue in row upon row of chairs make it less easy to foster friendships or mutual support. However, the less formal ones with
— a clear welcome for newcomers
— chairs grouped in small circles
— toys for the children
— a volunteer who can
— help with the children
— make mothers a cup of tea
and where mothers are encouraged to tell each other of their experiences, are more likely to be successful in this direction.

The clinic, on the other hand, often lacks privacy and therefore does not provide a good place for health visitors to offer support over some of the greater problems parents can face. These are usually followed up in the home. In planning their work, health visitors need to have thought out how they will help parents who have particular problems, be they quite common or a rare occurrence. Parents whose baby has died suddenly and unexpectedly and mothers suffering from postnatal depression are given as two examples.

Postnatal depression

It is quite a challenge to plan to arrange supportive care for mothers with postnatal depression. It tends to manifest itself six weeks postnatally, by which time the health visitor is generally calling less frequently. Also it is thought to be very common and involve at least one in ten mothers. Besides helping parents become aware of its existence (Ch. 3, page 47) and discovering it early (see above, page 84), health visitors need to know about all the relevant helping agencies in the locality (Waumsley, 1983, pp. 30–31) and to have thought about what approach might best help the mother. There are no simple solutions, but just raising the issue by suggesting the self-assessment questionnaire shows the health visitor wishes to help in this direction. The same can be achieved, of course, by simply asking the mother how she feels and helping her express this.

Waumsley (1983, pp. 32–33, 35–36) has described how the supportive gestures of volunteers has helped depressed mothers, and she lists some suggestions for dealing with the feelings of anger and stress that people experience at this time. Jenifer Holden (1985) has described a study in which some health visitors have been given special training in non-directive counselling techniques. They visit for eight, weekly half-hour sessions, which the mothers spend talking about their feelings. The results are not yet available, but it is evident that the scheme is being appreciated.

In order to alleviate loneliness and depression, a 'walk-in unit' was set up by health visitors in Hertfordshire in which small children could come and play, with or without their parents. They are now planning to extend its facilities and its hours of opening. Group counselling sessions of six to eight weeks duration, to help mothers with emotional problems, were set up by three health visitors in Hampshire. Their success led them to recommend others to do something similar (Hennessy et al, 1978).

Sudden infant death

Cot death affects around two per thousand live births. Some of the difficulties parents face, such as feelings of guilt, considerable stress, sometimes involving problems within the marriage and with the surviving children, and the practical aspects of the death, are described by Woodward et al (1985) and Audrey Heycock (1984). They also suggest ways that health visitors can help. The Foundation for the Study of Infant Death is an organisation which supplies information to parents and professionals; it raises funds for research, and formerly bereaved parents, Friends of the Foundation, are able to give personal support to the grieving parents. The process of grief and bereavement visiting are discussed in Chapter 7 (pp. 125–126).

Health visitors can themselves need support (see Ch. 2, p. 19). In an attempt to 'help the helpers', a psychiatrist, Michael Clarke (1980), held a series of fortnightly seminars in which health visitors presented problematic cases. The psychological consequences for parents following the death of a child, was one of the four areas that health visitors found particularly difficult. Clarke remarked on the important role for health visitors in identifying distortions in parents' mourning and in aiming to prevent further complications.

This chapter has given an overview of work with families with babies and very young children, especially with regard to certain aspects of planning. By artificially dividing the work into guidance, surveillance and supportive care, we have been able to look more closely at some of the particular issues and schemes and at a few of the dilemmas that are involved. We have discussed the need to make special efforts for the underprivileged, to work in partnership with parents and to help them understand so they can be actively involved in health care decisions.

USEFUL ADDRESSES

Child Accident Prevention Trust
75 Portland Place,
London WlN 3AL
Tel 01 636 2545

Cry-sis, British Monomark Cry-sis,
London WClN 3XX
Tel 01 404 5011

The Foundation for Sudden Infant Deaths.
5th Floor, 4/5 Grosvenor Place,
London SWlX 7HD
Tel 01 235 1721 or 01 245 9421

Meet-A-Mum Association
3 Woodside Avenue, South Norwood,
London SE25 5DW.
Please enclose a stamped self addressed envelope

National Childbirth Trust
9 Queensborough Terrace,
London W2 3TB
Tel 01 221 3833

Parents Anonymous 6–9 Manor Gardens,
London N7
Tel 01 263 5672 (office), 01 263 8918 (Lifeline)

REFERENCES

Ahamed M 1982 A research project. Nursing Times Community Outlook 78:223

Atkinson D 1983 Postnatal depression (letter). Health Visitor 56:116

Balter D 1985 Working with a women's self-help group. Health Visitor 58:260

Barber J H 1982 Preschool developmental screening—the results of a four year period. Health Bulletin 40: 170–178

Barber J H, Boothman R, Stanfield J P 1976a A new visual chart for preschool developmental screening. Health Bulletin 34: 80–91

Barber J H, Department of General Practice, University of Glasgow with assistance from the Department of Child Health, University of Glasgow 1976b The Woodside system pre-school developmental screening: description of the tests. Econoprint, Edinburgh

Beech C P 1981 A new service for parents with crying babies. Nursing Times 77: 245–246

Bell A, Moules E 1985 The demographic factor. Nursing Times 81, 31:28–30

Black D 1980 Inequalities in health. Report of a research working party, Department of Health and Social Security, London. p 328–329 (Chairman Sir Douglas Black)

Bogie A 1981 A crying baby advisory service. Health Visitor 54: 535–537

Bryant G M 1980 Use of Denver developmental screening test by health visitors. Health Visitor 53: 2–5

Carpenter R G, Gardner A, Jepson M, Taylor E M, Salvin A, Sunderland R, Emery J L, Pursall E, Roe J, Sheffield Health Visitors 1983 Prevention of unexpected infant death. The Lancet I: 723–727

CETHV 1977 An investigation into the principles of health visiting. Council for the Education and Training of Health Visitors, London

Child Development Project 1984 Child development programme. Early Childhood Development Unit, Senate House, University of Bristol, Bristol BS8 ITH. p 12

Clarke M G 1980 Psychiatric liaison with health visitors. Health Trends 12: 98–100

Community Outlook 1982 Fact sheet. Nursing Times Community Outlook 78, 32: 220–221

Community Outlook 1984 Which should you choose? Nursing Times Community Outlook 80, 27: 250–253

Colver A, Pearson P 1985 Safety in the home: how are we doing? Health Visitor 58: 41–42

Connolly P 1983 The health visitor's contribution. Nursing Times 79, 38: 30–32

Court Report 1976 Report of the Committee on Child Health Services, Fit for the future. Cmnd 6684. HMSO, London

Cox J 1986 Postnatal depression. A guide for health professionals. Churchill Livingstone, Edinburgh

Cranshaw S 1984 Remarkable changes in parents' competence. Nursing Times Supplement 80, 42:8

Darbyshire P 1985 Thumbs up for dummies. Nursing Times 81, 38: 40–42

David T J, Parris M R, Poynor M U, Hawnaur J M, Simm S A, Rigg E A, McCrae F C 1983 Reasons for late detection of hip dislocation in childhood. The Lancet II: 147–149

Davies D P, Williams T 1983 Is weighing babies in clinics worth while? British Medical Journal 286: 860–863

Dening F 1983 Tackling breast cancer. Nursing Times 79, 34:13

DHSS 1980 Prevention in the child health services. Department of Health and Social Security, London

Delvin D 1984 Is he really hyperactive? Mother and Baby December: 61–62

The Economist 1984 Some doctors still eat salt. The Economist 292, 7355: 67–68

Elliman A M, Bryan E M, Elliman A D, Palmer P, Dubowitz L 1985 Denver developmental screening test and preterm infants. Archives of Disease in Childhood 60: 20–24

Fairs J M 1984 A more caring family approach. Nursing Times Supplement 80, 42:8

Field S, Draper J, Kerr M, Hare M J 1983 Babies'

illnesses from the parents' point of view. Maternal and Child Health 8: 252–256

General Medical Services Committee of the British Medical Association 1984 Handbook of preventive care for pre-school children. General Medical Services Defence Fund Ltd and the Royal College of General Practitioners, London

Golding J, Limerick S, Macfarlane A 1985 Sudden infant death. Patterns, puzzles and problems. Open Books Publishing Ltd, Shepton Mallet, Somerset

Green C 1984 Toddler taming. A parents' guide to the first four years. Century Publishing Co Ltd, London

Habgood J 1985 Exposing the blues . . . Nursing Times Community Outlook 81, 33: 4–6

Harvey D, Wallis S 1978a Children of short stature: part 1. Midwife Health Visitor and Community Nurse 14: 136–139

Harvey D, Wallis S 1978b Children of short stature: part 2. Midwife Health Visitor and Community Nurse 14: 177–178

Health Education Council 1981 Play it safe! A guide to preventing children's accidents. Health Education Council and Scottish Health Education Group in association with the BBC

Hennessy D 1983 Parents support groups. Nursing 2, 19: 552–554

Hennessy D, Holgate B, Marr J 1978 With a little help from my friends. Nursing Times Community Outlook 74: 103–106

Heycock A 1984 Coping with a cot death. Nursing Mirror 158, 4: iii–viii

Holden J 1985 Talking it out. Nursing Times Community Outlook 81, 41: 6,10

HVA 1985 The health visitor's role in child health surveillance: a policy statement. Health Visitors Association, 36 Eccleston Square London

Illingworth R S 1981 The importance of knowing what is normal. Public Health, London 95: 66–68

Illingworth R S, Illingworth C M 1984 Mothers are easily worried. Archives of Disease in Childhood 59: 380–384

Ingalls A J, Salerno M C 1983 Maternal and child health nursing, 5th edn. Mosby, St Louis, p 328–360

Johnson A M 1984 Visual problems in children: detection and referral. Journal of the Royal College of General Practitioners 34: 32–35

Johnson L, Silman A 1985 Ready salted. Nursing Times 81, 32: 34–35

Jones I H 1984 Colic enough to make you scream. Mother July: 30

Kitzinger S 1985 Why do babies cry? Parents March: 37–38

Knight B 1983 Sudden death in infancy. The 'cot death' syndrome. Faber and Faber, London

Kumar R 1982 Neurotic disorders in childbearing women. In: Brockington I F, Kumar R (eds) Motherhood and mental illness. Academic Press, London

Latham A D, Haggard M P 1980 A pilot study to detect hearing impairment in the young. Midwife, Health Visitor and Community Nurse 16: 370–374

Laurence V 1983 An alternative approach. Nursing Times 79, 12:14

McCormick B 1983 Hearing screening by health visitors: a critical appraisal of the distraction test. Health Visitor 56: 449–451

Moore J 1982 Can they be prevented? Nursing Times, Community Outlook 78, 32: 212–214

Morris J B, Hird M D 1981 A neurodevelopmental infant screening programme undertaken by health visitors—preliminary report. Health Bulletin 39: 236–250

Moulds V, Hennessy D, Crack P 1983 Innovations by a primary health care team. 2. A postnatal group for first-time mothers. Health Visitor 56: 296–297

Nichols S 1983 The Southampton breast study—implications for nurses. Nursing Times 79, 50: 24–29

Owen C M 1982 How Surrey implemented the Court Report. Nursing Times 78: 673–675

Percy P 1984 Disturbingly poor levels of nutrition. Nursing Times Supplement 80, 42:9

Powell J 1984 Cot deaths—can they be prevented? Journal of the Royal Society of Health 104: 203–205

Powell J 1985 Keeping watch. Nursing Times Community Outlook 81, 2: 15–19

Rajan L 1985 Time to avoid the clinic? Nursing Times 81, 32: 24–26

Rawdon-Smith J 1984 Introduction of seven-day health visiting cover in Peterborough. Health Visitor 57: 53–54

Ray G 1982 At risk. Nursing Times Community Outlook 78, 32: 217–218

Rayner C 1977 Family feelings. Understanding your child from 0 to 5. Hutchinson & Co Ltd, London

Richman N 1983 Management of sleep problems. Maternal and Child Health 8: 227–233

Robertson C A 1981 Evaluation of screening: an epidemiological approach. 1: Measuring the effectiveness of health visitors. Health Visitor 54: 20–21

Robertson C A 1984 Preventive health care for infants. In: Houston M J (ed) Maternal and Infant Health Care. Churchill Livingstone, London

Robinson R J 1982 An evaluation of health visiting. Council for the Education and Training of Health Visitors, London

Robinson K 1983 The scandal of late diagnosis of deafness in children. Health Visitor 56: 452–453

Robinson R J 1982 The child who is slow to talk. British Medical Journal 285: 671–672

Rowden R 1983 Talking about taboos. Nursing Times 79, 50:12

Rowe J 1985 Supply and demand. Nursing Times 81, 4:52

Royal College of General Practitioners 1982 Healthier children—thinking prevention. Royal College of General Practitioners, London

Royal College of Nursing Health Visitors' Advisory Group 1983 Thinking about health visiting. Royal College of Nursing of the United Kingdom Society of Primary Health Care Nursing, London

Royal College of Nursing Health Visitors' Advisory Group 1984 Further thinking about health visiting. Royal College of Nursing of the United Kingdom Society of Primary Health Care Nursing, London

Sheridan M D 1975a Children's developmental progress from birth to five years: the Stycar sequences. NFER Publishing Company Ltd, Windsor

Sheridan M D 1975b The developmental progress of infants and young children. HMSO, London

Snaith R P 1984 Birth of the first child (letter). British Medical Journal 288: 2000–2001

Snaith R P, Constantopoulos A A, Jardine M Y. McGuffin P A 1978 A clinical scale for the self-assessment of irritability, depression and anxiety. British Journal of Psychiatry 132: 164–171 (THESE QUESTIONNAIRES ARE AVAILABLE, WITH A CHARGE FOR POSTAGE AND PRINTING, FROM LEEDS UNIVERSITY THROUGH R P Snaith, Senior Lecturer in Psychiatry, Department of Psychiatry, St James University Hospital, Leeds LS9 7TF Tel 0532 433144)

Social Services Committee 1984 Children in care. Second report from the Social Services Committee, 1983–84 Vol I. House of Commons Paper 360–I, London (Chairman: Renee Short)

Stretch C 1983 Does mother know best? Nursing Times 79, 10:14

Swaffield L 1984 Cry babies. Nursing Times 80, 31: 16–17

Tanner J M 1985 Catching them early. Nursing Times Community Outlook 81, 15: 19–22

Tanner J M, Whitehouse R H 1973 Height and weight charts from birth to 5 years allowing for length of gestation. Archives of Disease in Childhood 48: 786–789

Trick N 1985 Forming a new baby group. Health Visitor 58: 78

UKCC 1984 Code of professional conduct. United Kingdom Central Council for Nursing, Midwifery and Health Visiting, 23 Portland Place London W1N 3AF. paragraphs 13,14

Ware S 1984 A clicking hip in a newborn baby should never be ignored (letter). The Lancet I: 1184–1185

Waumsley L 1983 Mothers talking about postnatal depression. National Childbirth Trust, London

Webb P 1985 Someone to talk to directory 1985. A directory of self help and community support agencies in the UK and Republic of Ireland. Mental Health Foundation, London

Wood C B S, Walker-Smith J A 1981 MacKeith's infant feeding and feeding difficulties, 6th edn. Churchill Livingstone, Edinburgh. p 15

Wood T 1985 Formal and informal support systems for mothers with newborn. Midwife Health Visitor and Community Nurse 21: 42–49

Woodward S, Pope A, Robson W J, Hagan O 1985 Bereavement counselling after sudden infant death. British Medical Journal 290: 363–365

Zigmond A S, Snaith R P 1983 The hospital anxiety and depression (HAD) scale. Acta Psychiatrica Scandinavica 67: 361–370 (THESE QUESTIONNAIRES ARE AVAILABLE, FREE, THROUGH Mr D d'E Panrucker, Professional Communications Manager, Upjohn Ltd, Fleming Way, Crawley, West Sussex RH10 2NJ Tel 0293 31133)

Chapter 6 gives a second and more simple example of the use of the prevention model. Again, it provides a way of thinking about the role of the health visitor, this time with regard to families with children of around the age of three onwards. In this phase, thought is given to preparing the child for his/her school years and to continued surveillance and support for the family.

6

Pre-school visiting

CONTINUING EDUCATION, SCREENING AND SUPPORT

In the two years immediately prior to school entry, the aim is to continue to prevent the occurrence, development and deterioration of problems (see Table 6.1). This is done by encouraging parents to think ahead and prepare their children for their experiences and needs at school, by continuing the search for early signs of health problems and by offering support and/or referral to appropriate services where problems are already established.

A health visitor with a normal caseload would probably expect to visit most families only once or twice in this time. In Portsmouth, for example, they plan for one visit during the third year and then another between three and a half to four and a half years (Powell, 1985). In general, visiting from eighteen months onwards is much less frequent than that during the first year.

It was found by Mayall and Grossmith (1985) to be important that mothers should feel their health visitor was still accessible. They were sure a flying visit was not the answer: to some mothers it could be more irritating than helpful. Mayall and Grossmith suggested that during these years, when the health visitor calls less frequently, families should be sent a regular letter, letting them know or reminding them of where their health visitor can be contacted. They also felt that when

Table 6.1 Pre-school visiting: the work of the health visitor

Aspect of prevention	Examples of activities	
Preventing occurrence of condition (Anticipatory guidance)	*Discussion of*: booster immunisation, diet, sleep and stimulation, footwear, ability to dress, creative and social play, head lice, dental care and safety	
Preventing development of condition (Surveillance of family health)	*Screening re* gross motor and fine movements social attainments speech: sentence at 3, articulation at 4 hearing: especially after otitis media vision: especially re amblyopia height on centile chart	
Preventing deterioration of established condition (Supportive work)	*Sympathetic listening Information about services Encouraging self-help groups*	*re:* childhood problem behaviour, marital stress e.g. sex problem, divorce, finance, housing, unemployment, alcoholism in the family, maternal incontinence

Table 6.2 Example one: the Manners family

Aspect of prevention	Examples of activities
Preventing occurrence of condition (Anticipatory guidance)	Booster immunisation mentioned Safety mentioned Head lice discussed in depth Creative and social play discussed
Preventing development of condition (Surveillance of family health)	*Screening re:* gross motor and fine movements social attainments speech hearing vision, referred to orthoptists height on centile chart
Preventing deterioration of established condition (Supportive work)	*Encouraging self-help groups Information about services Sympathetic listening* None needed

their health visitor leaves the post, parents should be notified in writing. This sort of measure becomes much more important in areas of underprivilege where there tends to be a high turnover of staff.

EXAMPLES OF PRE-SCHOOL VISITING

The first example follows up Nancy Manners, introduced earlier in the chapters on antenatal and birth visits. She has moved house and has managed to return to work. The second concerns Helen Voisey's work with Mrs Prince, who attended a 'pre-school preparation group' and also a self-help group which Helen had told her about. Outlines of the examples will be found in Tables 6.2 and 6.3.

EXAMPLE ONE: THE MANNERS FAMILY

Mrs Hannah Van der Haastrecht (HV) was planning the priorities in her caseload and, at the same time, attempting to evaluate what had been

Table 6.3 Example two: the Prince family

Aspect of prevention	Examples of activities	
Preventing occurrence of condition (Anticipatory guidance)	*Group discussion of*: safety and discipline preparation for independence head lice creative and social play dental care	
Preventing development of condition (Surveillance of family health)	*Screening re:* hearing and language vision height, on centile chart gross motor movements fine movements social	stimulation discussed
Preventing deterioration of established condition (Supportive work)	*Sympathetic listening Information about services Encouraging self-help groups*	*re:* occasional incontinence: informed about I.I. group, reported as successful

achieved in recent years amongst the families with children soon to be going to school. She came to the Manners family's cards and found it difficult to believe that Pauline was now nearly five years old.

Miss Nancy Manners had had a very difficult time in getting new accommodation. In the end, when Pauline was two and a half, she had been given a council flat. Three months later she had been able to return to work because she had found, living in the same block of flats, another nurse with a child who wanted to work. Mrs Smith, her husband and Nancy were able to work between them a scheme which allowed them all to work full time. They had checked with the Social Services Department about whether they were obliged to register as a babysitter, and all was well.

When HV had called at the flat for the three year visit, Nancy had shown her how much easier it was now to maintain a safe environment than in the large-roomed bedsitter with an open plan kitchen. They had discussed preparation for school. Pauline was attending the same playgroup as the Smith's son, Eric. Mrs Manners was paying the playgroup fees. Head lice was mentioned and Nancy was very amused by HV's nit in a bottle. It seems that they had had 'trouble' at the nursery but that they had not given good instructions on how to deal with, or how to avoid, infestation. The health visitor made a mental note to mention to her colleague attached to that playgroup, that they needed some guidance.

At the next visit, when Pauline was four and a half years, Nancy had reported that the nursery's new approach had been successful and that they now had only a minimal and occasional problem with head lice. Booster immunisations were discussed at that visit, as were the exercises that Pauline had to do for her squint.

The squint had been brought to light at the three and a half year clinic assessment session for height, weight, hearing, vision and developmental attainments. Nancy had said she was not happy about the way Pauline responded to games entailing covering up her right eye. The child was referred to the orthoptists' secondary screening clinic, where she was confirmed to be an early case of straight-eyed amblyopia. Having been caught in good time, the problem was already beginning to be resolved.

Nancy had brought to that clinic her HMSO Sheridan (1975) booklet, marked with all of the attainments at each stage over the years. It had

evidently caused both grandmother and mother a great deal of amusement and, HV gathered, a fair amount of effort to cover the full test each time. They had been fascinated to see how consistently Pauline attained about three quarters of each stage in total, but sometimes more heavily in one of the four sectors and sometimes in another at each stage. The centile charts were completed as planned.

During these past two years, Nancy had been in no need of 'supportive' work. She had always known where to contact HV when she wished to. Nancy's accommodation, child care and occupation problems had been solved. Her general outlook and her very clear understanding of her daughter's developmental needs and potential, meant she had been able to cope competently with the normal child behaviour problems. The health visitor felt pleased that deficiencies in Pauline's vision, like several other possible problems, had been prevented from developing (or occurring) on account of the surveillance and information service she had offered. It had seemed relevant to the mother and had been used by her.

EXAMPLE TWO: THE PRINCE FAMILY

Miss Helen Voisey (HV) was looking through the health visitor records of the families who had a child due to attend the pre-school medical examination for the spring term. She was making a special note of children whose developmental surveillance had shown any unusual pattern, in order to bring it to the attention of the school nurse and the doctor.

On looking through the notes of the Prince family, she was reminded of how Daniel had 'faltered' in a social assessment test at three years. He had not needed to be referred, either at that stage or later. Christine had been aged one when Daniel had attended that clinic assessment session. Vera Prince had reported that he was not yet washing his hands, nor was he pulling his pants up and down. He had, until then, always attained either one or two of the items at each stage of the (Barber) developmental centile chart. There had not been much time for discussion at the time, as other people were waiting for their appointments.

Miss Voisey made an appointment to call on the Princes the following week, in order, sensitively, to make sure that Vera was in no way worried by the absence of a mark on the chart, and also to discuss stimulation and play for Daniel. At that visit they had discussed the sort of social behaviour, play and fine movements that Daniel would be likely to be capable of and what he might be able to do by the age of four and by five years of age. Vera said later that she had realised then that she had been leaving Daniel to his own devices whilst she was so busy with the new baby. He had consequently benefited from the attention that both she and her husband had given and they had been very proud of his ability, particularly to draw, at the four years test.

Also, the health visitor suggested Vera and the children attend the mothers' pre-school preparation group held at the health centre. She was pleased to be invited: one of her friends had attended an earlier course and had evidently enjoyed it. It had been a lively group.

Always at the first meeting of the pre-school preparation course there was discussion about which topics should be covered, and a plan for the six sessions was drawn up. This group had included two other mothers from the same multi-storey block as the Prince family and they were all very keen to discuss what to do about the lack of safe play areas in their locality. Their local councillor was now attempting to have one created. Besides safety, the group had chosen to discuss preparation for independence, head lice, tooth care, creative play and, in the final session, discipline. Vera Prince had made very confident contributions, particularly at these later meetings. Some retired ladies from a nearby church came in and looked after the children and made tea for the mothers.

The most significant feature of the most recent home visit was, in response to the question 'Do you ever lose urine when you don't intend to?', Mrs Prince said that she did, but only occasionally and did not need a pad. She had requested complete confidentiality about the issue. She was very sensitive about it and had not told anyone before. Being busy with the new baby meant her postnatal exercises had been given low priority and she attributed her problem to this.

Helen Voisey had told the young mother about a group she and another health visitor had helped set up which was now self-sustaining. It was whimsically referred to as 'Incontinence Inonymous', met fortnightly and all the members aimed to encourage each other to do the

necessary exercises. The local incontinence adviser attended when requested to do so. When HV had met Vera in the street four months later, Vera had indicated that after some hesitation she had attended the group and was very pleased with the outcome.

The health visitor thought about what had been achieved. Developmental assessment had played only one, though an important, part in her preventive work. The groups and the clinics had been very valuable, but she felt that it was at home that the instigatory enabling work was done.

THINKING AHEAD

Anticipatory guidance for families preparing a child for school can cover an enormous number of topics; a few, such as safety, dental care and head lice, are mentioned here as examples.

In these few pages it is not possible to present many subjects. Equally, it is not possible to talk over many items in a 20 minute or half-hour call. A large number of health educational matters can only be fitted in when the health visitor 'switches into automatic', rattles off a well-rehearsed speech and checklists queries and items of advice. This leaves very little time to take account of parental views, and the disadvantages of this sort of autocratic approach have already been touched on in earlier chapters. It seems likely that a two-way discussion of a few points, which are chosen and seen as relevant by the parents, will be more acceptable and more educational overall. This is, of course, provided they know what is 'permissible' (Robinson, 1983).

Time is at a premium, but health visitors may be able to give extra help to disadvantaged people by setting up a discussion group over a few weeks to which mothers are invited to exchange ideas on aspects of preparing young children for their schooling. Some of the issues that may be discussed, both at home visits or at groups meetings, might be
— pre-school immunisations
— diet

— footwear
— stimulation and creative play
— play with other children and playgroups
— toilet training
— ability to dress and undress
— head lice
— teaching small children about sex
— dental care and first visit to dentist
— safety, particularly road drill
and any special queries raised by any of the mothers.

Learning independence and sharing

The practical knowledge that children need in preparation for school includes, for example, experience of being away from their mother, sharing things and putting them away where they belong when not in use, taking care of their clothes, knowing left from right shoes and also recognising their name on their coat, wellingtons and other clothing.

This sort of experience is gained by children whose parents choose to and are able to send them to playgroups or nursery classes. A health visitor's knowledge of criteria for admission, waiting lists for places and any subsidised places that may be available, is invaluable, as is personal contact with local groups and classes. An ex-health visitor, Jeanette Clifton (1983), has described her work as chairman of a playgroup committee and has shown how, in a good playgroup, parents can be involved in practical and pleasant ways.

Safety

Home safety was discussed in the previous chapter (p. 76). As children grow more inquisitive, mobile, venturesome and independent, a very wide variety of safety factors needs to be considered. By this stage road safety is particularly important. Parents need, now, to be teaching by example and by showing their children the Green Cross Code (Health Education Council, 1981).

It seems that there has been a worldwide increase in fatal traffic accidents for children, so marked that it has hidden what have, in fact, been declines in other unnatural causes of child death. Dr Sunderland (1984) studied the child traffic accident figures in Sheffield. He has shown that readily available information can be used for planning for prevention and suggests that programmes should start prior to school age.

A significantly greater proportion of deaths were among underprivileged children living in 'accident prone' areas, those with crowded dwellings and often near to main roads. Dr Sunderland made a plea for attractive and safe play areas to be built in high risk zones and says these are now being provided in Sheffield. He says other studies have shown

the main difference between areas with a high accident rate and other areas was the lack of safe play areas.

Perhaps this is a matter over which health visitors would be able to 'influence policies affecting health' (CETHV, 1977; Phillips, 1986) in their locality. They might do this by liaising with voluntary and any statutory agencies involved in such interests. A pre-school mums' discussion group, of the sort described above, might have some constructive suggestions and be prepared to help.

Teaching children about sex

Pre-school children benefit enormously from being told stories and being read to, from being encouraged to talk about what they feel, do, see and hear and, of course, having their questions answered. Parents sometimes wonder how to respond to 'where do babies come from?' The Health Education Council (HEC) have some very helpful little booklets. One, 'Answering a child's questions' (L13), provides general guidance on what approach to take at the various stages of a child's development. It has a list of relevant inexpensive booklets and information about where further literature can be obtained.

Under four years of age it is suggested that parents give simple answers with small amounts of information which is repeated from time to time. The HEC booklet, 'How we grow up' (SE2), makes quite a useful visual aid to explanations as the child gets a little older, for example, how the baby grows and the abdomen expands. There are some colourful and well-presented, but rather more expensive, books. These, such as Claire Rayner's (1978) '*Body Book*', could be borrowed from the library. Group discussion might be particularly helpful to mothers unsure of how to discuss sex with their children. If the group is sympathetic and supportive, sexual problems that the parents have, might also be raised.

Head lice

As young children begin to find other young children to play with, to attend playgroup and later go to school, there is an increased risk that they will come into contact with head lice. This problem has grown in recent years, particularly in middle class communities. Young children work and play with their heads very closely together. It can be very useful, therefore, in these pre-school years to draw parents' attention to the situation and to the simple preventive measures they and their children can take.

Silky-looking hair these days is achieved by using a shampoo. In the past, middle class parents tended to encourage their children to brush their hair until it shone, thereby injuring any louse that might be there. This regular habit, particularly last thing at night, prevented egg laying and colonisation. It seems to have been a significant factor in causing the lower levels of infection amongst the wealthier sections of society, and not, as they might have thought, their being 'rich' or 'clean'. Careful attention, therefore, to brushing and combing and the occasional check to see if there is any evidence of the louse, is the best approach to prevention (Wickenden, 1982).

Head lice and their eggs are very difficult to see. Head inspections reveal only very advanced cases, generally of some four months' duration (Wickenden, 1982). John

Maunder (1983) described how the distance of the nits from the scalp can give an indication of the length of an infection and, equally, of the duration of the cure. He provided a list of the publications which can be sent for. They are those associated with the regular courses on head louse control held at the London School of Hygiene and Tropical Medicine.

A fairly common problem is that little white hair muffs brought about by a skin condition, can be mistaken for nits. Professor Maunder pointed out that a hand lens makes it easy to distinguish between them. Showing parents photographs (Wickenden, 1982; Maunder, 1983) can give them at least an idea of what they are looking for. However, a specimen louse and nit in a bottle give a truer picture and have been found, when used in group discussions, to help overcome the taboo associated with this subject (Moore, 1982).

Treatment is simple but care has to be taken over the use of carbaryl and malathion shampoos and lotions to prevent a resistance developing (Maunder, 1981). The louse has already become resistant to two insecticides. Adrienne de Mont (1985) explains about and lists preparations currently available. She says the district pharmacist will be able to provide details of current recommendations on the policy of rotation of the use of these insecticides. The health visitor is in a good position to be able to back up the community health physician's communications by keeping in touch with local chemists over this issue.

Dental care

In the pre-school and early school years, children become increasingly receptive to health advice, including that of preventive dental care. Their parents will be the best educators that they could have. However, most of the public and many health professionals fatalistically accept dental disease as inevitable and neglect opportunities for prevention. Health visitors, throughout their contact with the family, are in a good position to help improve parental understanding of the essential elements of dental health.

A Community Outlook (1981) 'teeth sheet' may make a useful visual aid. Very practical advice has been provided by Hadley and Sheiham (1984, 1985). They have given clear accounts of how a low sugar diet allows remineralisation of the teeth and can arrest decay, and how fluoride helps in this process. Dosages of fluoride supplements are stated according to different ages and the amount of fluoride in the drinking water. It is suggested that the water authority should be contacted to find out local fluoride levels. Good literature is suggested, and advice is given on tooth brushing techniques and keeping free of plaque.

Hadley and Sheiham say that dental disease is the third most costly aspect of health care and recommend regular contact between health visitors and community dental officers. These officers can be encouraged to come to talk to local groups. Haringey's community dental clinics have taken on and been very successful with a preventive strategy for dental care (Haringey dental officers, 1984). Let us hope the tide is beginning to turn.

In this section we have looked at some aspects of anticipatory guidance for families in the pre-school period, and particularly at road safety, head lice, sex instruction and dental care, and the need for parents to feel their health visitors are still accessible.

CONTINUING THE SEARCH

The part the health visitor plays in child health screening differs significantly from place to place. There is a great deal of variation between Health Districts as to who is responsible for child health clinics and surveillance: in East Suffolk, for example, it is mostly health visitors; in some other places it is GPs or clinical medical officers (Macfarlane & Pillay, 1984).

In many child health schemes, for example Professor Barber's (1982; Robertson, 1984), the screening is shared between the health visitor and the GP. This fits in well with the Health Visitors Association (1985) (HVA) proposals.

The HVA suggestions for the pre-school years are that for the test at about three years of age the health visitor undertakes it alone, and that at the screening prior to school entry it is undertaken by the health visitor and/or the school nurse and the doctor together.

Close cooperation between the health visitor and the GP is required in Somerset in both their urban and their rural schemes. They achieve very high attendance levels at the pre-school test by making it a prerequisite for school entry and by using computerised administration (Bowie & Jones, 1984).

There are many screening and surveillance schemes available. Validated examples range between the time consuming, in-depth Sheridan (1975) approach and the neat, centile chart scheme by Barber et al (1976) discussed in Chapter 5 (pp. 85–87). There is a booklet for use with the Barber scheme which provides a clear description of how it is intended the tests should be undertaken (Barber & Glasgow University Department of Child Health, 1976). Each item is individually explained with the exception of the 'whisper' hearing test at four years of age.

Hearing

The explanation about this item is to be found in the introduction of the Reed hearing test booklet used in the test. This booklet is published by the Royal National Institute for the Deaf (RNID), whose addresses are given at the end of the chapter.

Deafness is liable to be a problem in the aftermath of recurrent ear infections. These infections are fairly common in young children and it therefore seems worth discussing with parents whether their child tends to suffer from them. Barritt and Darbyshire (1984) suggested that GPs examine children's ears six weeks after an attack of otitis media, as they found that children with abnormal eardrums at that stage were more likely to have a problem with deafness and warranted audiological testing. In their small study they found the appearance of the eardrum to be a more reliable indicator than parental opinion about their child's deafness. However, this should not deter health visitors from treating very seriously any concern expressed by parents.

Sight

Vision testing at four years in the Barber scheme uses very simple equipment. Some very small objects such as threads, small beads and pins are put on the table and, with each eye covered separately, the child is asked to pick some up, one at a time. This is likely to be an easier test in the home than the Stycar five letter test, which can present problems when space and light are inadequate (Robertson, 1981).

However, Hall et al (1982) studied various vision screening tests and found that their 'hundreds and thousands' test on older, more reliable six-year olds was able only to discover fairly severe reduction in visual acuity. Regarding squints they found that parents and other non-professionals were generally the people to notice the squint first. Also, it did not tend to be a cover test or corneal reflections but careful observation that led professionals to discover squints. Hall et al felt that earlier referral from the community was encouraged by the reduced ophthalmic outpatient waiting list due to the community orthoptist's secondary screening role. It is important to keep the wait between detection and diagnosis as short as reasonably possible and National Health Service opticians can also be very helpful in this.

A study of school entrants in London by Ismail and Lall (1981) found that two thirds of the children with visual defects had not been detected prior to going to school. However, this is not as bad as it might seem, as all the children with a severe impairment had been diagnosed. Their research led them to feel that the problem was lack of suitable visual screening techniques rather than lack of expertise. They recommended that screening should continue using currently available procedures, but that there should be further

investigation and a thorough search for more objective techniques for pre-school vision screening.

Minor and/or recently developed hearing and vision defects were discovered in some school entrants in Gwent. Lambert et al (1984) found some of the children with vision defects had not been tested at the three and a half year medical. They noted that health visitors need a reliable system to inform them of non-attendance. One child had been uncooperative at the test, which it is pointed out can be a sign of a possible problem. Ounsted et al (1983) felt that non-cooperation at the pre-school assessment should always be followed up.

Speech

The expectation that a child at three years of age would be able to use three word sentences was mentioned in the previous chapter (p. 36). At four years, a child with poor articulation, perhaps omitting or substituting consonants, would also need to be referred on for investigation by a speech therapist, and by a doctor if necessary. Margaret Pollak (1984) feels that speech problems are not taken seriously and not dealt with early enough. She explained causes of speech problems, described diagnosis and treatment and demonstrated the value of early referral.

Physical measurements

Parents will be interested to see, as the years have passed, the sort of picture that has emerged on the centile height, weight and head circumference charts (see Ch. 5, page 89). It is easier to measure the weight and height of children attending a clinic equipped for these procedures. Measuring children who do not attend needs a little more ingenuity.

Height can be measured in the home against a doorway (or a wall) where there is no skirting board, so the child can stand absolutely upright. A carpenter's/DIY collaps-

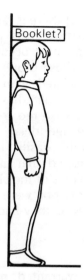

Fig. 6.1 Tape measuring, at home.

ible wooden rule or a metal expandible tape could be used. The RNID hearing test booklet or a block of wood could be used to ensure a right angle with the doorway (see Fig. 6.1). Accuracy also depends on the child standing with heels together, touching the ground and against the doorway. The head should be looking straight forward, eyes on a level with the tops of the ears, and, perhaps, with a very gentle upward pressure on the back of the jaw, as shown by Harvey and Wallis (1978). Parents may feel it is worth noting the child's weight at regular intervals at the chemist, and would be particularly encouraged to do so, should there be any concern.

A school nurse in Oxford, Jill Moss (1985), described how she measured children in primary schools and found a number of cases with unidentified growth problems. She used Whitehouse and Castlemead Publications' portable wall chart. Routine measuring in schools was later discontinued there, as it was undertaken in the pre-school period by health visitors at child health clinics, though in many places this measuring is continued into the school years.

The last visit or clinic session before school entry is a good time to check with the parents that they have a complete personal record, not only of immunisations, including the pre-

school booster, but also of centile height and weight charts for future reference should they ever be needed.

Maintaining contact and continuity

One of the problems in child health screening and surveillance can be that children sometimes remain unscreened because it is difficult to make contact with the family. A large number of mothers with pre-school children go out to work and their children are minded. Sue Owen (1984) surveyed Area Health Authorities to find out if they had special liaison arrangements between health visitors and social services regarding child-minders and the children who were minded. She asked, too, whether there were special arrangements for health visitors to meet the minders and whether evening child health clinics were available for working mothers.

It was found that most social service departments sent lists of child-minders, but did not state which children were placed with them. However, in three areas health visitors were notified about where children were being minded, one of them very helpfully on a weekly basis. This service depends on the local authority having a scheme which requires weekly returns from the child-minders.

Health visitor contact with child-minders varied. Sue Owen found that geographic patch-based health visitors tended to be in contact with and visit child-minders in their patch. In some health authorities, child-minders were being visited by the health visitor from the practice of the minder's own GP. The health visitor then notified colleagues about the children being minded there. Evening clinics were held in only six health authorities, others relying on evening visits by health visitors and/or assuming parents would ask the minder to take their child to the clinic.

An improvement in health visitor contact with child-minders and the children they care for is much needed. Liaison with the social services department and explanations about the potential benefits to the health of the children being minded, might trigger the appropriate cooperation between a larger number of social service and health departments.

Government advice (DHSS, 1980) is that the results of early childhood surveillance should be made known to those responsible for screening in the school years. Systems of notification and liaison arrangements will vary from place to place. There is an obvious advantage if the height and weight charts can be passed on to and continue through the school medical notes.

Parents who want to know about school medicals, will find a brief outline in Elizabeth Forsythe's (1981) *Preparation for School. A Medical Guide for parents*. It could also be useful for explaining about some of the common health problems that might be found at these examinations or encountered during the schooldays.

In this section we have looked at some aspects of screening and surveillance in the immediate pre-school years, in particular hearing, vision and speech, and we have looked at the need for liaison with social service departments in order to keep in contact with children who spend their day with a child-minder.

CONTINUED SUPPORT

Supportive work where problems are already established can be very important. By giving people a chance to talk out their problems and by telling them of help and services available, health visitors may be able to help prevent greater difficulties arising out of the current situation. Examples given here of this supportive work are child behavioural difficulties, marital difficulties such as sexual problems and impending separation and divorce, and young women's urinary incontinence. These types of problems might, of course, be encountered at earlier visits too.

Problem behaviour

Studies of children's behaviour up to school age have found that there is far more problem behaviour in the two years prior to school than in babyhood, most occurring at around the age of three. These problems were found to be often associated with mental health problems of the mother (Bax & Hart, 1976). They were also discovered to correlate with speech and language delay (Jenkins et al, 1980). They could easily be overlooked because it was found that mothers did not tend to take problems of the children's behaviour to the doctor, nor were they attending the clinic regularly as they had done.

Assessment

Early attention is warranted, not only to help the mothers' mental state but also on account of the association between speech and language delay with slow attainments in reading and writing and this, in turn, with deviant behaviour later on. The studies found that around a fifth or more of the children seen had behavioural problems in these pre-school years, half of the problems being classed as moderate or severe.

A chart has been provided by Ruth Brink (1982) which can assist in assessing whether or not a child's problem is serious. Some parents might find it a reassuring document. Parent counselling was discussed by Peter Tucker (1985a, 1985b). He stressed the importance of being able to see the problem from the parents' viewpoint and of having counselling skills that include effective listening.

What can be done

The most disruptive problems for the family and the most difficult to deal with in South Glamorgan research were found to be sleep problems and hyperactivity. A study of the records of eleven health visitors showed that the families with this problem had received more visits than other families, but that over a year little improvement had been achieved. Behavioural techniques developed by South Glamorgan psychologists had been used very successfully, achieving improvements in just a few weeks. It was therefore felt that health visitors should have the opportunity to train in these methods. To use them health visitors would need to change their visiting pattern a little, as the programme needs two or three weekly contacts initially (Thomas et al, 1982).

Practical guidance has been provided by a clinical psychologist, Hewitt (1981a, 1981b), on what help health visitors can give to families with pre-school children who have sleeping problems and those whose children are over-active. Bowler & Watson (1984) described the outcome of a workshop set up to help health visitors gain a better understanding of behavioural techniques. It was very successful. This course and lunchtime follow-up group discussions, enabled more help to be given to families with problems, without referral to the psychology department. Of course, consultation with Child Guidance is always a possible option.

One health visitor, Mavis Maureen Raper (1985a, 1985b, 1985c), made a special study of hyperactive children. She described common characteristics of these children and, by providing a case history, demonstrated the way play therapy is planned. Nicky Milligan (1984) put forward the particular case of 'gifted children'. Both of these writers gave the addresses of support groups. Frieda Painter (1984) has written a parents' guide to *Living with a Gifted Child*, which some parents may find helpful as it offers guidance on a range of problems, ways of coping and of assessing the child.

There is much greater understanding now of the correlation between stress in the mother and pre-school childhood behaviour and illness problems. Parental emotional status is therefore an important priority (Bax et al, 1980).

Marital stress and problems

It is generally felt that one of the advantages for areas where health visitors remain with the same caseload and the same families for a long time, is that very delicate issues which trouble the family may more easily be brought into discussions. This is because trust has been built up over the years. However, a health visitor with the appropriate manner, training and skills should be able to establish a good counselling relationship relatively quickly.

Jack Dominion (1982) saw the health visitor as being in a good position to be able to help couples in the early, vulnerable years of their marriage. He said that when a problem is identified, the couple should be persuaded to seek expert help, but that this is not always acceptable to them. In this case, he suggested the health visitor should try to help them 'as best she can'. He provided some helpful tips on counselling style and approach. Health visitors can also turn to people such as family planning or marriage guidance counsellors for consultation on the general principles of how to help.

Sexuality

Health visitors sometimes feel inadequately educated for helping a couple with sexual difficulties. Those finding themselves the confidant of couples with problems who are unable or unwilling to seek expert advice, may feel the need to attend a course on psycho-sexual counselling like the one described by Jennett Caldwell (1982). It may be very helpful to consult with and/or involve the GP with a couple's problem, if they wish this.

Sometimes couples can find that a book provides the answers. One that is intended to enable people to help themselves is David Mace's (1972) *Sexual Difficulties in Marriage*. Another approach which can be helpful is to invite several couples facing problems to come to the clinic one evening to see the film, 'Sexuality and Communication'. The film demonstrates the important part played by communication and gives a clear explanation, often demonstrated through role play, of common difficulties. It is very useful as a trigger film to encourage discussion. It can be hired free of charge from Ortho Pharmaceutical (address at end of chapter).

Divorce

Marital problems may have got to such a pitch that the parents are considering separation and divorce. They will be facing all the feelings associated with grief, so well described by Tony Lake (1984), and have the same need to talk about their problems and feelings. The Divorce Conciliation and Advisory Service (Health Visitor, 1983; Harris, 1983) or the Marriage Guidance Council may be able to offer help. Self-help groups, such as Gingerbread and Families Need Fathers, tend to be turned to later (Richards, 1982).

Dr Richards and Ann Mitchell (1985) both studied the effect of separation and divorce on children and found that they tend to fare better if they are able to talk about it, if they have the family situation explained to them and are able to keep in touch with both parents from very early on. Ann Mitchell feels her book might help parents contemplating divorce, and wider family members associated with it, to see how other people's children have felt, and to better understand the problems of their own children. Dr Richards saw support for parents and children as important preventive work for health visitors. He said simple counselling can be very effective and felt discussion might help parents to see their children's needs as separate from their own.

Incontinence

Urinary incontinence has been shown to be a very common problem. Jennifer Sleep (1984) in her study of the effects of episiotomy on around a thousand women found that three months after the birth of a baby 22% of the multiparae and 15% of the primiparae suffered from it. Some 6% were needing to wear a pad. Perhaps it is something health visitors should routinely ask about, very sensitively, as part of their surveillance of mothers' health.

In explaining about assessment and the promotion of continence, Christine Norton (1984) said that it is still not generally believed that most sufferers can regain continence. A physiotherapist, Sheila Harrison (1984), has described how weakened muscles can be re-educated by regular practice and how assessment and instruction are an essential feature of treatment.

Feneley and Blannin's (1984) well-written book gives a short, optimistic and clear account of the problem and is very much to be recommended. It is likely to improve the quality of many people's lives. However, a group of mothers may find it particularly helpful to see the tape/slide presentation, 'The management of incontinence' by Camera Talks Ltd (1982), with a health visitor explaining, as necessary, some of the more technical jargon. They might also find useful some of the literature from the Paddington and North Kensington Health Education Departments with Victoria Health Education Department (1986) catalogue, 'Health Education Resources on Women's Health'. It is not always easy to maintain the necessary level of exercises by oneself, and a small self-help group may be the best answer.

Although the main thrust of health visiting is generally aimed towards preventing the occurrence and the development of problems, supportive work can be an important feature. We have looked at examples such as marital problems of a sexual nature and of impending separation and divorce. Incontinence may occur more widely and also be more amenable to treatment than is generally thought.

This chapter on pre-school visiting provided another example of the way the role of the health visitor can be thought about and described. As before, it has been done by artificially dividing the work into three aspects of the prevention of health problems. Examples were provided of preventing the occurrence and the development of conditions and of preventing deterioration in the case of known problems.

USEFUL ADDRESSES

Ortho Pharmaceutical Limited
The Administrator, Department of
Educational Services,
Ortho Pharmaceutical Limited,
P.O. Box 79,
Saunderton, High Wycombe,
Buckinghamshire HP14 4HJ

Royal National Institute for the Deaf
9a Clairmont Gardens, GLASGOW
Tel 041 332 0343
105 Gower Street,
LONDON WC1E 6AH
Tel 01 387 8033

REFERENCES

Barber J H 1982 Preschool developmental screening—the results of a four year period. Health Bulletin 40: 170–178

Barber J H, Boothman R, Stanfield J P 1976 A new visual chart for preschool developmental screening. Health Bulletin 34: 80–91

Barber J H, Department of General Practice, University of Glasgow with assistance from the Department of Child Health, University of Glasgow 1976 The Woodside system of preschool developmental screening: description of the tests. Econoprint, Edinburgh

Barritt P W, Darbyshire P J 1984 Deafness after otitis media in general practice. Journal of the Royal College of General Practitioners 34: 92–94

Bax M, Hart H 1976 Health needs of preschool children. Archives of Disease in Childhood 51: 848–852

Bax M, Hart H, Jenkins S 1980 The health needs of preschool children. Thomas Coram Research Unit, University of London, London

Bowie C, Jones A P 1984 Court come true—for better or for worse? British Medical Journal 289: 1322–1324

Bowler J F, Watson P L 1984 A child behaviour workshop. Health Visitor 57: 302–303

Brink R E 1982 How serious is the child's behaviour problem? American Journal of Maternal and Child Nursing 7: 33–36

Caldwell J 1982 On the right course. Nursing Times 78:58

Camera Talks Ltd 1982 The management of incontinence. Tape/slide: two parts. Camera Talks Ltd, London

Clifton J 1983 What's your view of a playgroup? Health Visitor 56: 342–343

Community Outlook 1981 Teeth sheet. Nursing Times Community Outlook 77, 33: 272–273

CETHV 1977 An investigation into the principles of health visiting. Council for the Education and Training of Health Visitors, London

DHSS 1980 Prevention in the child health services. Department of Health and Social Security, London

Dominian J 1982 Marital stress in the early years. Health Visitor 55: 146–149

Feneley R C L, Blannin J P 1984 Incontinence. Help for an unmentionable problem. Churchill Livingstone, Edinburgh

Forsythe E 1981 Preparation for school. A medical guide for parents. Faber and Faber, London

Hadley A, Sheiham A 1984 Smile please! Nursing Times 80, 27: 28–31

Hadley A, Sheiham A 1985 Guidelines for promoting better dental health in children. Health Visitor 58: 133–134

Hall S M, Pugh A G, Hall D M B 1982 Vision screening in the under-5s. British Medical Journal 285: 1096–1098

Haringey dental officers 1984 Making sure the children don't have a caries in the world. Health and Social Services Journal XCIV: 322–323

Harris P M 1983 Coping with divorce. Health Visitor 56: 98–99

Harrison S M 1984 Re-education of pelvic floor muscles. Nursing Times Supplement 80, 14: 13–14

Harvey D, Wallis S 1978 Children of short stature: part 1. Midwife, Health Visitor and Community Nurse 14: 136–139

Health Education Council 1981 Play it safe! A guide to preventing children's accidents. Health Education Council and Scottish Health Education Group in Association with the BBC

Health Visitor 1983 The Divorce Conciliation and Advisory Service. Health Visitor 56:97

Health Visitors Association 1985 The health visitor's role in child health surveillance: a policy statement. Health Visitors Association, London

Hewitt K E 1981a Sleeping problems in pre-school children: what to ask and what to do. Health Visitor 54: 100–101

Hewitt K E 1981b Overactivity in young children: how health visitors can help. Health Visitor 54: 276–277

Ismail H, Lall P 1981 Visual acuity of school entrants. Child: Care, Health and Development 7: 127–134

Jenkins S, Bax M, Hart H 1980 Behaviour problems in pre-school children. Journal of Child Psychology and Psychiatry 21: 5–17

Lambert C, Miers M, Edwards J, Farrow 1984 Hearing and vision screening in preschool children. Health Visitor 57: 329–331

Lake T 1984 Living with grief. Sheldon Press, London

Mace D 1972 Sexual difficulties in marriage. The National Guidance Council, Rugby

Macfarlane J A, Pillay U 1984 Who does what, and how much in the preschool child health services in England. British Medical Journal 289: 851–852

Maunder J W 1981 Treatment for head lice (letter). Nursing Times 77:995

Maunder J W 1983 The head louse resurgence. Maternal and Child Health 8: 51–56

Mayall B, Grossmith C 1985 The health visitor and the provision of services. Health Visitor 58: 349–352

Milligan N 1984 Gifted children—how to help in the preschool years. Health Visitor 57: 22–23

Mitchell A 1985 Children in the middle. Living through divorce. Tavistock Publications, London

de Mont A 1985 Don't let your hair down. Nursing Times Community Outlook 81, 37: 16–17

Moore P M 1982 Message-in-a-bottle (letter). Health Visitor 55: 629

Moss J 1985 Measuring up. Nursing Times Community Outlook 81, 15: 24–26

Norton C 1984 The promotion of continence. Nursing Times Supplement 80, 14: 4–10

Ounsted M, Cockburn J, Moar V A 1983 Developmental assessment at four years: are there any differences between children who do, or do not, cooperate? Archives of Disease in Childhood 58: 286–289

Owen S 1984 Childminders' contact with health visitors results of a nationwide survey. Health Visitor 57: 171–172

Paddington and North Kensington Health Education Departments with Victoria Health Education Department 1986 Health education resources on women's health. Victoria Health Education Department, 1a Thorndite Close, London SW10

Painter F 1984 Living with a gifted child. Souvenir Press ltd, London

Phillips S 1986 A centre for change. Nursing Times Community Outlook 82, 7: 15–17

Pollak M 1984 Speech problems in childhood. Health Visitor 57: 334–335

Powell J 1985 Keeping watch. Nursing Times Community Outlook 81, 2: 15–19

Raper M M 1985a In perpetual motion. Nursing Mirror 160, 10: 16–17

Raper M M 1985b Food—the unknown enemy. Nursing Mirror 160, 11: 35–37

Raper M M 1985c Play therapy. Nursing Mirror 160, 12: 19–21

Rayner C 1978 Body book. Deutsch, London

Richards M 1982 Do broken marriages affect children? Health Visitor 55: 152–153

Robertson C A 1981 A review of vision screening in pre-school children. Health Visitor 54: 52–57

Robertson C A 1984 Preventive health care for infants. In: Houston M J (ed) Maternal and Infant Health. Churchill Livingstone, Edinburgh

Robinson K 1983 Talking with clients. In: Clark J, Henderson J (eds) Community health. Churchill Livingstone, Edinburgh

Sheridan M D 1975 The developmental progress of infants and young children. HMSO, London

Sleep J 1984 Management of the perineum. Nursing Times 80, 48: 51–54

Sunderland R 1984 Dying young in traffic. Archives of Disease in Childhood 59: 754–757

Thomas J A, Bidder R T, Hewitt K, Gray O P 1982 Health visiting and pre-school children with behavioural problems in the County of South Glamorgan: an exploratory study. Child: Care, Health and Development 8: 93–103

Tucker P 1985a The scope and practice of parent counselling: part 1. Midwife Health Visitor and Community Nurse 21: 282–286

Tucker P 1985b The scope and practice of parent counselling: part 2. Midwife Health Visitor and Community Nurse 21: 310–313

Wickenden J 1982 'Nurse, why are the kids always getting nits?' Health Visitor 55: 469–476

Both the prevention and the family health needs frameworks are used in this chapter to describe health visitors' work in preventive health care for the elderly. The chapter ends with two visits given as examples of these activities.

7

Work with the elderly

THE FRAMEWORKS

In this chapter both of the perspectives demonstrated in the previous four chapters are used. In the first three sections we use the prevention model to describe ways in which the health visitor can help prevent the occurrence and the development of problems and a deterioration in established conditions.

The fourth section takes a brief look at an old person's requirements in daily living, using a form of the family health needs model which includes physical, emotional, environmental and social aspects of health. Two examples are given in this format, but running through them are also concepts from the prevention framework of the earlier sections.

The three aspects of prevention

Attachment to general practice has brought health visitors into closer contact with the elderly, but for most this is only once a crisis has occurred. A good preventive service, however, depends on making contact early. For example, increasing people's awareness of health needs in retirement is best undertaken much earlier in life. To be effective, a screening programme needs to bring to light potentially incapacitating problems well before they reach serious proportions. Also, where a crisis such as bereavement has occurred, care should be offered in good time. The prevention framework can draw attention to each of these three aspects of the role of the health visitor in this field.

Preventive health care for the elderly is becoming more and more necessary, but there are many constraints (Robertson, 1984a). For example, care of the elderly has traditionally been given low priority. Also, a special approach is needed, especially with regard to screening. Here the aim is to maximise on an old person's ability to overcome and minimise socio-functional problems rather than to cure disease.

Many examples of activities with the elderly are given in these first three sections. It is *not* the intention to draw up an 'ideal model' of health visiting practice in this field. The aim is to discuss its potential and to present possibilities by looking at a range of schemes

currently undertaken. However, a health visitor working only with the elderly may be able to cover quite a number of the points raised.

EDUCATION AND ACTION

Work aimed at avoiding the occurrence of problems and at promoting the health of old people, as shown in Figure 7.1, can involve health visitors in a variety of activities. This might be in clinics and teaching sessions both before and during retirement, in individual and general discussions and sometimes in negotiations in the community to try to improve the environment and local facilities.

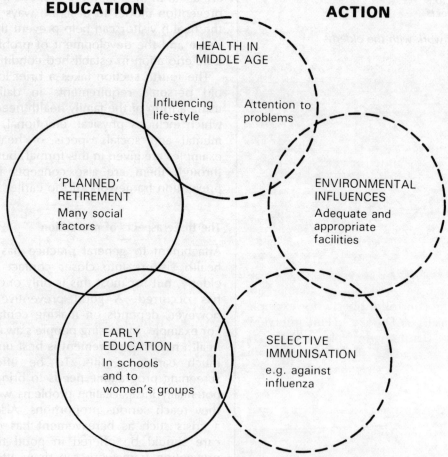

EDUCATION　　　　　　　　　　　　**ACTION**

HEALTH IN
MIDDLE AGE

Influencing
life-style

Attention to
problems

'PLANNED'
RETIREMENT

Many social
factors

ENVIRONMENTAL
INFLUENCES

Adequate and
appropriate
facilities

EARLY
EDUCATION

In schools
and to
women's groups

SELECTIVE
IMMUNISATION

e.g. against
influenza

Fig. 7.1　Aspects of primary preventive care—to prevent problems occurring in retirement.

EDUCATION

Health education in schools

It could be argued that really effective health education in preparation for old age should be started in the school years. Many significant diseases are affected by life-style, for example, obesity, pulmonary and cardiovascular. Habits established in youth, like eating habits, smoking and exercise, can set patterns for health in later years. Health visitors may be able to help young people become aware of these factors by giving talks in schools or, alternatively, by acting as advisers to teachers.

Health education and screening in the middle years

In the middle years problems can emerge which may be troublesome in old age (Burkitt, 1977). This may also be the best time to start thinking, more specifically, about retirement. Health visitors may be able to become involved at well women or well men clinics like those described by Kerr (1975), Pike (1975) and Antrobus (1981). It seems that the health visitor at the Antrobus clinic covers the more emotional and social aspects of care, whilst the district nurse and the SEN concentrate upon the physical aspects of screening like urinalysis, blood pressure and breast palpation. They back up the examination with health education, using leaflets provided by the local health education department. Mrs Antrobus says the aim is to detect and overcome hidden disease at an early stage and to encourage people to adopt a suitable life-style, over the control of obesity for example. The health visitor at Dr Pike's clinic interviews and discusses retirement plans with the middle-aged people who come (Dodsworth, 1976).

Pre-retirement talks and discussions

A happy retirement involves many factors such as those shown in Table 7.3 in the fourth section: adequate finance and housing, friendship, interesting things to do and satisfactory health, both physical and emotional. Retirement can, however, bring the need for enormous, and often sudden, adjustments to accustomed patterns of daily activity and companionship. Early planning and preparation is a great advantage.

Health visitors may have the opportunity to conduct pre-retirement courses or, alternatively, to encourage local employers to undertake them. The Pre-Retirement Association and the Workers Educational Association help employers organise the classes in various parts of the country. It seems that only 6% of those about to retire currently receive formal pre-retirement preparation (DHSS, 1981).

Stott (1982) and Clapham (1980) have shown how a health visitor with a normal caseload can undertake classes. Denise Stott describes how high levels of redundancy inspired her to start a '50-plus club', eight week pre-retirement course for the over-50s. She used films and other visual aids, tape recordings and visiting speakers to help cover the following topics:

— adjustment to retirement
— bereavement
— diet
— finance
— accommodation
— accidents
— leisure and
— exercise.

A questionnaire completed by the participants at the end of the course proved very useful in helping to plan subsequent sessions. Stott listed the books, films and organisations found to be particularly helpful.

Joyce Clapham found that in addition to teaching on topics such as:

— diet
— constipation
— teeth
— sleeping
— keeping warm
— care of the feet
— influenza and
— home nursing,

she was able to help participants increase

their mobility by introducing them to gentle exercises in her 'Keeping Fit in Retirement' classes. After a very disappointing beginning, (only one person came to the first session) there was a gradual increase in numbers, levelling out at attendances of around 17 at each session.

There is widespread ignorance about the financial and support services available to people in need (Equal Opportunities Commission, 1980). Knowing how to get this help and awareness of the value of seeking it early may help to avoid potential crises and to enable people to maintain an independent style of life. Health visitors who are asked to give talks to groups such as the Women's Institute, Townswomen's Guild, Ladies Circle and old people's luncheon clubs, may be able to draw attention to these benefits and find this a useful approach to increasing local understanding of health and social needs in retirement.

ACTION

Immunisation

Shukla (1981) has suggested that some measure of illness amongst old people could be prevented if those who were particularly vulnerable were given influenza vaccine. Special attention might be given to people over 75 years, those living in old people's homes and those with chronic chest complaints, and health visitors might become involved in this activity by explaining the scheme to those who would qualify for it.

Provision of facilities

Individual preparation for retirement is nullified for some people by their poverty, by lack of local meeting places and by traditional attitudes.

Townsend (1963) has drawn a very sad picture of working class men in their late 60s and early 70s. They showed considerable apprehension about retirement as, once they ceased to work, their status would be lowered in the eyes of their family and they would have little or no spare money for hobbies. After a lifetime where friendships were formed through work or the pub, the prospect of retirement appeared particularly bleak.

Such people need help of a practical nature once retirement has begun. Townsend suggested the need for occupational provision for the retired, a sentiment vaguely reflected in a DHSS (1981) White Paper. This mentioned a range of voluntary occupations, the need for clubs, recreational facilities, low cost holidays, libraries and adult education.

Health visitors may need to step outside their day-to-day visiting role in order to use their influence over the provision of suitable facilities. Liz Day (1981) is a health visitor who is gradually achieving an effect in this way (Day & Mogridge, 1981). At her suggestion, a local vicar incorporated a workshop for the elderly into his community centre and she had plans to set up meeting places which would bring the isolated together as well as providing services such as health education, keep fit and screening. Her appointment is as a specialist health visitor. It is unlikely that a generalist appointment would leave much time for going out and helping to organise community facilities.

In this section, we have looked at health visitors' primary preventive work for the elderly, which tends mostly to be through health education: helping to make people aware of risks to health in old age. The aim is to try to encourage people to pursue suitable life-styles and to organise their environment and their social relationships in order to minimise health risks and to promote good mental and physical health. Activities such as screening for physical, social and emotional difficulties in the middle years and schemes to improve local facilities, can also play an important part.

SCREENING THE ELDERLY

A socio-functional approach

Effective health visitor screening for the

elderly is aimed, not at a search for specific medical conditions, but at discovering *functional disabilities*, basically the *effects* of disease and of social circumstances. Health visitors seek, in particular, the factors which influence people's *ability to cope* (see Fig. 7.2). It is hoped these can be attended to early and old people helped to maintain the independence and mobility they desire—despite the presence of disease.

Questions similar to those considered in Chapter 5, such as those about monitoring the programme, the availability of services (in this case mostly social services) and whom the screening might not be reaching, need to be covered in both planning and evaluation of the programmes. These questions, along with an early example of health visitor geriatric screening, have been discussed elsewhere. They have, of course, a range of different answers (Robertson, 1984b).

Designing programmes

Every Health District will have a different and particular health and welfare profile of its elderly and ought, therefore, to have a specially designed programme to meet those needs. For this reason I have not put forward a prescribed format. Instead, some illustrations and references are provided, so that health visitors can investigate further and map out a scheme which suits their special circumstances.

A variety of methods have been described in the professional journals and Figure 7.3

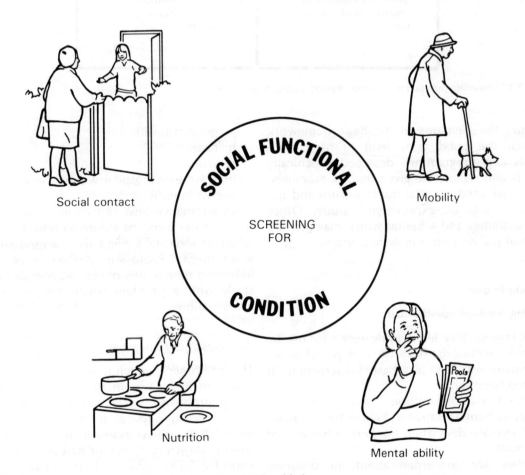

Social contact

Mobility

Nutrition

Mental ability

SOCIAL FUNCTIONAL CONDITION

SCREENING FOR

Fig. 7.2 The main concern in health visitor screening for the elderly.

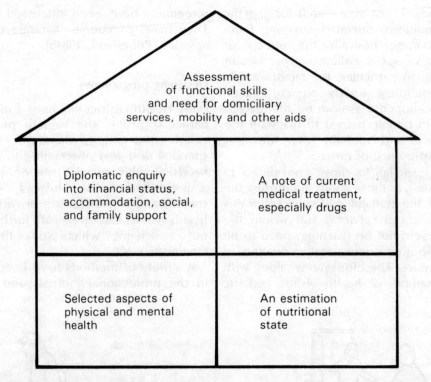

Fig. 7.3 Screening programmes for the elderly: a basic framework.

shows the elements of the basic framework which the good ones tend to have. Two screening programmes designed specifically for health visitors are given here as examples. The first used a postal questionnaire and the second was an experimental study. Other programmes and schemes which may provide useful pointers are mentioned briefly.

Example one

Using a postal questionnaire

In Glasgow, a system was designed for use by health visitors (Barber, 1981). A postal questionnaire was used as a basis for screening. It asked whether:
— the person lives alone
— is without a relative to help in time of need
— there are days when the person has no hot meal
— they are concerned about, or suffering from, a problem with

a. general health
b. hearing
c. vision
— they were in hospital within the previous twelve months.

An affirmative answer to any of the questions on the form, or failure to return it, was taken to indicate a need for comprehensive assessment. Professor Barber says this identified nine tenths of the old people in his study with a problem which needed more investigation.

An assessment interview

The assessment, which took the health visitor about an hour, was in three parts: medicosocial problems; social service needs; and questions on physical health. A sample of each of the three assessment record cards used is shown in Professor Barber's article. A checklist format was used. The health visitor referred people with previously undisclosed medical symptoms to the GP and other problems to appropriate members of the health care team. Averaged over a year, it was estimated that it took the health visitor some four and a half hours a week to undertake the scheme, including the associated administrative work.

Example two

An experimental study

The most fully reported screening format is the one undertaken by Karen Luker (1982), who studied the effect of health visiting-intervention in the context of care for the elderly. A problem-oriented format was used for recording, with a separate sheet to show changes in the situation. The interview schedule (pp. 73–88) included:
— a life satisfaction index
— a mental impairment measure
— housing
— finances
— children and social contacts
— health
— cooking and dietary history
— shopping and housework
— mobility
— bathing and dressing
— dentition
— weight
— heating
— sleep
— medication
— vision
— hearing
— balance.
Also listed (pp. 89–94) were the health visitor's responses to some of the problems that were found.

Other programmes and schemes

The Kilsyth Questionnaire (Powell & Crombie, 1974) is an early example of a scheme devised for health visitors to screen old people in their own homes. It included assessment of the ability to do everyday tasks, physical and

mental health, a nutrition test and an investigation of current drug therapy.

Screening programmes for use by the primary health care team have been described by Williams (1979, Ch. 8), Dodsworth (1976) and Douglas-Jones (1980). Neil (1982) has reported on one undertaken by a health visitor and SEN.

The Williams programme was explained in great detail and many useful ideas were included. One was the checklist for assessment by Barlow and Matthews (pp. 45–46) to help discover old people's need for domiciliary services and is outlined in Table 7.1. Another was the way some old people were selected for regular contact by someone from the primary health care team because they were considered to be 'at risk'. Williams' (pp. 114–115) criteria and some suggested by Stanton (1979) include people
— living alone
— housebound

Table 7.1 Checklists for assessment of old people's functional ability and need for domiciliary services

Aspect	Examples
Personal	
Involving the whole body	Cutting toe nails; climbing stairs and using public transport
Mobility in the home	Getting around the house; getting in and out of bed and getting to the lavatory
Manipulation of the hands	Shaving, combing the hair, washing and being able to feed self
Mobility outside	Ability to get out of doors
Domestic	
Heavier tasks	Decorating, cleaning windows on the outside and undertaking minor household repairs
Moderate tasks	Cleaning windows inside, washing floors and washing clothes
Lighter tasks	Sewing, cooking, unscrewing jars, using a frying pan and making a cup of tea

(From Williams, 1979, pp. 45–46 (Barlow and Matthews))
N.B. A person experiencing difficulty with one task is likely to have difficulty with others in the same group. The list of domestic tasks needs to be used with care, as some tasks will not be undertaken, more for reasons of the traditional male and female roles than of functional inability (Williams, 1979, p. 79)

— recently bereaved
— liable to hypothermia
— vulnerable to poor nutrition
— liable to fall
— with locomotor difficulties (whatever the cause)
— showing signs of mental impairment
— recently discharged from hospital especially if showing signs of self-neglect on admission)
— socially isolated.

Health visitors may find helpful the questionnaire which Dodsworth published. It aimed to cover the more important systems of body function and bring out difficulties often met with in the middle and later years. McCabe (1985) described simple tests to discover old people at greatest risk of falling.

Harwin (1975) described the assessment of old people's mental health and included two questionnaires which, he suggested, GPs might use to find out whether or not an old person is suffering from dementia or depression. The test for dementia amounts to a few simple questions to check on memory and orientation and uses a scoring system. The presence or otherwise of anxiety or depression is gauged by noting the old person's replies to a specially designed series of questions. Harwin found that with a sympathetic approach the questioning had been acceptable to his patients. Other tests are also available (Gilleard, 1984, p. 109; Wilcock, 1982).

Assessment of old people's nutritional

Box 7.1 Inadequate diet—ten 'at risk' factors (from Louise Davies (1981. p. 135))

```
'At risk' factors

 (i)  Less than eight main meals, whether hot or
      cold, that are eaten in a week
 (ii) Less than half a pint of milk each day
(iii) Almost no fruit or vegetables
 (iv) Food wasted, e.g. uneaten meals on wheels
  (v) Lengthy spells in a day without food
 (vi) Loneliness and depression
(vii) Unexpected and significant weight gain or loss
(viii) Problems with shopping
 (ix) Low income
  (x) Other difficulties or disabilities, including
      alcohol consumption
```

status, based on Louise Davies' (1981, p. 135) ten 'at risk' factors, is shown in Box 7.1. A questionnaire for estimating need for meals on wheels and other relevant services incorporating these factors is now available (Davies et al, 1982).

RESULTS

The results of several studies have been reported. Some researchers have been more concerned with validation of health visitors' ability to discover medical and social conditions, whilst others have concentrated on trying to ascertain the extent to which old people have problems and how they might benefit from screening.

a. Validation

The researchers generally agree that there are a large number of unreported functional, social and medical problems amongst the elderly which are amenable to 'treatment', and that health visitors are competent to discover them. Several studies have compared the health visitors' assessments with those of medical and other specialists in the field (Williamson et al, 1966; Player et al, 1971; Powell & Crombie, 1974) and showed high levels of agreement in functional, social and physical conditions, but a little less so with regard to mental health. Williamson et al pointed out that the health visitors in the study were given no practical instruction for the screening programme and that, like many other medical personnel, they would benefit from specific guidance in psycho-geriatrics.

One small study used psychologists and psychiatrists to check health visitors' assessments and showed that out of a sample of forty people they were able to recognise the four with moderate disability. The health visitors failed to identify mild cases, which is, anyway, an area in which disagreement is not unusual (Player et al, 1971). Perhaps much depends on the quality of the guidance notes and the questionnaire itself.

Using the Kilsyth Questionnaire and guidance notes, health visitors were able to identify 83 old people said to be at risk with regard to mental ill-health. In five of these cases, the health visitors' diagnoses differed from those of the psychiatrists'. As Powell and Crombie point out, this is not important. Health visitors aim, in screening, to identify the need for further investigation or care, not to provide a medical diagnosis.

b. Outcome

Some research reports on the benefits of screening have looked not only at the number of problems discovered and attended to, but also at the morale boosting effect the programme had for some old people.

Barber (1981) studied long-term effectiveness by reassessing a hundred old people nine months after the original appraisal. Of the 641 functional, social and medical problems discovered in the first assessment, he found improvements in a third. The reassessment brought to light a further 79 previously unknown problems that would become the object of further attention.

Williams (1974) grouped his sample of 297 old people according to their 'effective health': those coping well (60%); those with restricted movements but managing to deal with their problems (36%) and a small number (4%) who were unable to care for themselves. He followed up his original sample a year later. 75% were revisited. Most of those thought to have needed social services had been able to receive them. Of the original 297 old people, 27% were said to have improved. The percentages in the broad categories according to ability to cope had remained largely unchanged, even though, over time, a decline might have been expected.

These studies had no matched control group against which to compare results, a necessity for more reliable evaluation. There are, however, some difficulties in using a control group in this sort of research. For example, it is difficult to explain to a large number of people that they are to be denied a service and are to be used merely for comparison. Karen Luker's cross-over experiment (see Ch. 2, p. 28) shows one way of avoiding that problem.

Dr Luker (1981a) was able to compare the state of 60 old ladies' problems after 6 months when no health visitor had come, against 60 where the health visitor had visited. Table 7.2 shows the results. With no health visitor intervention, the problems remained very much the same. There was a significant degree of improvement where the health visitor had called, just as there was in the control group when it crossed to become the experimental group and received health visitor attention. The group that received no visits in the second six months showed that the effect of the health visitor's intervention lasted after the withdrawal of the service—indicating that such intensive visiting need not be maintained indefinitely.

Table 7.2 Karen Luker's experiment: Assessment of elderly women

	After 1st 6 months	After 2nd 6 months
1st group of 60 elderly women	*Health visitor visiting* Improvement	*No visits* Improvement maintained
2nd group of 60 elderly women	*No visits* No particular change	*Health visitor visiting* Improvement

Effect upon morale

Karen Luker (1981b) also attempted to estimate the old people's opinions about the visits and their degree of satisfaction. Most, though not all, felt the visits to be beneficial and many positively looked forward to them: 'therapeutic anticipation'. Remarks were made such as:

. . . it was nice to think people were taking an interest in you . . .
. . . you knew that somebody was paying attention to how you were and they would be there if you needed them.
It helped. It gave me something to look forward to . . .

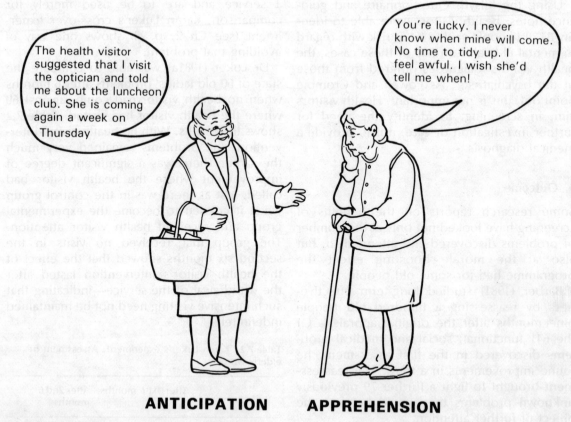

ANTICIPATION   **APPREHENSION**

Fig. 7.4 Appointments and 'therapeutic anticipation'.

. . . and knowing that she is coming it does something for you—it gives you a lift.

Dr Luker feels this may encourage health visitors to adopt the habit of making appointments, the basic message in Figure 7.4.

Williamson says that the effect upon morale is an aspect of assessment which is often neglected. He suggested the type of questions asked by Karen Luker and shown in Box 7.2 could be incorporated into the assessment of screening programmes. Williams (1974) felt that his survey itself had had a beneficial effect upon some of the people seen, making them more outgoing and better able to cope. Neil (1982) was aware of a psychological benefit for some of the old people in her screening programme.

To summarise, outlines and references have been given for a variety of screening

Box 7.2 Assessing satisfaction with the service (Karen Luker (1981a))

Questioning elderly women's opinions
Whether or not they: — enjoyed the health visitor visiting   — thought it helped them   — thought it a good idea   — had previously met health visitors   — would like the visits to continue
Probing with 'how', 'what', 'why', 'where' and 'when'   — to encourage a full report

programmes. These schemes are designed to find old people's socio-functional disabilities so that timely help can be given, the aim being to maintain or improve these people's ability to cope, to maintain their independence and to improve their quality of life. We have looked, too, at some reports of results: at the way some researchers have concentrated on validating the health visitors' contribution whilst others have tried to discover the benefits of screening.

SUPPORTIVE WORK

The aim in this aspect of the work, is to avoid deterioration in known problems and to try to bring about an improvement. It is quite often a crisis in the old person's life which precipitates his/her referral for this supportive care. Health visitors are notified through a variety of sources (Robertson, 1984a), for example from GPs, fellow nurses, social workers or the local hospital.

In preparing for the first visit following the referral, just as in any other aspect of their work, health visitors are at a distinct advantage if they can consult any previous notes, GPs', social workers', previous health visiting documentation, and find out as much as they can from the person referring the case. During the visit, health visitors are then able to add their own impressions of the practical home situation. More importantly, they can listen carefully to the old person's own view of his/her circumstances, the crucial factor in an assessment of the situation and for decisions on how to help.

Sometimes people merely need some information on appropriate facilities and entitlements. In other cases, follow-up and liaison with other health and welfare services is beneficial. For some people, a listening, supportive approach is more appropriate, especially in bereavement. We shall look at each of these three in turn.

REFERRAL TO SERVICES

One of the more difficult things for health visitors is the problem of keeping sufficiently knowledgeable and up to date on the enormous range of health and welfare services which exists in the community. Trying to find out if any particular service is available can be very time consuming, unless there is some local scheme for getting reliable information quickly. Mostly, there is none and health visitors are left to devise their individual ways of coping.

It is, naturally, those taking up a new post who face the greatest problem. There is so much to be learned in so short a time. One health visitor (Neil, 1982) used a notebook to list all the agencies which had been of help to the elderly. Local addresses and telephone numbers might usefully include:

— the Department of Health and Social Security
— local authority officers for rent and rates rebates
— luncheon clubs
— meals on wheels
— home helps
— good neighbour schemes
— day centres
— chiropodists
— dentists
— opticians
— Gas and Electricity Boards' customer service departments
— Citizens Advice Bureau
— Legal Aid Committee secretary
— Age Concern
— Red Cross Society.

These addresses tend to stay the same over time. However, many health visitors find, like Louise Davies (1981, p. 137), that much of the information they get is incomplete or out of date. Details on groups such as:

— Darby and Joan Clubs
— local church facilities
— delivery services
— shopping assistance schemes

listed in good faith in the local town hall, public library or Citizens Advice Bureau, go quickly out of date. It took the Davies team several days to visit or telephone these local services in order to find out the basic information they needed:

— costs
— hours of opening
— provision of transport

— organisers' names and addresses and telephone numbers, before they could get on with their study!

Keeping up to date

Good record keeping includes making a note of which services have been recommended to individual retired and elderly people. It provides a reminder to ask how, or whether, the old people found them. Health visitors and social workers might be able to help each other keep up to date by meeting at lunchtime from time to time, to tell each other about changes they have heard of and new and useful self-help groups that are emerging.

The Wessex Library-based service, funded by the NHS, which provides an up-to-date and wide-ranging information service was mentioned in Chapter 2 (p. 18). Anyone can ring or contact them. Help for Health need only to know what service is sought and they can give details on what is available. Health visitors are saved hours of work on the telephone and following up false starts.

Use of the services

Not all people will want to follow up health visitors' suggestions, however accurate and up to date, and it is difficult to discover what deters them from using the services. To some extent, health visitors are caught in a cleft stick. They hope to disseminate knowledge— not to try to lead people's lives for them. On the other hand, some individuals may feel shy about venturing into a luncheon club where they know no one. They may intend to go to an optician, but not get round to it. Should health visitors make the first appointment? Should they arrange for someone from the luncheon club to come and offer to take them? Maintaining the delicate balance between being as helpful as possible and yet respecting old people's right to make no use of the service needs great sensitivity.

The growing popularity of the idea of self-help groups for the retired and elderly has already been mentioned. But enthusiasm should be tempered with caution. Self-help services can vary in quality. They depend upon the particular skills that the volunteers happen to have. Opportunities for selection and training are sometimes minimal. However, when old people come across a scheme which does not seem to give them what they need, they can, for the most part, simply stop attending. The same does not necessarily apply to old people whose problems are of an emotional nature. They may be in no position to differentiate between good and bad. For example, a bereaved person visited by a volunteer who misuses these visits to work out his/her own personal emotional problems (Milne, 1982) is less likely to see exactly what is happening.

Health visitors trying to discover more about the quality of the service provided by self-help groups and other agencies, may find information from the elderly people referred to them the most useful source. There may also be opportunities to meet some of the personalities involved or, better still, to attend one or two of their meetings. Judgement, however, is necessarily subjective and is always difficult.

LIAISON

There is a large measure of overlap between workers in the community care of the retired and elderly, particularly between health visitors and social workers, district nurses, GPs and some people from voluntary agencies. Personal contact can be very important. It is one way to get to know the particular emphasis, style and approach of other workers. It can help to cut down duplication of services or, at the other extreme, to minimise the number of people who are missed altogether.

Health visitors who are new to a Health District have many people to meet, but it is a sound investment in time. The understanding established between workers means that on many subsequent occasions even the briefest of telephone calls can be very helpful.

Voluntary agencies

Most contacts are with other professional workers. However, it is important to keep in touch with the voluntary agencies, to find out what they do, to tell them of people who would benefit from their service and for feedback on how those people are faring. But there is another side to it. These agencies need encouragement; they face many difficulties, sometimes working on very limited funds. Their workers give their time for little more reward than the satisfaction of seeing things turn out well. Health visitors may be able to offer background support from time to time—if an agency requests it.

Social workers

The work of health visitors and social workers frequently overlaps in supportive, preventive care: trying to help people through problems. There are disadvantages in this overlap, but it can certainly be used to advantage if the work is taken up in a logical way.

Whether it is the primary health care team or social services who deal with an old person's problem mostly depends on which agency has been contacted. When problems come to the attention of GPs, they sometimes deal with the matter themselves; they may notify the health visitor or the geriatric visitor or, rarely, a social worker attached to the practice. When the matter is brought to the attention of the social services department, it is likely to be taken on by an assistant social worker. Liaison with the health visitor may be of benefit where health considerations put limitations on what their client can do. Conversely, health visitors or geriatric assistants often need to know to what extent local authority services are likely to be available. They may like to talk about the relative priority which might be given to certain needy cases.

If it is possible to meet key workers such as the home help supervisor and the meals-on-wheels administrator, and get to know each other's problems, it can simplify future communications on the allocation of these services. Furthermore, should old people find themselves facing further difficulties once a service is being provided, these key workers are likely to be the first to hear of it when the workers actually delivering the service report in. They would find it much easier to alert the health visitor to what is going on, once good liaison is established.

District nurses

The main overlap between district nurses and health visitors in supportive preventive care is in their listening role and in the information they give their patients about services and facilities that will be useful to them. Some district nurses prefer to take on the bereavement counselling of the families they have been visiting. Some like to take, from the beginning, hospital discharge referrals when, in the long run, it looks as if there is likely to be a need for home nursing. It makes for continuity of care. In many cases the old people are referred directly to the district nurse. Sometimes both the the nurse and the health visitor visit the home (Wilson, 1970). With good liaison, a scheme can be worked out which suits each of their particular skills and circumstances and, more importantly, which benefits the old people they care for.

The changing structure of the ageing population is making people wonder how district nurses and health visitors are going to be able to cope. In *A Happier Old Age* (DHSS, 1978), it is pointed out that 50% of district nurses' cases are elderly, against 15% of health visitors'. The question is raised as to whether there is scope for adjusting community nursing roles. This, it was suggested, could be done by providing auxiliary staff within the district nursing service. The discussion document has provided health visitors and district nurses with a stimulus to think about their role in the future.

One new approach has been piloted in Manchester. A geriatric team has been set up within the health visiting service. The aim is to maintain the health and independence of old people in their own homes. A health visitor helped by two staff nurses and two nursing auxiliaries follow up hospital discharges and bereaved spouses. They help with screening, give support and advice to families with elderly relatives and visit some old people living alone (Halladay, 1981). Working in concert like this in the field of prevention may have great potential.

Liaison health visitor

A very useful link between hospital and the community can be forged by a liaison health visitor who has opportunities for regular meetings and detailed discussions, both with staff in the hospital and with community colleagues.

Sometimes health visitors with a normal caseload can spend half a day a week in the geriatric day hospital, for example, whilst another visits outpatients or the wards. Wallis (1982) describes a full-time liaison post which included opportunities to establish relationships with staff in the hospital and in the community, to contact consultants about queries, to encourage health visitors to send information to the hospital, to talk to relatives and to devise appropriate forms for conveying information. Several of the activities are summarised in Box 7.3.

Telephone calls can be made when information is complex or needs to be conveyed speedily. Where one health visitor undertakes this go-between work, it makes it easier for

Box 7.3 The liaison health visitor

Aspects of hospital liaison work

Convey information
— in person
— by phone
— written message
Devise appropriate forms
Explain role of health visitor
Regular meetings with hospital staff
Attend staff meetings in community
Establish relationships
Contacting consultants
Meet relatives
Encourage community staff to give information to hospital

health visitors and district nurses in the field to identify and use the service.

Parnell (1982a, 1982b) reported that hospitals had greater contact with district nurses than health visitors. A liaison health visitor has the opportunity to explain the health visitors' role and encourage their involvement in appropriate cases.

In general terms, however, liaison can often be difficult to achieve. Pressures of work, the distance between offices and the inevitable elusiveness of people working out in the community, make communication difficult. Often even telephone contact is hard to make. It may not be easy, but it is well worth trying to get to know other workers in the field. When health visitors, district nurses, social workers, voluntary agencies and GPs work closely together, they are much more likely to provide a rational and effective service for the retired and elderly.

SUPPORTIVE LISTENING

As in other aspects of their work, health visitors will sometimes find that by listening they can enable old people to talk through their problems, to sort out their thoughts and feelings and to adjust to their circumstances. They may, alternatively, decide on another line of action.

Some old people can benefit from reminiscing. Through reminiscence they may be able to come to terms with their past and find a new equilibrium (Rowlings, 1981). Few generalist health visitors with a busy caseload feel able to become involved in this sort of work. This would be much more likely to be undertaken in casework by a social worker.

Health visitors sometimes meet very lonely elderly people with a great need to talk. The health visitor's role in the case of someone whose problem is basically loneliness, is to act as a referral agent, sensitively arranging for a volunteer visitor or a relevant service to be contacted—if this is acceptable to the old person.

Bereavement visiting

There is one aspect of this supportive role in which health visitors are becoming increasingly involved. This is bereavement visiting. There is now sufficient evidence of high rates of mental and physical illness during or due to bereavement (Grindel, 1981; Godber, 1980) to convince many health visitors that they should be involved at an early stage, to enable people to work through the normal mourning process, especially those people lacking the support of relatives and friends. The aim is to prevent people from becoming locked into one of the earlier stages of grief and, therefore, from being able to arrive at eventual full adjustment.

Bereavement can, of course, affect any group. It is because it is so much more likely to affect the retired and elderly that a description of the sort of commitment and visiting schedule it can involve is included in this chapter.

Pre-requisites

Firstly, in order to be of any help the health visitors need to have come to terms with the idea of their own death. Those who have, themselves, suffered a bereavement, need to have achieved readjustment. These people offer a bonus. They can empathise: they have a fuller understanding of how the bereaved person is feeling.

It is also necessary to have studied and understood the complex processes and components of grief: shock, searching, disorganisation, denial, depression, guilt, anxiety, aggression and, finally, resolution, acceptance and reintegration (Parkes, 1972; Hodgkinson, 1980; Nuttall, 1980; Parkes & Weiss, 1983).

Thirdly, what is needed is the ability to show acceptance of bereaved people's need to pour out their anguish and grief. This also applies to the bitter anger which may, on occasions, be directed against the health visitor or some other member of the primary health care team.

When should visits begin?

Dr Parkes (1972, Ch. 10) suggests that this may be best in the week after the funeral because this often coincides with the greatest intensity of grief. By this time, the supporting relatives have mainly dispersed. Sometimes bereaved people are more able to pour out their feelings to an 'outsider' than to relatives who are themselves involved.

A health visitor described how she arranged to visit cases of known terminal illness during the course of the disease (Wilson, 1970). As the district nurse where she worked stopped visiting when the patient died, this scheme provided continuity of care. She felt she had a much better opportunity in the early stages to encourage the relatives to let the old people show their grief as they felt inclined.

What should be said?

It is not easy to find the right thing to say when visiting a bereaved person. Parkes says that pity is unwanted and that there is no 'proper thing to say'. It is bound to be painful for both the visitor and the bereaved: neither is able to give what the other wants. The visitor cannot bring back the person who has died. The bereaved person cannot give the visitor the satisfaction of appearing to be helped.

The important thing is to let bereaved people express their feelings in their own way and in their own time. Interpersonal skills (see Ch. 2, pp. 25–26) are crucial in this context.

Practical advice may be requested. A DHSS (1979) leaflet *What to do after a death* is a useful source of information on the more immediate problems following a death. The addresses of several very helpful and supportive organisations such as Cruse, The Compassionate Friends and Age Concern are included. Some members of the St Christopher's Hospice Bereavement service have brought out an excellent book (Dyne, 1981) as a guide for other people thinking of undertaking this sort of work.

Where health visitors know of reliable bereavement counselling services locally, such as through the church or the bodies mentioned above, they may tend to refer people on to them, if it is wished, and play a rather more background role themselves.

Indicators of vulnerability

In a very useful and succinct article, Paddy Yorkstone (1981) lists risk factors in bereavement, the factors that make people more likely to face problems later on if they are unsupported in the critical, early stages. Included are bereaved people where there has been an unexpected death, especially of a young person, child or still birth; those who have no supportive family; people who spend all day at home; and those with financial and housing difficulties. These and the factors below are listed in Box 7.4 as trigger signals for action by the health visitor.

It has been suggested (Parkes, 1972, p. 165) that the visitor should not be afraid to ask direct questions about suicide. People seriously contemplating it tend to admit it. Psychiatric help is needed in such cases.

Other people who need special help are those who suffer from excessive guilt or anger; those who show no grief when it would be expected, or, at the other end of the

Box 7.4 Some trigger signals in bereavement visiting (from Parkes (1972) and Yorkstone (1981))

People needing action or attention

---

1. Extra *vulnerable* if:
   death unexpected
   — young person
   — child
   — still birth
   have demanding dependants
   no supportive family
   at home all day
   financial difficulties
   housing problems
   history of inadequate personality
2. Extra *help* needed if:
   serious contemplation of suicide
   excessive gult or anger
   no grief shown when expected
   intense grief, abnormally long time

scale, suffer from intense grief for an abnormally long time. These people need to be brought to the attention of their GP.

When should visiting stop?

Bereavement usually lasts from 6–18 months. Visits generally stop when the health visitors feel they have fulfilled their part in helping a person through to the stage of acceptance and reintegration into society. The anniversary of the death is an important date for a bereaved person. A visit on this day is found to be helpful by many people.

In these three sections, we have looked at work with the elderly from the viewpoint of the sort of activities health visitors might undertake in order to provide a preventive health service. This can involve education and work in the community. Screening programmes were discussed in the second section. Work which involves informing old people about available services, liaising as necessary with other agencies and listening, especially in bereavement, were covered in this last part. In the next section the perspective is changed towards the individual old person's health needs from the standpoint of his/her daily life.

ENVIRONMENTAL, HEALTH AND SOCIAL NEEDS IN RETIREMENT

There is now a wide range of practical and sensitive guidance written for the elderly and those who care for old people (Skeet, 1982; Hooker, 1981; Gray & McKenzie, 1980), though some is written more specifically for the carers (Dartington, 1980; Brown, 1982). It is not possible or necessary, here, to repeat all this information already available to health visitors.

In this section we use a derivative of the family health needs model to provide a way of categorising basic requirements in retirement, in order to help in the mental planning for individual care. The model is later demonstrated in two examples of visits, through which also run themes from the earlier sections.

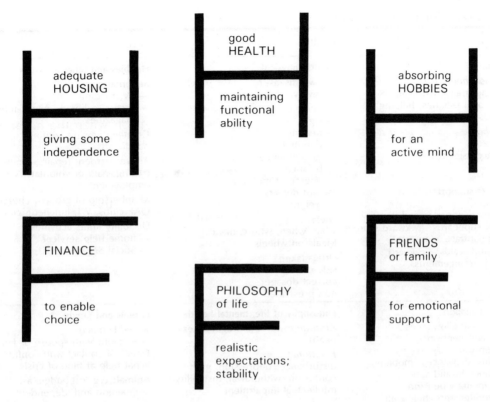

Fig. 7.5 Some factors affecting retirement.

The suggested categorisation of day-to-day needs in retirement is shown in essence in Figure 7.5. The six factors are expanded into the tabular format in Box 7.5 and classified under environmental, health and social needs, some of which are considered below. The Box is not intended to provide an ideal model: health visitors' experience and individual reading will enable them each to develop their own mental listings of matters affecting old people which might require attention or discussion.

ENVIRONMENTAL FACTORS

Housing

Research shows just how important a part housing plays in the provision of old people's welfare (Tinker, 1984). It is the key to the highly-treasured independence and, like all needs for old people, is best planned for prior to retirement. Warmth and accident hazards can be a problem to many old people.

Falls constitute a large proportion of accidents in the elderly (Abrams, 1985), and there is a growing interest in alarm call systems (Geriatric Medicine, 1981; Butler, 1982). Wild et al (1981; Isaacs, 1981) said the greatest risk factors associated with falling are:
— being female
— over 75 years
— having fallen previously
— difficulties in mobility and gait
— impaired balance
— blood pressure problems and
— the effects of some drugs.
Hazards include things like slip mats, trailing flexes, and inadequately lit stairs (Mitchell, 1984). Frances McCabe (1985) studied some 110 housebound old people said to be at risk of falling, and concluded that careful forethought was necessary for the prevention of falls. She found many seemingly useful ideas

Box 7.5 Family health needs—the elderly

Environmental	Health	Social
Housing	**Health, physical**	**Hobbies and other activities**
Neighbourhood	Known disease?	Sedentary:
shopping, transport, health &	— involves handicap?	— TV, reading
recreational facilities, helping	*Check* e.g.	— access to library, newspapers,
agencies and friends	— sight	magazines
Household	— hearing	Creative: sewing, writing,
Heating:	— dentition	handicrafts
type, accessibility	— incontinence	Active: garden, repairs, rambling,
Safety	— balance	cycling, paid or voluntary
Falls:	— degree of mobility	employment
— steps: supports,	— foot defects	Membership of groups: church,
— lighting	— weight	OAP clubs, WI, luncheon club
— floor covering: frayed/slippery	Diet:	Disability limits activities?
— high cupboards: awkward storing	what, when, who cooks it	— home help service?
— bath: surface, supports	Meals on wheels	— Social Services aids?
Burns and scalds: fireguard,	Drugs taken:	
cooking arrangements	side-effects?	
	correct dosage?	
	non-prescribed	
Financial support	**Philosophy of life, mental health**	**Friends and family**
Benefits and allowances	*Attitude* towards old age, illness,	*Social contacts*
Retirement pension	death	Lives alone/with spouse or family
War pension	*Emotional*	Extent of contact with confidant(e)s
Disability allowances: mobility,	disturbance: depression, grief,	What help at time of crisis
attendance invalid care	confusion, withdrawal, instability,	Animal: e.g. cat/budgie as
Supplementary pension	intellectual impairment	companion and 'dependent'
extra entitlements: help with		Possible cause of voluntary
heating costs, dental and other care		isolation:
Local authority rent rebates, grants		— incontinence
for insulation		— fear of falling
Occupational pensions		

were not acceptable to the old people in her study, and she pointed out that any interventions must be in line with old people's 'felt needs', the way they perceived the problem. She described how a simple test of balance and discussions about their recent falls, history and the drugs they take, can help draw old people's attention to ways they may avoid falls. RoSPA (1981) have a very good self-assessment safety checklist for old people, which could stimulate a wide range of thought and discussion.

Nora Saddington (1983) made suggestions as to how professionals can help with inexpensive aids to prevent a person falling and, as a consequence, becoming extremely cold. She also described how to recognise and deal appropriately with hypothermia. Warmth has

been shown to be a basic problem in this country in winter. Within two days of a cold spell, deaths from coronary disease and, soon after, deaths from other diseases increase significantly. It seems that governments have failed to make these facts known for fear of pressures on resources being created by public demand to overcome these problems (Taylor, 1982).

Financial support

Advice on financial help with heating, together with advice on matters like insulation, payment schemes for gas and electricity and what to do in case of disconnection, is provided by Age Concern (1985). This organisation has produced some very useful and readable booklets for old people, particularly *Your Rights* (Age Concern, 1983), which explains about local authority rent rebates, supplementary pensions and the various allowances available. Health visitors would probably find it very helpful to have this booklet available in their bag. The address for Age Concern's publications list will be found at the end of the reference section. The Department of Transport (1982) has printed a guide to the transport benefits which are available to disabled people, which some older people may find useful.

HEALTH FACTORS

Physical aspects

The aim in preventive care for the elderly is to maintain the best possible level of functional ability rather than to cure disease. Urinary and mobility problems tend to be under-reported, endured and accepted, wrongly, as an inevitable part of the ageing process (Williamson, 1981). Also, the effects of drugs can be misunderstood. If neglected, these problems can severely limit a person's ability to cope and remain reasonably independent in the community.

The elderly can be specially sensitive to certain drugs and their side-effects (MacLennan, 1981; Bliss, 1981). Many have difficulties in being able to see and differentiate between tablets (Hurd & Blevins, 1984). These factors and evidence of old people's lack of understanding about drugs, together with a correlation between reduced compliance with instructions and increased complexity of dose schedules (Kiernan & Isaacs, 1981), show a need for special care to be taken. It is a nursing as well as a medical problem and old people will benefit where the primary health care team work together to find a scheme to monitor what drugs their elderly population are given and are taking. Literature such as the Family Doctor booklet on medicines (Lewis, 198(2)) may help some individuals understand the drugs they need (or need not) take.

The ability to be independent can be helped in many ways. There is now an increasing amount of interest in exercise for old people to improve their physical condition (Copple, 1983; Clapham, 1980; Hooker, 1981, p. 133–139; Lawrence, 1981; Fentem, 1981) and in helping people prevent and overcome foot problems (Collyer, 1981; Turnbull, 1981; Foulston, 1981) in order to maintain their mobility. However, whatever their basic skills in this field, if old people suffer from incontinence they will be liable to loneliness and isolation through fear of going out. Dr Trimmer (1982), Vivien Rooney (1984) and Sally Robbins (1984) describe how important it is to have a clear history of an old person's incontinence problems and how a clear picture can lead to some very beneficial progress. This topic was also discussed in Chapter 6 (p. 108).

Mental health

It is said that to be forewarned is to be forearmed. Some older people may find very helpful two booklets that describe how to cope with death, both from emotional and practical points of view (Parkes, 1981; DHSS, 1979). These booklets would probably be particularly useful in pre-retirement discussions or classes.

If the primary health care team can have early warning of problems for old people such as the onset of dementia (see p. 118), it means that support services can beneficially be provided in good time (Williamson, 1981). Gilleard (1984, p. 62) describes the gradual stages of decline, the carers' bewilderment and then adjustment with each stage of dementia. They need sympathetic and practical support. The community psychiatric nurse (CPN) may be able to help. Age Concern have some booklets, such as the one providing advice for carers on 'reality orientation' for their relative (Dowdell, 1982), which can provide useful and practical ideas. Another problem of mental health is depression. This is relatively common amongst the elderly. There are, of course, many causes, one of them being the medication that old people take. Josephs (1982) lists some of the drugs, including alcohol, which can tend to precipitate depression.

SOCIAL ASPECTS

Hobbies and other activities

The sort of activities people choose or are able to undertake in old age will, of course, depend on many of the factors already touched on—finances, accommodation, physical health and mental attitudes. They are likely to reflect the earlier chances in, or style of, life and the interests developed prior to retirement. We have already considered, in the section on screening the elderly, the importance of looking out for incipient functional disabilities, in order to maintain old people's activities at the best possible level.

Friends and family

Loneliness can be a problem. It has been suggested by Dorothy Walster (1982) that owning a pet can help and can bring significant therapeutic benefits, mentally, physically and socially. She says the caring professionals

and other visitors call and leave, whereas the pet provides 24-hour companionship.

Full-time companionship, however, can have its problems. When an old person has become dependent and moves in with a member of their family, it can sometimes cause significant tensions and, from time to time, can involve 'granny abuse'. Eastman and Sutton (1982) quote Green's observations that there is a correlation between high dependency and abuse where:

— increasing disability sours an originally loving relationship
— the care-giver accepted the old person reluctantly when s/he was unable to continue to live alone
— the family is, anyway, under stress.

Eastman (1982, 1984) suggested that factors that should alert professionals to the possibility of abuse are a cluster of any of those characteristics listed in Box 7.6. If a number of these features apply to a household, then he feels the situation warrants further investigation. He says the most important thing is for there to be available emotional support and someone prepared to listen.

There is evidence of the great problems these carers face with little or no help from

Box 7.6 Signs of strain and, perhaps, violence (derived from Eastman (1984))

A number of factors *occurring together* in a household caring for a dependent old person should trigger the health visitor into considering further investigation and *increased support* for the family. Significant factors are, for example:
Where the old person:
— is dependent upon the key care-giver
— is known to be shouted at by the care-giver
— has frustrating behaviour, e.g. incontinence or shouting at night
— has a history of falls with vague explanations
— is sleepless
— has facial bruising
When the care-giver:
— has been obliged to change her life-style significantly
— is responsible for another family member
— has a history of mental ill-health
— frequently visits GP for 'nerves'
— is drinking heavily
— suffers from sleeplessness
Where there is evidence of:
— role reversal between adult child–parent
— family isolation and lack of emotional support
— inadequate accommodation
— financial problems
— marital conflict or divorce
— unemployment in the family

the services (Equal Opportunities Commission, 1980; Wright, 1983; Walker, 1983), often on account of ignorance of what is available to help them. Heather McKenzie (1984), of the National Council for Carers and their Elderly Dependants, has described how her organisation has now been emulated by others in sending out information packs to their members. They now also provide a granny-sitting service in various parts of the country. Dinah Tedman (1982) offers advice on supportive 'care for the carers' and emphasises the need for professionals to listen, to offer suggestions and emotional support and to keep any promises they make.

A health visitor, Geraldine Drummond (1984) and someone from Age Concern, worked together to set up a relatives' support group. The phases and stages through which the group went are described. It was found to be very helpful and went on to become an independent self-help group. This sort of proactive work will, hopefully, be widely emulated.

In this section, we have looked at some of the factors listed in the health needs format in Box 7.5, some of which have already been mentioned in the earlier sections. The chapter concludes with two examples of visits to elderly people.

EXAMPLES OF WORK WITH THE ELDERLY

Of the two examples given, one shows how a person may be encouraged to take timely action over problems: secondary prevention aimed at maximising functional ability and maintaining independence. In the second, the health visitor was not involved until problems had reached crisis proportions. Preventive care, mainly tertiary at this late stage, was fortunately successful in this case.

EXAMPLE ONE: MRS PERKINS

Miss Helen Voisey (HV) has planned and is now undertaking an assessment scheme aimed at contacting all the elderly people listed in a suburban group practice. She started by contacting all the over-80s and is now gradually meeting all the over-75s. The aim is to make 70 the routine age of contact within a year or two.

Mrs Bella Perkins, a 77-year old, was identified through reference to the age–sex register. An introductory, explanatory letter suggested a day when the health visitor would call.

Having introduced herself and checked that the visit was in fact convenient, HV found herself warmly welcomed and invited in. After some slight initial apprehension, Mrs Perkins showed a great deal of interest in the assessment scheme. She was shown her record card. She was very cooperative and chatty as they gradually worked through the prescribed format. Much of the relevant information on Mrs Perkins' circumstances will be found listed in Box 7.7.

Mrs Perkins walked with evident discomfort. Her health though was generally good. However, she had not been to the optician for 12 years and her dentures were painful, ill-fitting and 15 years old. She said her friends had had to 'pay a fortune' for their replacement spectacles and dentures. She did not 'have that sort of money'. There was a tendency for Mrs Perkins to be somewhat fatalistic about her problems, especially about her painful feet and loss of mobility, and to assume it was to be expected in old age.

Mrs Perkins was asked if she considered her finances too private a matter for discussion. She did not. There ensued a lively conversation about the advantages of being on supplementary benefit—especially with regard to free optical and dental care. Mrs Perkins decided to make appointments for treatment.

Waiting list places for chiropody were some 3 or 4 months long. As Mrs Perkins was then liable to remain relatively housebound for a while, visitors from Age Concern and the local school OAP Aid Scheme were suggested to supplement her social contacts. The schoolchildren would be keen to help in practical ways, for example by gardening and shopping.

On parting it was agreed that HV or the geriatric assistant would call monthly for a while, hoping to see Mrs Perkins soon with better glasses and dentures (and improved nutrition). The date of the next visit was arranged. It was suggested that, if possible, Mrs Perkins should wear open-toed sandals instead of slippers and her laced or barred shoes to hold the foot back and avoid further friction.

Box 7.7 Example one: Mrs Perkins

Environmental	Health	Social
Housing	**Physical health**	**Activities**
Home: owner occupied	Reports poorer vision Ref. optician	Reads and sews less than previously
Shops and other facilities: 1/2 mile	Painful dentures:	Limited mobility
Garden unkempt, referred to local school OAP Aid Scheme	no longer wearing lower one for eating	— feet
Safety:	Ref. dentist	Copes with housework
Carpet wall to wall	Feet:	Shopping mainly delivered to door
Reports hand rails	thickened nails, painful corns and calluses	OAP Luncheon Club monthly
— stairway	Ref. chiropody	
— bathroom	(Might need voluntary car service)	
Fireguard available	No regular medication	
	Enjoys cooking: concentrating on softer foods	
Financial status	**Mental health**	**Friendship networks**
National Insurance retirement pension: currently being collected by friend	Scored well on tests	Lives alone
	Seems well adjusted to death of husband and to daughter's move away	Small group of friends of own age gradually dwindling
Says would be entitled to supplementary benefit—too small to bother: 30 p per week: advantages explained	No regular medication	Next of kin: daughter in Scotland, three grandchildren
		Welcomed idea of visitors
Rate rebate applied for: advised by neighbour		OAP Aid Scheme may provide regular contact with young
		Age Concern visitor

The health visitor left feeling there was a good chance that Mrs Perkins would follow up most of the ideas that had emerged during the assessment and that her independence and health would be maintained on account of it. This proved later on to be so.

EXAMPLE TWO: MRS DEAN

Mr Harold Vosper (HV) is attached to a group practice where there was not, at the time, a scheme for initiating contact with their elderly.

Mrs Dean, a 76-year old with osteo-arthritis, was referred to HV by one of the doctors. Mrs Farley, an only daughter with whom she lived, had come to the surgery saying that her mother would 'have to go into a home'. The doctor had listened as she talked about her problem. He visited Mrs Deal at home. The basic problem was the demands that caring for the mother and her constant presence in their small house was making on the Farleys. It had been brought to a

head by a recent row between the couple. They had not yet reached a decision on what they hoped to do and seemed to have very little knowledge about what services might be available.

A visit by Harry Vosper was arranged. Some of the family's circumstances are outlined in Box 7.8. Mrs Dean described pain in her wrists, hips, knees and neck and chose to take no drugs for it. She tended to remain inactive. HV encouraged her to talk about her circumstances and feelings. She was resentful about her situation but gradually showed, more and more, her sympathy for her daughter's predicament. Mrs Dean was very anxious not to be cut off from her family. The nearest 'home' was many miles away and far from a bus stop. She responded positively to the ideas of a day centre place and volunteer visitors.

Before he returned downstairs, HV called Mrs Farley so he could witness their management difficulties in getting Mrs Farley to the toilet. He demonstrated lifting techniques. The manoeuvres gave HV an opportunity to follow up a hunch he

Box 7.8 Example two: Mrs Dean

	Environmental	Health	Social
	Housing	**Physical health**	**Activities**
M	Bedroom in daughter's home since death of husband 5 years ago, Warm, well kept Bathroom adjacent Safety factors: no loose mats or unguarded fire; rails in bathroom	Osteo-arthritis: reported significant deterioration in recent years Uses walking sticks Bedbathing service not wanted Refuses medication Possible deafness: ref. GP	Sedentary: reads, radio and TV Said to spend most of day in bed or in chair by window Difficulty in walking to toilet Occasionally carried downstairs in a wheelchair
D	Owner-occupied 2 bed home, thro' lounge Near shops and other facilities Transport: no car, bus—1/2 mile	Some backpain since frequent lifting of mother: liaison with Soc Services about aids	Gave up work 2 yrs ago to be with M Activities home based No holidays away Pops out to shops
S	Circumstances as above	Reportedly good	Clerk DIY redecoration
	Financial status	**Emotional health**	**Friendship networks**
M	Retirement pension collected by son in law Attendance and invalid care allowances not applied for— leaflets NI.205, NI.212 and SB1 given	Described as difficult, uncooperative and demanding Alert mind Deeply resentful of 'being treated like a child' and loss of useful role	Main contact by banging walking stick to summon daughter Few local friends, moved from 10 miles away No 'grannie sitter' Day centre and holiday schemes suggested
D	Significant drop in income now no longer contributing to family budget	Frequent arguments with mother—uses avoidance tactics to minimise tension Strong feeling of responsibility for mother	Neighbours call in Fears relationship with husband deteriorating Now considering minding service
S	Full-time employment	Said to be resentful of wife's absorption in her mother	No longer socialising with same friends as wife

Key: M = Mother; D = Daughter; S = Son in law

had had during his earlier conversation. He had suspected some deafness and found that Mrs Dean did not respond to low voice sounds when her head was turned. Both ladies were somewhat surprised at the idea of deafness and happy that the GP should follow it up.

Mrs Farley listened earnestly to what services and benefits might be available for the family. She was anxious to discuss some of the suggestions with her husband and her mother. It was important to her to have her mother nearby. She was beginning to feel it was much more possible to keep her mother with her, but did not yet want to commit herself. She remarked on how helpful it had been to talk about her problems. There was a discussion about the extent to which Mrs Dean's 'uncooperativeness' might be due to misunderstandings on account of hearing loss. Mrs Farley reminisced and recalled

that they had not had these problems in the early years. Aids were discussed. A hoist, a zimmer frame and a commode were suggested. HV undertook to make tentative enquiries about this and other equipment that might be helpful, such as the loan of a stair lift.

The next few visits were made as the family requested—weekly for a month, and were mainly of a supportive nature. Mr and Mrs Farley decided that, with the aids and hospital day care, and later day centre support, with volunteer visitors, grannie sitters, holiday schemes and National Insurance allowances, they would be able to manage. The discussions at the primary health care team meetings on this and other cases has led to the decision to try to contact old people in the practice before their situation reaches crisis proportions. An assessment scheme is now being prepared.

USEFUL ADDRESSES

The Pre-Retirement Association
19 Undine Street, Tooting,
London SW17 8PP
Tel 01 767 3225/6; 01 767 3854

Workers Educational Association,
Temple House,
9 Upper Berkeley Street,
London W1H 8BY
Tel 01 402 5608

Age Concern England,
Publications Department,
Bernard Sunley House,
60 Pitcairn Road, Mitcham,
Surrey CR4 3LL
Tel 10 640 5431

RoSPA, Cannon House,
The Priory Queensway,
Birmingham B4 6BS
Tel 021 233 2461

REFERENCES

Abrams M 1985 Falls in the home. New Age Winter: 22

Age Concern 1983 Your rights, llth ed. Age Concern, Mitcham, Surrey

Age Concern 1985 Fact Sheet on Help with Heating. Age Concern, Mitcham, Surrey

Antrobus M 1981 Self-care in sickness and in health. Nursing Times Community Outlook 77, 42: 342–350, 357

Barber J M 1981 Screening and assessment: a challenge to GPs. Geriatric Medicine 11, 4: 39–45

Bliss M R 1981 Prescribing for the elderly. British Medical Journal 283: 203–206

Brown P 1982 The other side of growing older. Macmillan Press Ltd, London

Burkitt A 1977 Life begins at forty. Hutchinson Benham, London

Butler A 1982 Alarms that reassure. Health and Social Services Journal XCII: 734–736

Clapham J 1980 Keeping fit in retirement. Health Visitor 53:532

Collyer M I 1981 Maintaining the elderly patient's mobility. Geriatric Medicine 11, 12: 27–30

Copple P 1983 The concept of exercise. Nursing Times 79, 32: 66–69

Dartington T 1980 Family care of old people. Souvenir Press (E & A) Ltd, London

Davies L 1981 Three score years—and then? A study of nutrition and wellbeing of elderly people at home. William Heinemann Medical Books Ltd, London

Davies L, Holdsworth M D, Purves R 1982 Who needs meals on wheels? Community Care 407: 12–13

Day L 1981 Health visiting the elderly in the 1980s—do we care enough? Health Visitor 54: 538–539

Day L, Mogridge J 1981 Health visitor who stayed. Health and Social Services Journal XCI: 1114–1115

Department of Transport 1982 Door to door. A guide to transport for disabled people. Department of Transport, London

DHSS 1978 A happier old age. A discussion document on elderly people in our society. HMSO, London, p 33

DHSS 1979 What to do after a death. D49/Aug 79 Department of Health and Social Security, London

DHSS 1981 Growing older. Cmnd 8173 HMSO, London

Dodsworth A J 1976 Screening the elderly. Nursing Times 72: 909–910

Douglas-Jones A 1980 Screening for a healthy future. Geriatric Medicine 10, 5: 67–68

Dowdell T 1982 Forgetfulness in elderly persons. Advice for carers. Age Concern, London

Drummond G 1984 Laughter is better than medicine—a support group for caring relatives. Health Visitor 57: 201–202

Dyne G (ed) 1981 Bereavement visiting. King Edwards Hospital Fund for London

Eastman M 1982 'Granny battering' a hidden problem. Community Care 413: 12–13

Eastman M 1984 Old age abuse. Midwife Health Visitor and Community Nurse 20: 162–165

Eastman M, Sutton M 1982 Granny battering. Geriatric Medicine 12, 11: 11–15

Equal Opportunities Commission 1980 The experience of caring for elderly and handicapped dependants: survey report. Equal Opportunities Commission, London

Fentem P 1981 Do you ever prescribe exercise? Geriatric Medicine 11, 8: 53–56

Foulston J 1981 Make the best use of your chiropodist! Geriatric Medicine 11, 7: 44–49

Geriatric Medicine 1981 Alarm call systems: an aid in emergencies. Geriatric Medicine 11, 3: 45–47

Gilleard C J 1984 Living with dementia. Croom Helm, London

Godber C 1980 Complications of bereavement. Geriatric Medicine 10, 5:81

Gray J A M, McKenzie H 1980 Take care of your elderly relative. George Allen & Unwin, London

Grindel P 1981 Help for the bereaved. Health Visitor 54: 330–333

Halladay H 1981 A geriatric team within the health visiting service. Nursing Times 77, 38: 1039–1040

Harwin B 1975 Psychogeriatric screening. In: Hart C R (ed) Screening in general practice. Churchill Livingstone, Edinburgh

Hodgkinson P E 1980 Treating abnormal grief in the bereaved. Nursing Times 76: 126–128

Hooker S 1981 Caring for elderly people, 2nd ed. Routledge and Kegan Paul, London.

Hurd P D, Blevins J 1984 Aging and the color of pills (letter). New England Journal of Medicine 310:202

Isaacs B 1981 Why do the elderly fall? Geriatric Medicine 11, 3: 17–13

Josephs C 1982 Depression. Geriatric Medicine 12, 12: 24–25

Kerr I F W 1975 Women in the middle years. In: Hart

C R (ed) Screening in general practice. Churchill Livingstone, Edinburgh

Kiernan P J, Isaacs J B 1981 Use of drugs by the elderly. Journal of the Royal Society of Medicine 74: 196–200

Lawrence N 1981 Age and exercise. Geriatric Medicine 11, 1: 78–79

Lewis R J R 198(2) Is your medicine really necessary? British Medical Association, London

Luker K A 1981a Health visiting and the elderly. Nursing Times Occasional Paper No 35 77, 51: 137–140

Luker K A 1981b Elderly women's opinions about the benefits of health visitor visits. Nursing Times Occasional Paper No 9 77, 12: 33–35

Luker K A 1982 Evaluating health visiting practice. Royal College of Nursing, London

McCabe F 1985 Mind you don't fall. Nursing Mirror 160, 26: 52–56

McKenzie H 1984 Viewpoint. New Age, Autumn: 24

MacLennan W J 1981 Drug side-effects and the elderly patient. Geriatric Medicine 11, 9: 52–58

Milne J 1982 Care-less. The Guardian April 21st: 17

Mitchell R G 1984 Falls in the elderly. Nursing Times 80, 2: 51–53

Neil M 1982 It's nice to know that someone cares. Nursing Times Community Outlook 78, 37: 243–246

Nuttall D 1980 Bereavement. Health Visitor 53: 84–86

Parkes C M 1972 Bereavement: studies of grief in adult life. Tavistock Publications, London

Parkes C M 1981 Facing death. National Extension College, Cambridge

Parkes C M, Weiss R S 1983 Recovery from bereavement. Basic Books, New York

Parnell J 1982a Continuity and communication—1. Nursing Times Occasional Paper No 9 78, 13: 33–36

Parnell J 1982b Continuity and communication—2. Nursing Times Occasional Paper No 10 78, 14: 37–40

Pike L A 1975 Men in the middle years. In: Hart C R (ed) Screening in general practice. Churchill Livingstone, Edinburgh

Player D A, Irving G, Robinson R A 1971 Psychiatric, psychological and social findings in a pilot community health survey. Health Bulletin XXIX: 104–107

Powell C, Crombie A 1974 The Kilsyth Questionnaire: a method of screening elderly people at home. Age and Ageing 3: 23–28

Robbins S 1984 Incontinence in the elderly mentally infirm. Nursing Times Supplement 80, 14: 25–27

Robertson C A 1984a Health visitors and preventive care. Nursing Times 80, 34: 29–31

Roberston C A 1984b Screening for health. Nursing Times 80, 35: 44–45

Rooney V 1984 Incontinence in the elderly in the community. Nursing Times Supplement 80, 14: 13–14

RoSPA 1981 Safety in retirement HS/108/1981. The Royal Society for the Prevention of Accidents, Birmingham

Rowlings C 1981 Social work with elderly people. George Allen and Unwin, London, p 63

Saddington N 1983 Winter of discontent? Nursing Times 79, 43: 10–11

Shukla R B 1981 The role of the primary care team in the care of the elderly. The Practitioner 225: 791–797

Skeet M 1982 The third age. Darton, Longman and Todd, London

Stanton A 1979 A first experience of planning in a group practice. Health Visitor 52: 310–319

Stott D 1982 Running a pre-retirement course. Health Visitor 55:360

Taylor G 1982 Cold comfort. Nursing Times 78:181

Tedman D 1982 Carers need care. Nursing Times Community Outlook 78, 10: 71–76

Tinker A 1984 Health and housing. Nursing Times 80, 18: 57–59

Trimmer E 1982 About incontinence. Midwife, Health Visitor and Community Nurse 18:386

Townsend P 1963 The family life of old people. Penguin, London, Ch. 11

Turnbull E M 1981 The practical problems of footwear, hosiery, and aids. Geriatric Medicine 11, 12: 33–36

Walker A 1983 Care for elderly people: a conflict between women and the state. In: Finch J, Groves D (eds) A Labour of Love. Women, Work and Caring. Routledge and Kegan Paul, London

Wallis M 1982 An extended talking service. Nursing Mirror 155, 10: 24–28

Walster D 1982 Why not prescribe a pet? Geriatric Medicine 12, 4: 13–19

Wilcock G K 1982 A review of dementia. Midwife Health Visitor and Community Nurse 18: 378–384

Wild D, Nayak U S L, Isaacs B 1981 How dangerous are falls in old people at home? British Medical Journal 282: 266–268

Williams I 1974 A follow up of geriatric patients after medico-social assessment. Journal of the Royal College of General Practitioners 24: 341–346

Williams I 1979 The care of the elderly in the community. Croom Helm, London

Williamson J 1981 Screening, surveillance and casefinding. In: Arie T (ed) Health Care of the Elderly. Croom Helm, Beckenham, Kent

Williamson J, Lowther C P, Gray S 1966 The use of health visitors in preventive geriatrics. Gerontologia Clinica 8: 362–369

Wilson F G 1970 Social isolation and bereavement. The Lancet II: 1356–1357

Wright F 1983 Single cares: employment, housework and caring. In: Finch J, Groves D (eds) A Labour of Love. Women, Work and Caring. Routledge and Kegan Paul, London

Yorkstone P 1981 Bereavement. British Medical Journal 282: 1224–1225

The health visitor cycle is the framework used to highlight important aspects of record making. Examples of records schemes are given, using case histories from earlier chapters. Evaluation is considered from three viewpoints: the clients', the health visitors' and by looking at quantifiability. A discussion about confidentiality concludes the chapter.

Stating what has happened

Records
  The health visitor cycle
  SOAP derivations
  SSD records
  SOAP (E) records

Evaluation
  Families' evaluation
  Assessment by health visitors
  Quantification

Confidentiality

8

Records and evaluation

STATING WHAT HAS HAPPENED

Records are necessary for communication and investigation. The basic essentials that should be recorded to provide for these requirements are suggested as follows: firstly, key matters that have been reported by the family members or observed by the health visitor; secondly an indication of the service given by the health visitor; and thirdly an evaluation, through what the family has reported and changes the health visitor has noticed. Arrangements undertaken between visits, or at the next visit, can also be noted.

Evaluation can take many forms (Luker, 1985). Here it has been classified into three ways it might be experienced by a practising health visitor: firstly, trying to gain an understanding of the family's perspective and the way they value the work; secondly through self- and peer group assessment; and thirdly, by looking at ways in which aspects of the work can be quantified.

Record making and monitoring the work have implications for confidentiality. Particular care with regard to people's personal information and family dynamics is recommended and also that the clients should be enabled, if they wish, to be aware of what is written in their health visiting records.

RECORDS

BASIC REQUIREMENTS

Communication and investigation

Some of the many reasons why records are needed are listed on this page, Box 8.1. They are needed as a means of communication with self and, potentially, with others. Firstly, they help health visitors recall what has happened at previous visits and, on account of this, aid both planning and the actual provision of the service. They make an excellent aide-mémoire when reports and referrals are needed in communications with other health and welfare workers, and can act as a source of inspiration when health visitors want to publish descriptions of the sort of work they do by providing (anonymously, of course) specific types of real life examples.

Secondly, good records help to demonstrate to (the very few) other people who have a right to see the notes, the key issues emerging from a visit. For example, they can help show clients how the health visitor has interpreted each encounter and help to improve their understanding of the purpose

of health visiting. As another example, they can show a health visitor's successor, or anybody temporarily standing in, what has happened to date.

Records are invaluable when the work is being investigated in any way. This applies when health visitors are looking at and evaluating their own work as well as when others are undertaking the research. These matters are considered in the next section of this chapter. There are also other situations in which health visitors need good notes in order to be able to describe the work that was undertaken. Records can be used as a memory aid in a law court, providing they were written up contemporaneously.

Records are also needed because health visitors are accountable to their employing authority to provide some evidence of their work. Health visitors also provide various facts and figures for their nurse manager, their Health District and/or for the Department of Health and Social Security. Furthermore, if ever the Health Services Commissioner were requested to investigate a case, or a health visitor's conduct were called into question in any way, full, clear and contemporaneous notes would be an obvious advantage (Whincup, 1981).

What should be included?

It is not always easy to know how much to write in the records. Health visitors know of the need for full notes. However, it is obvious that it would be impossible, for example, to record on paper everything that one would be able to see and hear in a video recording of a twenty or thirty minute visit, and even less possible to show a full picture of the environment in which the family lives. It is a question of trying to select out that which is felt to be important and to portray the key issues.

The problem of inadequate recording is well known. It has been a common fault amongst health visitors and is partly associated with the structure of their work, the fact that they see so many people in a day and do not always have the clerical support they need (Robertson,

Box 8.1 Reasons for keeping records

A. **Accurate communication**	1. As aide-mémoire:
	  a. basis on which to plan work
	  b. and aid implementation
	2. To inform others:
	  a. client
	  b. successors/stand-in
	  c. co-professionals: referrals and reports
	3. Publish, to tell:
	  a. professions—health and welfare
	  b. public

B. **Investigation**	1. Evaluation of own work: individual cases, group sessions, clinics, aspects of caseload
	2. Data for research: own/other
	3. Accountability:
	  a. in law—memory aid, if immediate recording
	  b. to health authority NM; DHA/DHSS
	  c. to public—Ombudsman

Notes

1 February 1988

Children seen, speech satisfactory. Playing with bricks.   HAV

Fig. 8.1a Hazel Vickery's visit to the Trent family.

Notes   Action
                                                                           req'd   (√)
                                                                           done   (X)

1 February 1988

TRENT FAMILY - Transfer in

PARENTS
Decorating new home: short visit. Father has constructed wide safety gates to
provide large, safe play area. Mother given HV visiting care and list of clinics
and mothers' groups. Mother enjoyed previous HV's mothers' groups: seeks similar
"educational" group.
NB - contact "Help for Health" re educational groups in area.   ✗

CHILDREN - Mary, 3; Ann, 2.
Playing together with bricks. Mary building towers and bridges; asking many
"what, where, who" questions. Ann's two-year assessment at next visit.   √
Toddler negativism discussed.

REVISIT - Monday 15 February, am.   √

Dictated 1 February, am.   Signed/date H.A.Vickery.....4-2-88..

Fig. 8.1b Visit to the Trents: alternative case notes.

1982). June Clark (1985) says health visitors tend to write only what they have observed and not what they have done. An example of poor notes, written up very sparsely, is given in Figure 8.1a. It is a record of the visit making contact with the Trent family from Chapter 2. It will be seen that a picture of the key issues within that visit is demonstrated much better by the record of that same visit shown in Figure 8.1b.

The question is, what, in general terms, are these key issues that should be noted down? There are innumerable family health needs, potentially of importance in health visiting, that might be worth a mention, as can be seen from a quick glance at the various chapters of this book. There is no simple formula for choosing, and each individual health visitor has to use his or her professional judgement as to which actual/potential need/problem and what action taken are important enough to warrant a mention.

THE HEALTH VISITOR CYCLE

It may help a little, however, to look at writing records from another point of view. By returning to the health visitor cycle we can consider which of its thought processes and stages might be the most informative and the most logical to record. It will be recalled that the health visitor cycle, introduced briefly in Chapter 1 and developed in Chapter 2, is a development of the nursing process which concentrates on the data on which decisions are made: (a) background knowledge, (b) information available prior to the visit, (c) information available at the visit and (d) that available as a consequence of the visit.

This model has been extended a little to show, in Figure 8.2, the factors that most need to be recorded. The stages seen in the Figure in capital letters are suggested as those which provide the best vehicle and the simplest approach to drawing out the necessary key issues. Those in brackets are the parts of the cycle which do not seem to need, specifically, to be stated in the notes.

Key points: what has been 'Said, Seen and Done' (SSD)

1. The most important items to record after any visit are those matters which the family members have raised as issues, be they, for example, any worries they may have, reports of developmental attainments or any special requests.

2. Also important to mention are any significant observations by the health visitor, which might be, for example, that an old lady had difficulty in walking, a child's developmental attainments seen or the evident anxiety of a mother.

3. The next thing that needs to be made clear is what service has been provided: in effect, the action taken on immediate objectives (see Ch. 2, pp. 29; 31), for example, 'A range of strategies for sleeping problems discussed: book lent' or 'Baby's hearing tested'.

If what has been said, seen and done is made clear, then the 'assessment' and 'plan' that lie behind the action decided upon should be able to be logically deduced, particularly by other health visitors. They are trained to have a similar background knowledge and would therefore be expected to go through similar thought processes. If the records are very clear and the factors involved are simple, then even a layman should be able to work out the underlying assessment and plan. It is proposed, therefore, that it should

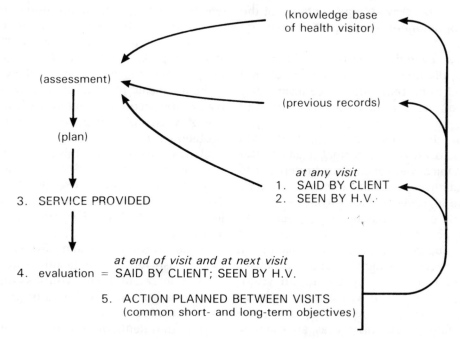

Fig. 8.2 Records and the health visitor cycle.

not really be necessary to make these factors explicit in the vast majority of cases.

4. Evaluation, in terms of how the family members see the outcome of any strategies and ideas that were tried, and any significant observations by the health visitor on what has been achieved, are important to record. However, much of this information will not be available until the next meeting. It can then be recorded as 'what has been said' and as 'what has been seen' within the normal recording of that (following) encounter.

This information is needed, anyway, for assessment and planning that meeting and, although labelled under a separate heading in the model shown in Figure 8.2, does not necessarily need to be separated in the notes. What is important is that a note should be made of the results of the activities emanating from the previous contact.

5. Conclusions as to what activities, if any, the health visitor should undertake between visits, notions that evolve out of evaluation and deliberations during a visit, should also be included: for example, 'Promised to contact bereavement service' or 'Liaison with midwife'. Any arrangements about the next appointment should, of course, be noted.

Ordinary, everyday short- and long-term objectives, discussed in Chapter 2, should not really need to be recorded. Once again, they are part of the shared basic knowledge of practising health visitors and, as the subject matter of this book shows, are far too numerous to list out in normal health visitor records. Objectives which have turned out to be particularly important at any visit should be able to be logically deduced from the rest of the records of what has been said, seen and done, as above. However, this information could be supplemented by, for example, a note of particular thoughts about or promises for further care made by the health visitor with regard to future visits. This style of recording is demonstrated below using the Manners family case history as an example (see p. 143).

Exactly what is written in any given case depends, of course, on each individual visit, and varies according to the issues the family members have raised and their responses to health visitor led ideas. It is not always easy to find the right balance. The level of content of the records should convey enough information to another member of the health visiting profession, to enable him/her to take over in the absence of the current health visitor. The aim is for succinct notes containing key 'factual' indicators: opinions could be more confusing than informative.

To summarise, it has been suggested here that the basic and key points that should be mentioned in records of a home visit are: what has been said, seen and done and, where necessary, what is intended. The ideas have been mapped out on the health visitor cycle depicted in Figure 8.2 and the reasons for the selection of these particular factors have been outlined.

SOAP DERIVATIONS

There is, of course, no absolute or set way in which records should be presented, and there are some very interesting experiments being undertaken in this field (Marsden, 1985; Clark, 1985; Rogers, 1982; Hendy, 1983). Some people feel it is important to draw out and make a specific point of an assessment and a plan in the records, sometimes advocating the use of written objectives set out as a needs or problems list.

Many of the ideas for this approach evolved from the basic SOAP or SOAPE model used as a guide for recording (Hendy, 1983; Clark, 1983; 1985; Luker, 1985). In these models, the letters S, O, A, P and E signify, more or less, as follows:

— S: subjective data (client history)
— O: observed (by the health visitor) data
— A: assessment (health visitor's conclusions)
— P: plan/goal for each need or problem
— E: evaluation.

The equivalents of 'S' and 'O' in the health visitor cycle will be found on the right in

Figure 8.2, as what is *said by client* and what is *seen by hv*. Under either model, as Kate Robinson (1983, 1985) has made quite clear, the health visitor's data is no less subjective than the client's. The equivalents in the health visitor cycle of 'A', 'P' and 'E' are, of course, '(assessment)', '(plan)' and 'evaluation' on the left side and at the bottom of the model. In the SOAP(E) approach to recording, each of these stages is supposedly made explicit and recorded. A list of problems and needs are listed, frequently on a separate sheet.

One disadvantage of a needs list is that it might prevent abandonment of impressions (and prejudices) of a previous visit. Also, a full written list of objectives brings with it the implication that something needs to be done about each of these particular issues. It could, then, tend to act as a muzzle to further thought, rather than as a vehicle for creative ideas, a tool to help respond to what seem to be the most important and relevant *current* needs from the family's point of view.

On the other hand, a needs or problems list could encourage follow-up of earlier worries. It might also help give to clients a better idea of the purpose of health visiting. This latter benefit assumes, of course, that the contents of the records are, in fact, shared with or shown to the clients, a matter returned to below.

Open records

An open and frank approach to health visiting is made much easier when contents of records can be made known to the families being visited. June Clark (1985) used her notes in conjunction with her clients. It can be done in many ways. The records might, for example as in Figure 8.3, physically be shown to the people being visited, or alternatively, written on site with the health visitor speaking aloud whilst writing. Everyone develops their own style in these things. This open approach, however, is very demanding and might be time consuming. Not all health visitors, nor the families they visit, feel confident enough

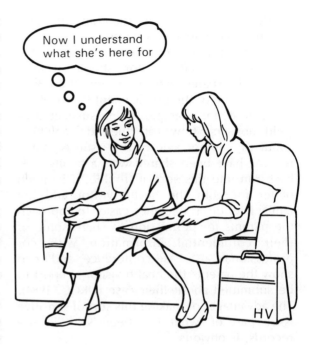

Now I understand what she's here for

Fig. 8.3 Open records: for education and trust.

to be able to take part in this style of communication.

One important factor in whether or not the records are shared will be the health visitor's style and approach to recording. For example, recording certain aspects of the health visitor's assessment could act as a distinct disincentive to open records. Asking health visitors to set down their view of the situation and their impressions may encourage them to write down a personal view of, for example, family dynamics, which might tend to be derogatory or patronising. This they would obviously prefer not to share with their clients. Either way, they should not be writing about these aspects of family life.

A statement of what has been heard, seen and done, on the other hand, is based on matters which should provide the client with no surprises and, if properly written, no insult. As a basic principle, nothing in the notes should cause offence, with or without open records. A clear description of what has happened, as advocated above, should provide evidence enough of anything that really worries the health visitor: recording the facts on which any concern is based.

The moral question, of course, arises: if it worries the health visitor should it not, anyway, be shared with the client? If a family are not aware of the predicament they may be in, such as, for example, being suspected as child abusers, how can they do anything about it? Another side of the issue is that if records have been shared with a family who have run into this sort of trouble, it is much better for both the health visitor and the family later on. It becomes easier to approach the parents for permission to share some of their confidential information with co-professionals at a case conference, and/or to show the parents the health visitor's report to be submitted about their case (UKCC, 1984). The advantages of making this sort of sensitive issue part of 'what has been said' in the records, is obvious.

Sharing the contents of notes with clients, as shown in Figure 8.3, is helpful, both educationally and for trust. When a client can see the matters which a health visitor selects as important enough to record, it probably demonstrates better than anything else the areas of interests within health visiting, and its purpose. Centile charts for a child's development and weight, a questionnaire for post-natal depression and so on, can all add to the understanding and, as mentioned in earlier chapters, lead to useful questioning and discussion. Trust is likely to be enhanced. By seeing the actual range of concern of health visitors and what they write, people will more readily comprehend that the intention is for support and education and not for social policing.

Parent-held records

Sharing child health records is facilitated by a booklet specially designed by the Society of Area Nurses, Child Health (Owen, 1980). This booklet and another developed in Oxford were distributed to over 300 mothers attending clinics in Oxford (Green & Macfarlane, 1985). There was a high level of both parental and professional approval of both booklets from those who responded at the end of the survey, and helpful suggestions were made for improvements.

Further research is now being undertaken on giving parents custody of the normal type of child health clinic records (Green & Macfarlane, 1985; Saffin, 1985). This has been welcomed by most parents. Improvements to the records to help with educational aspects of the notes are under way. In her study Pauline Pearson (1985) found that a proportion of the doctors and health visitors involved with parents holding the small booklet failed to fill it in. This, as Kate Saffin pointed out, is not a problem when parents hold the primary document.

Whether they are parent-held or not, notes designed for a schedule of complex and regular child health medicals may discourage parents from contacting the doctor when they first suspect a problem. Dr Nicoll (1983, 1984) said the implications of the old MCW46 forms, universal and frequent examinations for all children, led to an overcrowded and rather cursory service at the clinics. Attendance levels decreased as the likelihood of a problem occurring increased. Oversight by health visitors and a flexible system were found to be a much better method in which to identify difficulties. We should be warned not to be hedged in by records systems, and always to be questioning whether we are actually achieving our objectives rather than merely filling them in!

RECORDS IN ACTION

We conclude this section by looking at examples of ways in which health visitor recording can be undertaken, and indicate some of the experiments and schemes currently in progress.

SSD RECORDS

An example

First is what we shall call the 'Said, Seen and Done' (SSD) approach to recording, the one advocated earlier in this chapter. The illustrations in Figures 8.4a and 8.4b show how the antenatal visiting and birth visit to Nancy Manners, examples from Chapters 3 and 4, might have been recorded under this scheme. The visit notes alone are shown. The face card is not reproduced in this example.

Explanation of the example

We can now demonstrate the rationale of this simple system by looking at the SSD records in Figure 8.4 in the context of the features of the health visitor cycle in Figure 8.2:

1. and 2. What said by client and seen by HV

In these records, what the *mother said*, for example, about her diet, benefits, housing and crèche plans and arrangements are noted, as is *health visitor observation*, for example, that the cooking facilities were available and the baby's condition.

3. What done: service provided

The assessment and plan could be derived from reading what had been said and observed and from what *service* had been *given*: in this case, for example, the need for and plan to give information on breastfeeding, the attempt to assess attitudes towards 'mothering' and the need for and plan to give information on potential friendship networks.

4. Evaluation: what said and seen

The *evaluation* can be found in what the *mother reported* at the following visit, for example, having found *The Breastfeeding Book* (Messenger, 1982) very helpful, and what the *health visitor observed* in her manner, i.e. being now more confident about breastfeeding and about being able to continue for a while after starting back at work. In the October visit it was reported that the referral to the Gingerbread Group seemed to be providing a useful friendship and self-help network. This was reinforced in the visit of 12th November, the birth visit, as Nancy stated she intended to join their babysitting circle.

5. Action planned between visits

There was, in this example, no action planned between visits. However, there *might* have been a plan to contact the secretary of the Gingerbread Group after the visit of 3rd September, to arrange for a member of the group to visit Nancy and take her to the meeting and introduce her round. This action was not undertaken here, either because Nancy did not feel it was necessary or, perhaps, as the health visitor did not feel it was worth suggesting.

Objectives

A note of a particular short-term objective which Hannah Van der Haastrecht wanted to remember is seen, for example, in the records of the 5th August visit, in the reference to the promise 'to tell about organisations—Gingerbread and National Council'. Another can be found at the end of the notes on the birth visit (12th November) regarding Nancy's seeing breastfeeding as an important factor to be covered at the next meeting, scheduled for the following week. Ticks in the action column draw attention to the items/objectives needing to be followed up. These are subsequently crossed through to show they have been attended to.

Other everyday health visiting objectives, for example concern over nutrition and the intention to explain about immunisation programmes, have not been given a special mention as objectives for further visits. However, the presence of such objectives can be derived from the fact that these matters were included in the conversations and hence in the notes of subsequent visits.

Open records

If this health visitor had shared the content of the records with her client, then Nancy would

```
Notes                                                        Action
                                                             req'd  (√)
5 August 1988                                                done   (X)

NANCY MANNERS - antenatal: 28 weeks
Nancy says is 'keeping off baccy an' booze' and has been using hospital dining
room for main meals.  Cooking facilities in bedsitter.  Will claim benefits;
on housing list: expects flat - one year.  Hopes to use hospital creche.
Seeking information on breastfeeding whilst at work: discussion and Messenger
and Garner books recommended.  Not attending A/N classes.
Nancy's mother (lives Mychester) said to have been 'moderately firm; listened
to reason':  Nancy hopes to be same sort of mother.  Personnel department and
nursing friends 'supportive' but says her mother's attitude was the key to her
decision that she could cope as a single parent.
I promised to tell about organisations - Gingerbread and National Council.    X

APPT - Tuesday 6 September, am.                                               X

Dictated 5 August, am.           Signed/date H.S. Van der Haastreht 8.8.88


6 September 1988

NANCY MANNERS - ANTENATAL: 32 weeks
Nancy says studying hard to help when she returns to training and more busy
with baby.  Eating well, especially salads.
Had discovered full time creche charges everywhere far too expensive for her:
bitterly disappointed.  Says her mother will care for baby (half by coming
to Overhampton and half in Mychester) on the days Nancy works, just until she
qualifies.  Nancy plans to stop work then until child care becomes possible.
She talked at length: fully aware of current difficulties re free nursery
places.
Messenger breastfeeding book found helpful; discovered several books at library.
Now more confident about breastfeeding.
One-parent family organisations discussed.  Gingerbread address, meeting place and
time provided.  Immunisation programme discussed.  Hesitant about whooping cough:
literature given.  Says does not intend to attend A/N classes - anticipates
prejudice; midwife very informative.

APPT - Tuesday 3 October, am.                                                X

Dictated 3 September, am.        Signed/date H.S. Van der Haastreht 6.9.88
```

Fig. 8.4a The 'said, seen and done' records scheme: an example—visit notes for the Manners family.

have been able to see what points the health visitor saw as key issues during the conversation. She would also have been able to further her own understanding and give the health visitor an opportunity to explain about her work and intentions, by asking about the content of the records. For example she could have asked, if it had not already been explained during the conversation, why the remarks about her relationship with her mother were included.

Had our fictitious health visitor felt, as many health visitors seem to, that matters of family dynamics are too sensitive and too private to be recorded, then the conversations associated with the attempt to assess attitudes on 'mothering' and potential for depression or stress, might have been left out. The health visitor's understanding of the family interactions from such conversation would then simply be stored in her memory.

Pre-requisites

It can be seen that no specially printed record cards are needed for the 'said, seen and done' scheme of recording. The pre-requisites are for enough space to record full notes, and preferably with a dictaphone and an audio-typist clerical support system to help neaten and speed up the record-making (O'Connor & Willis, 1985).

```
Notes                                                       Action
                                                            req'd   (√)
3 October 1988                                              done    (X)

NANCY MANNERS - antenatal: 36 weeks
Garner book found reassuring.  Has visited Gingerbread 3 times: establishing
friendships.  Immunisation discussed.  Nancy thinks her baby will 'have the lot'.
List of clinics given.
Developmental assessment discussed.  Local scheme shown.  HMSO Sheridan
booklet lent.


Dictated 3 October, am.          Signed/dated ..H.S.Van.der.Haastrecht. 4.10.88    X

11 November 1988

Birth visit with midwife for 'handover'.  Nancy has her mother, Mrs Manners,
staying to help.  Caesarian delivery and 'bonding' discussed.  Nancy feared
inadequate bonding.  Rayner booklet used: lent till next visit.           √ √
Mrs Manners intends to buy HMSO Sheridan for monitoring baby ' for fun'.
Developmental assessment discussed.  Local scheme shown. Local clinic
described.  Nancy talked of friendship networks; intends to join Gingerbread
babysitting circle.

PAULINE - 2 weeks
Breastfeeding 3 to 4 hourly: midwife's support appreciated.  Pauline wakeful
in evening: not seen as a problem.  Hearing tested with hand clap: startled.
Eyes clear; umbilicus dry.  Passing urine; stools loose.  Baby looks well;
colour good, fontanelles normal.  Making eye contact.  Weight 3 kg.
Visit  next week requested: especially re breastfeeding.                  √

APPT - Tuesday 15 November, am.                                           √

Dictated 11 November, am.        Signed/ dated ..S.Van.der.Haastrecht 14.10.88
```

Fig. 8.4b Visit notes for the Manners family, overleaf.

SOAP (E) RECORDS

DIY formats

Problem-oriented recording as proposed by Karen Luker (1985, pp. 149–153), does not need specially designed new record cards either. She explains how this approach to record making was pioneered by a doctor in the late 1960s for medical records and gives an example of how it can be modified for and used in health visiting.

Experimenting with a more complex system is also possible without specially printed record cards. June Clark (1985) has described how she ruled up A4 paper and photostatted it in order to have the ability to classify her records as she wished. She designed assessment/plan sheets for the family and the child and for the neonatal visit, and a problem/needs list for when several problems emerged and

needed to be clarified and sorted out. A contact record card was used for for short-term plans and records of telephone conversations and contact with other agencies. She felt her structured approach helped her find problems she had previously missed. The limiting effect that can be associated with the checklist approach, incorporated to some extent in Dr Clark's scheme, were discussed in Chapter 2 (pp. 30–31).

Tailor-made formats

Specially designed cards were described by health visitors from Portsmouth and South East Hampshire (Rogers, 1982; Wilson & Cowan, 1982; Hedley et al, 1982). Record cards Mark I and II (Rogers, 1982) are now superseded by Mark III. Interest in their work has been so great that they are preparing to market a work pack on their method of recording.

Developments by Portsmouth's neighbours in Southampton and South West Hampshire have been described by Marjorie Marsden (1985). They have devised a family history card and a child record card. In this latter, on one side they have set out four columns in which they state:

1. a pre-visit reason for making contact and observations
2. objectives
3. action taken and short- and/or long-term objectives
4. whether or not objectives have been achieved

An example

Experiments with schemes derived from the problem-oriented approach to recording are beginning to emerge elsewhere. Richmond, Twickenham and Roehampton Health Authority health visitors have produced an interesting one. On their records, the series of visits to the Manners family, our example from Chapters 3 and 4, might be recorded as shown in Figures 8.5a to 8.5d.

In this scheme, there would also be other cards. For example, there would be one for a confidential household profile which describes the family circumstances. There would be another recording information about the type of birth and the reasons for it and other matters, such as the general appearance and condition of the baby when newly born. This card also has space for screening tests undertaken, prophylaxis and childhood illnesses.

This records system is versatile and has space to show, in the way that the writer chooses, what
— the client said
— the health visitor saw
— was done
— was intended to be done
— what has been achieved.

Detailed notes about any encounter between the family and the health visitor can easily be contained in records systems such as these.

However, actually getting the notes written up is another matter. In many authorities, health visitors still have no clerical support and no access to the services of an audio-typist able to transcribe tape-recorded messages from a small handbag-sized dictaphone.

Writing full, clear and neat records by hand and, conversely, deciphering tightly packed handwritten notes to try to find the key issues, can be very time consuming. When multiplied by the hundreds of people seen in their homes and at clinics each year, it is potentially quite an encroachment on possible home visiting time. However beautiful and accommodating any records scheme may be, there may well be a tendency towards skimping on records, both in reading them and writing them, in order to protect time to visit. In the end it comes down to choosing whichever system the health visitors and their employers feel is most appropriate for their area and for their circumstances.

To summarise, when choosing a scheme for recording, be it SSD, SOAP or some derivative of them, there are some key questions to be asked such as: is it *simple to use* and does it help enable:
— health visitors to note down and take into consideration the families' aims and wishes?
— families to understand the purpose and make good use of health visiting?
— key observations and the service given by health visitors to be clearly noted?
— results of the work to be shown, not only as the health visitor sees it, but also as the family report the situation?
In effect, does the chosen system of record making facilitate good communication and enable appropriate investigation?

EVALUATION

Three approaches

Overlapping meaning in commonly-used terminology scuh as evaluation, assessment and measurement, masks some of the differing concepts involved. 'Value', 'assessment' and 'quantification' are terms used in

NAME MANNERS

ADDRESS Room 2, 14 Mountgrove Road, Overhampton

ASSESSMENT AT FIRST VISIT — DATE 5·8·85

A visit was made to Nancy – a student nurse, who is 28 weeks pregnant and is at present living in a 'bedsit' with cooking facilities. She is hoping to resume her nursing training postnatally. Nancy has given much thought, both to her practical arrangements for the expected baby and her capabilities and attitudes towards being a single parent. She has a very supportive mother who has encouraged her to look after her own baby. Her landlady, her nursing colleagues and the Personnel Department have also been supportive. Nancy appears to have a very positive attitude and is keen to find information that will help her be a good mother.

DATE	LONG TERM AIM	EVALUATION	SIGNATURE
5·8·85	(1) To enable and encourage Nancy to accept and enjoy the responsibility of being a mother. To support her through the difficulties of being a single parent so that the bonding between her and her baby will be established, thus enabling her child to develop emotionally and physically within a secure environment.		
	(2) To detect as early as possible any signs of ill-health, or abnormalities through regular visiting, developmental checks and health education.		
	(3) Promotion of health through health education, immunisation and regular visiting.		H.S. Vander Haastrecht 5th Aug. '85

Fig. 8.5a Problem-oriented records: an example. 1. Health visitor care plan.

FAMILY NAME: MANNERS

CODE: H = HOME VISIT   C = CLINIC
T = TELEPHONE   S = SURGERY
O = OTHERS

DATE AND TIME	CODE	NEED AND OBSERVATION	PLAN/ACTION	REVIEW	SIGNATURE
5.8.85	H	Nancy is now 28 weeks pregnant and is hoping to continue working. Concerned regarding her future accommodation and is hoping to be rehoused by the council in one year. She will claim social security benefits when baby is born and hopes to use Hospital crèche. Nancy says she is "keeping off (racey) and booze" and is eating hospital meals.	① Check place on housing list. ② Advice on diet. ③ Invitation to A/N classes. ④ Information given on health education literature for pregnant mothers and support groups ie. Gingerbread and National Council.	3.9.85	HS vander Haastrecht 5.8.85
3.9.85	H	32/40 Nancy more confident and eager to talk. Is studying hard to alleviate pressure when she returns to nursing, postnatally. Is eating well, especially salads. Is bitterly disappointed that crèche charges are too expensive and that there is a shortage of free nursery places. Has decided to stop work after qualifying until suitable care can be arranged. Has decided against A/N classes as she anticipates prejudice. Midwife and mother very supportive.	① Encourage attitude towards breastfeeding ② Encourage interest in reading material regarding immunisation programmes ③ To discuss with mother the arrangements for looking after the baby until Nancy has completed her training.	1.10.85	HS vander Haastrecht 3.9.85

Fig. 8.5b Problem-oriented records: an example. 2. Health visiting record—family.

DATE/TIME	CODE	NEED AND OBSERVATION	PLAN/ACTION	REVIEW	SIGNATURE
1·10·85	H	36/40 Nancy has found Garner book reassuring and has made three visits to Gingerbread meetings; establishing friendships.	① Immunisation and developmental checks for baby discussed. ② Information given re clinics in area. ③ Local assessment schemes described and discussed.		H. S. Vander Haastrecht 1·10·85
2·11·85	H	P/N visit with midwife. Maternal grandmother Mrs Manners staying to help Nancy with baby Pauline. Midwife very supportive. Long discussion re- Caesarian delivery and bonding as Nancy anxious re "inadequate bonding".	① Developmental assessment and clinic described. ② Appointment for developmental check. ③ Ongoing encouragement re bonding with baby Pauline. ④ Rayner booklet lent. ⑤ Encouragement and support over breastfeeding. ⑥ Encouraged to join Gingerbread babysitting circle.	19·11·85	H.S. Vander Haastrecht 12·11·85

Fig. 8.5c Problem-oriented records: an example. 3. Health visiting record—family, overleaf.

HEALTH VISITOR CARE PLAN — GIRL

NAME **MANNERS** Pauline   ADDRESS **14 Mountgrove Road.**

CODE: H - Home Visit   C - Clinic   O - Other
            T - Telephone   S - Surgery

DATE/TIME	CODE	NEED AND OBSERVATION	PLAN/ACTION	REVIEW	SIGNATURE
2·11·85	H	2/52 'Handover' visit with midwife. Breastfeeding 3-4 hourly. Wakeful in evening - not seen as a problem. Maternal grandmother helping and intends to buy HMSO Sheridan for monitoring for 'fun'.	① Hearing tested : hand clap ✓ ② Eyes clear ③ Vision : eye contact ; responds to facial expression. ④ Umbilicus dry ⑤ Buttocks ✓ ⑥ Passing urine ; stools loose ⑦ Baby's colour good ⑧ Fontanelles ✓ ⑨ Weight 3 kg	19·11·85	H.S. vander Haabrecht 12·11·85

Fig. 8.5d Problem oriented records: an example. 4. Health visitor care plan—girl.

this section to try to draw out three approaches to evaluation in which health visitors can become involved in their day-to-day work. Figure 8.6 shows a cartoonised and very simplistic version of these three viewpoints: the clients', the health visitors' and that involved in wider management and planning.

The best judge of the *value* of a service is, for the most part, the person who actually receives it. The people who give the service can only make a guess at its value to their clients and try to find out from them to what extent it is helpful. The providers can, of course, think about what they have planned to offer and about their overall aims. They can then try to *assess* the degree to which their goals and tactics seem to have been effective and, more importantly, decide whether the chosen goals and tactics were, in the event, the most appropriate. It may be felt that these

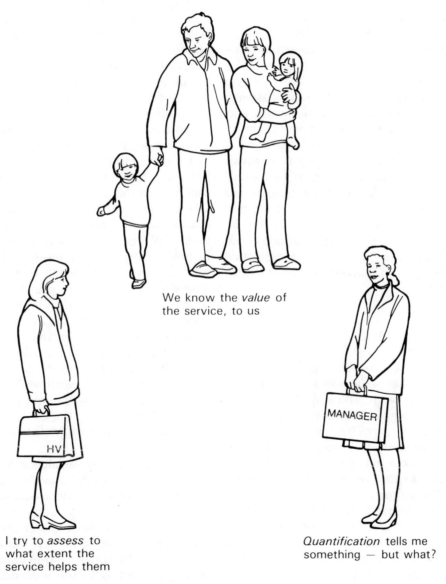

We know the *value* of
the service, to us

I try to *assess* to
what extent the
service helps them

Quantification tells me
something — but what?

Fig. 8.6 Three approaches to evaluation of health visiting.

two viewpoints are too subjective, but, as Karen Luker (1985) shows, all evaluation carries some measure of subjectivity.

The third approach to evaluation, *quantification*, involves numerical measurement of certain aspects of the service provided, such as the number of babies or old people discovered to have defective hearing, the number of health visitors employed or homes visited. These measures can vary significantly in the extent to which they are able to show what has been achieved in the work.

Both of the first two approaches, investigating the value of the service and critical self-assessment by health visitors, mostly involve a broad-based descriptive or narrative approach. They have the advantage of being able to encompass consideration of all aspects of the current service, potential aspects and a range of possible alternatives. Quantification, on the other hand, in measuring a range of specific items, covers a narrower field and is, of course, restricted to current practice or practice at the time it was carried out. However, such measurement can, when founded on soundly-based criteria, be an extremely useful tool. A well thought out combination of the three ways of evaluating the work is likely, in practice, to give the most helpful view.

FAMILIES' EVALUATION

The value of the service to the families receiving it is a key issue and seems the most important to research. The way the service is seen as, for example, instructive, supportive and courteously provided or not, directly influences whether it is received either as relevant and acceptable or is rejected and amounts only to misdirected and wasted effort by the health visitor.

We have referred in earlier chapters, particularly in Chapter 2, to some important studies of client opinion undertaken by health visitors. It will be recalled, for example, that about 70 mothers with their first babies were interviewed by Jean Orr (1980). As a conse-

quence of her investigations, she was able to give some very useful advice to health visitors on important features of the provision of the service. The study involving in-depth interviewing by Jane Robinson (1982), who was seeking reasons for non-use of the service, was also very instructive. Although undertaken with very few families, it was able to show how people can feel about the different styles within health visiting and to draw attention to some of the factors that seem to affect take-up of the service.

In Chapter 7, we looked at Karen Luker's (1982) scheme for finding out old ladies' opinion of the service. This sort of format, outlined on page 120, Box 7.2, could be used by other health visitors to find out what people think of their work. It could be used for getting people's opinions about clinic or group work as well as about home visiting.

An investigation does not necessarily have to be on a large scale to be useful. Pauline Pearson (1984) tape recorded her conversations with the parents of sixteen babies. She asked open-ended questions and discovered a wide range of needs and views. She found quite divergent opinions about a similar style of health visiting. One mother, for example, was grateful that the health visitor did not say 'you should do this and you should do that', whereas another mother was yearning for 'an honest bit of advice': two very different responses to a non-directive approach. This sort of research does not provide simple guidance on exactly what to do or how to do it. It is, however, well worthwhile. It can give some useful leads, is thought provoking and is, as we said above, the best way to get to know the *value* of health visiting to the families receiving it.

There is, of course, a value in health visiting of which the family may be unaware or, perhaps, discounts. For example, immunisation against whooping cough on a large scale helps protect the most vulnerable in society, the extremely young babies, from the consequences of the disease—providing a value to society as well as to the individual. Here we have been concerned directly with the viewpoint of the families on how they see the value of the service as it affects them.

ASSESSMENT BY HEALTH VISITORS

Health visitors, like the families they visit, are, of course, constantly assessing and coming to conclusions about each encounter they have. Here it is suggested that in addition to this everyday evaluation of each case, health visitors should make a conscious decision to step back from their work every so often and look at some individual cases and at their caseload overall, in order to think in a broader way about what has been achieved to date.

Peer group discussion can provide a very good environment for assessment of the work. It can encourage a wide-ranging view of possible alternative strategies for care. Brainstorming sessions in these groups could give health visitors courage to follow up and act on latent ideas for improvements in their service. Ann Stanton (1984) has described how 'peer group auditing' was set up in Edinburgh. She said that they had, unknowingly, followed Shirley Goodwin's (1983a) ground rules for success in starting and running such a group. It seems the group was very successful. The auditing was described as having become addictive and plans were being made for looking at and assessing even more aspects of practice.

Another side of peer group assessment can be seen in the time spent with the nurse manager talking about cases that are of concern or present some dilemma, or in discussing the relative merits of new ideas for promoting the health of the local community. In these deliberations and assessments, nurse managers and their health visitors will have many factors to consider.

The fundamental question will be, of course, whether the aspect of health visiting under scrutiny is making or is likely to make a contribution to fulfilment of the aims and objectives of the work.

If stated in terms of the prevention and family health needs models of this book, then the questions will ask whether the service being provided, or proposed, is likely to help

— *prevent the occurrence* of problems or conditions
— *prevent the development* of problems or conditions
— *prevent deterioration* in established problems or conditions

with regard to *environmental, physical, mental/emotional and social* aspects of people's health and welfare.

The well-known questions raised by the Children's Committee (1980) are very important, too. It was felt that they helped to indicate the extent to which the professional is practising in partnership with clients. The points raised were whether

— parents were seen as central to the life of their child and treated in accordance with this
— parents were encouraged to help each other and were enabled to do so
— the service was sensitive to the families' cultural and social norms
— the service was easily understood by the parents.

Other important basic factors are whether the service being provided or proposed

— allows for creativity and encourages innovation
— takes a proactive rather than a reactive approach
— is formulated and devised in relation to local small area OPCS evidence of social deprivation and other evidence of health need.

Records and evaluation

Health visitors wanting a peer support group or their nursing manager to help them assess certain aspects of their care, may find their records provide an important aide-mémoire about the details of individual family members' progress and problems (presented, of course, anonymously). However, using records the other way round, that is attempting to assess how health visitors are performing their work *solely* on an inspection of their records, has distinct limitations.

Although well-recorded and full notes can give an observer such as a nurse manager a professional picture of what health visitors have been doing on their visits, the records cannot necessarily show how appropriate these activities were in relation to other possible alternatives. One cannot tell the whole story (see p. 137) either on what did happen or what could have happened. Only the health visitors know what choice there was as they saw it, and as the family appeared to see it, at the time. Only they can make informed speculations as to what topics could, perhaps, have been discussed or expanded and what possible alternative approaches there might have been. However, nursing managers who have been community trained understand the possible innuendoes and complexities within a visit and can empathise when these matters are discussed.

Normal health visitor records necessarily show only an outline or provide an index of what happened at any encounter. Robert Dingwall (1977, p. 113) observed that

the major part of what a field health visitor knows about her clients is in her head.

For this reason, assessment by outsiders benefits from being founded, for the most part, upon discussions with the health visitor involved. Also, the records cannot portray the appropriateness or otherwise of a health visitor's style and approach. This, too, is probably best ascertained, where no client view can be gained, through conversation in a counselling sort of environment and, perhaps, using some of the eight criteria said to be associated with interviewing skills and listed by Karen Luker (1985, p. 137), for example 'willing to listen and empathises' and 'shows human warmth'. Another possible basis for discussion could be provided by health visitors tape recording their own visit (Robinson, 1986).

Peer group analysis, where it is supportive, constructive and creative, can be extremely helpful in enabling health visitors to share and

evaluate their problems and concerns, and can provide a very important back-up for individual health visitor's own attempts to stand back and *assess* their work.

QUANTIFICATION

There are an enormous number of measurable entities that are available to analyse and provide some guidance. Both health visitors and their managers need to understand the implications of what is being quantified and how it is being measured. Also of importance is what evidence is being particularly singled out and used to guide the allocation of resources and the choice of projects to be undertaken.

What quantified?

When some aspect of health visiting is being measured, it is important to know, for example, what are the particular entities that have been selected for measurement, whether these entities are being assessed against pre-set and validated criteria on a pre-selected group, whether there is also a control group or the research could be replicated, and if it is a prospective study.

The Child Development Project (1984) provides an excellent example of this sort of well thought-out and 'scientific' approach. The research involves assessment over a three year period of parental environment and children's development and how this correlates with a particular style of health visiting. The style is one in which the parent is encouraged to take the initiative with the health visitor acting as a resource, as opposed to the rather more traditional style which sees the parent as the recipient of 'expert' health visiting advice.

In this research, an enormous amount of information is being coded and computerised for analysis. A variety of aspects are being studied. For example, a child development profile is being built up on each child by using parental reports, the researcher's observations and researcher assessments of the child's ability to complete a wide range of tasks. A child activity level questionnaire, a child's progress form and a maternal self-esteem questionnaire are being used. A nutritional questionnaire, concerned with what the children are being fed and the environment in which they are fed, has been used in some districts. It will be some time before the study is complete and the results are made fully available, but early results are optimistic (see Ch. 3, p. 30 and Ch. 5, p. 76).

The most important aspect of this research is that it shows that, given the expertise and the resources, it *is* possible to monitor and evaluate practices in health visiting in terms of indicators, for example, of good and bad health, the quality of the home's developmental environment and the child's progress.

The information traditionally collected has not been so useful. Knowledge of the number of homes visited or classifications of clients seen, for example, may be useful for maintaining the status quo regarding the management of the work. However, it does not give any indication of what has been achieved and in what way the service could provide more effective care.

The Körner Committee (Steering Group on Health Services Information, 1984) information system for services to the community will help to give a better picture of a variety of aspects of health visiting—some, such as immunisation more successfully than others. Unfortunately, it looks as if educational aspects of the work will largely go unrecorded. The Committee expects greater use to be made of OPCS small area statistics and computerised age–sex population data as a guide to the need for the preventive service and how it should be allocated.

Hopefully, information about health surveillance and early detection of disease will identify people who have been missed by the normal provision of services, so that funds can be set aside for the more costly and time consuming follow-up of, for example, children of working mothers whose families can only be visited in the evening. A further study (para 2.8) is being undertaken on the preva-

lence and incidence of disease or disability, which will eventually provide further indicators against which to measure the need for resources and, to some extent, the degree of success of screening procedures (Robertson, 1981).

It has been suggested that there is a need for increased understanding of the benefits to the child, the health visitor and to management of centralised records for pre-school developmental screening to bring about improved reliability and validity of the central records. Under-recording has been shown to be associated with inefficient methods of data collection and lack of interest by staff who did not know the use to which such information could be put. This, it is suggested, would be as much of a problem with computerised as with handwritten data (Lambert et al, 1985). These factors will be important to remember as the new systems are implemented.

The Körner Committee recognised that the enormous variety of activities involved in services to the community meant that a count of contacts could not be taken as a measure of the work done. They said that the proposed broad classifications give only a general indication of activity during the contact (para 7.9) and that a deeper description of what happens during that contact is necessary. Sadly, the categorisation of activities they suggest in Annex III is still at a distinctly general level from a health visiting point of view. It does, however, provide at least a chance to expand on the 'main purpose' categorisation of the extremely simplistic 'surveillance' or 'professional advice and support'.

It is good that the Committee made such a clear statement about the inability to measure health visiting by a count of contacts. Health visitors do sometimes tend to feel that they are being judged on the number of visits that they make. Robert Dingwall (1977, p. 114) explained how he thought this comes about. During his study he observed that management stressed empathetically that the quality of visits and not their quantity was what was important. However, he noticed guidelines were proposed for the number of visits at various phases of a child's life. This and management's preoccupation with classification of visits for the weekly returns, gave health visitors the *impression* that work was being monitored from a quantitative point of view.

Records as quantifiable evidence

The sort of records kept in a study such as the Child Development Project or Karen Luker's (1982) research into the health needs of 120 old ladies, have to be very detailed, well planned and in accord with certain validated criteria. Health visitor records are not, for the most part, of this sort of calibre and such detail could probably only be justified in specifically planned experimental research or those few specific projects which it has been agreed health visitors should participate in. Normal health visitor records, however full and well presented, are not generally able on their own, to provide reliable, quantifiable evidence and are really only useful at the self- and peer-assessment level of evaluation described above.

Local statistics

Infant mortality figures in Sheffield and Gosport, Portsmouth, have improved remarkably (see Ch. 5, page 88). Health visitors there are undertaking special surveillance schemes aimed at lowering the rate of sudden and unexpected infant deaths. June Clark (1983) questioned whether it can be proven that it was the health visitor intervention that caused this to happen because the actual health visitor–client activities undertaken were not described. Only if described could they be tried out again, and only if repeated, and with similar results, could proof be assumed. However, since she wrote, Carpenter et al (1983) have given a detailed account in *The Lancet* defending their case that the factor that made the difference was, in fact, the health visitor contact. Also, the Portsmouth study (Powell, 1985) has become very well known and so it should be fairly easy to try it

out again and thereby verify the matter or not so far as this is possible.

In Chapter 2 (p. 17–18) we looked at the sort of local statistics that are available to help demonstrate where health visiting effort should be concentrated. Doreen Irving (1985) shows how scoring systems can be used. It seems the British Medical Association has decided to adopt an eight point scoring system to help identify areas eligible for special help in improving the services. It is described as a crude but 'good enough' device for identifying need. Doreen Irving says free copies of the figures for electoral wards in any specific district can be supplied by Peter Rice and that John Yates is producing analyses of district figures for health authorities.

Evaluation of health visiting outcome must go hand in hand with investigations of levels of health and ill health in the community. This is necessary to show, as far as is possible, not only the overall need for the work but also its overall effect, such as on infant mortality rates.

It will be interesting to see to what extent John Dobby's (1984) research can contribute towards this. He is experimenting with certain classes of information which may be able to help health visitors estimate both the effectiveness of and the constraints on their work and help decide priorities for health visiting activities in their area.

What evidence is chosen?

There is, then, an increasing amount of evidence currently and potentially available which can give some guidance on various ways in which health visiting services might be organised or allocated. Probably the most important question regarding evaluation of health visiting is 'To what use is the evidence being put and, of all that is available, which aspects do managers choose to guide their decisions?'

Are health visitor managers encouraging, for example, up-to-date monitoring of local mortality and morbidity statistics? Are they taking into account the evidence from recent research into health visiting, such as that from the Child Development Project? Perhaps even more significantly, are they prepared, where necessary, to change the structure of the traditional staffing patterns and work schedules, as is necessary for this programme (Child Development Project, 1984)?

Health visitors are, in general terms, the health workers most closely aware of social needs and situations in the various corners of their District. To what extent do they share this knowledge? Do they and their managers use the OPCS and other statistics available locally to demonstrate to people allocating the resources where need seems to be greatest and why and where they recommend special efforts to be concentrated?

Nora Saddington (Nursing Times, 1984) was quoted as warning that the minimum data collection recommended by the Körner Committee will not be enough to make informed decisions about priorities in health visiting. It seems she gave two examples of how, in Birmingham, health visitors had used social information in addition to the data assembled by the health authority managers and, in this way, had identified the whereabouts of the people most in need of intensive health visiting.

Discovering and deciding on 'need' in a community is a complex matter. Jean Orr (1985) has described many of the issues and difficulties involved and has advocated that health visitors should compile, and keep up to date, a community health profile from which to plan and provide health visiting activities.

These quantitative matters, that is looking at and using 'facts' and figures, are an important aspect of evaluation, as is, in the day to day work of the practising health visitor, self-and peer-assessment and attempts to understand what value the families put on the work.

CONFIDENTIALITY

Confidentiality is an important issue both in

recording and in the evaluation of our work. Trends towards records which are becoming increasingly geared for evaluation and, in some cases, pressures towards closer oversight of the records, bring the matter to the fore. In general terms, any information given to a nurse is given with the expectation that it will go no further. Matters of an impersonal and general nature are less likely to be categorised in this way, but clinical and personal matters are given to the nurse with the underlying assumption of confidentiality (Bailey, 1980).

There is a need for health visitors to be particularly sensitive to this issue and also to the vulnerability of their clientèle in this respect. Working in the informal way that we do in people's homes, on occasions using questioning techniques or some other approach to help people express how they feel, confidential information is often entrusted to the health visitor within the natural course of conversation. Personal information, however casually it appears to have been given, whether in the secrecy of the person's home, in a quiet corner of the clinic or anywhere else, should never be treated casually. This is one of the areas where 'full recording' and describing every activity and key issue at a visit become difficult, not for lack of space or time, but on grounds of confidentiality.

Individual health visitors have to make their own ethical decisions on this matter. Should health visitors note down, for example, how someone is quarrelling with his/her spouse or, perhaps, how a woman has revealed that the true paternity of her child is not the father thought by everyone else to be so? The important question is: what risks to confidentiality or what benefits for the family are likely to result from recording personal details? Is the better alternative to record 'Personal problem discussed'—or to write nothing?

In a small way, this problem was touched on with regard to Nancy Manners' relationship with her mother (p. 144). Would Mrs Van der Haastrecht have made a note of a poor relationship, where, for example, the mother was said to have beaten her? This would have implications for Nancy's need for extra support and, perhaps, her own tendency later to treat her child in the same way, an issue returned to in Chapter 11. In some cases it is no simple matter to gauge just what should be committed to paper. Perhaps 'when in doubt, write nought' should provide the final guidance.

Robert Dingwall (1977, p. 93) in his study, noted that the health visitor's records did not reflect the degree to which conversation at visits was in fact concentrated upon the mother's welfare and feelings. It could be that this tendency reflected the health visitor's intuitive protection of client confidentiality over personal issues. If it is not written then it cannot be leaked, for example, either to a manager or later by some subsequent health visitor working with the family.

The protection of confidentiality may mean that, from a records point of view, the work will inevitably portray a medical model, for example showing a bias towards surveillance of developmental progress and interest in physical aspects of adult health. Supportive aspects of the work associated with a relation-ship-oriented model and with health visitors' social awareness, may remain largely invisible and secret by being unrecorded. As Kate Robinson (1985) says, we do not yet have enough knowledge of what actually happens in health visiting to know what approaches and philosophies are actually involved. More-over, it seems that normal health visitor records are not going to tell us the whole truth about the work, whatever records scheme is invented.

With the moves to make health visitor records (a) more explicit and/or (b) more subject to review, comes an increasing need for these issues to be discussed at length, both between health visitors and between health visitors and their managers. Currently, general agreement seems the norm, presum-ably because managers with a health visitor background can empathise over the problems involved.

There may be difficulties, however, when an employing authority requests information which involves a breach of confidentiality. Joan Bailey (1980) suggests that if facing such a dilemma the nurse should seek advice. This could be, for example, from a professional organisation, such as the Rcn or HVA, and especially from the Professional Conduct Division of the UKCC who specialise in matters of confidentiality. Miss Bailey explains that in general it is felt that employers have no legal entitlement to confidential information and that it is therefore wrong for the nurse to provide it.

The Health Visitor Association has drawn up a useful guide on confidentiality (Health Visitor, 1980). Advice is given, for example, on disclosure at case conferences, obtaining clients' permission before handing on infor-mation and how to approach requests to break confidences in a court of law. Peter Godber (1981) said that requests to disclose case notes in court should be contested, and quotes a Court of Appeal decision which protects health visitors from having to surrender them. However, he advised that they should take their notes with them into the courtroom, in order to remind themselves of the facts and give more accurate evidence.

Guidelines on confidentiality are also avail-able from the Royal College of Nursing (1980). There will, however, always be grey areas where it is difficult to be sure what is for the best, and manager and peer group support and, perhaps, contact with the UKCC can clarify ideas and the issues involved.

Open records

Perhaps the best way to ensure having an appropriate and ethically acceptable balance of information, which is neither surprising nor offensive to the families involved and states reasonably clearly what happened at a visit, is to share the content of the records with them. The exercise of going through it together should help to crystallise out key matters. Furthermore, if clients are encour-aged to say what they think should be included from what has been observed, achieved or requested, it represents another move towards true partnership and gives one more opportunity to discover the families' viewpoint.

Shirley Goodwin (1983b) warned that sooner or later there will be legislation enabling people to have right of access to their records. She urges health visitors to think very carefully about what they are writing and its purpose. The Data Protection Bill is being put into force; the DHSS has issued a circular which states the general principles associated with people's rights to see their records in local authority social services departments (Health Visitor, 1983), and a circular is expected in the spring of 1986 on personal health information.

Health visitors can naturally be concerned by the prospect of notes and records, originally expected to remain unseen by their clients, becoming open for them to inspect (Anonymous, 1983). However, if all records are written by health visitors bearing in mind

to what extent they would blush to read them, not only in court but also to the families concerned, it may help them to find an appropriate balance between what is useful and what is invasive and/or offensive.

It has been suggested in this chapter that statements of facts about what has been said, seen and done at a visit are proper to record, and that it should generally be unnecessary to make a note, specifically, of the health visitor's assessment or opinion, particularly over family dynamics and personal details. Three aspects of evaluation—the way clients value the service, health visitors' attempts to assess what they have achieved and numerical measurement of aspects of the work—were considered, as was the use of statistical information in planning priorities. Records, evaluation and confidentiality are distinctly interlinked and are very important aspects of our work.

USEFUL ADDRESSES

United Kingdom Central Council for Nursing, Midwifery and Health Visiting (UKCC)
23 Portland Place,
London W1N 3AF
Tel 01 637 7181

The Royal College of Nursing of the United Kingdom (Rcn)
Henrietta Place,
Cavendish Square,
London W1M 0AB
Tel 01 409 3333

Health Visitors Association (HVA)
36 Eccleston Square,
London SW1 1PF
Tel 10 834 9523

REFERENCES

Anonymous 1983 Patients' access to records (letter). Health Visitor 56:319
Bailey J M 1980 The law and the community nurse. Cumbria Area Health Authority, Carlisle
Carpenter R G, Gardner A, Jepson M, Taylor E M, Salvin A, Sunderland R, Emery J L, Pursall E, Roe J, Sheffield Health Visitors 1983 Prevention of unexpected infant death. The Lancet I: 723–727
Child Development Project 1984 Child development programme. Early Childhood Development Unit, Bristol. p 17–20
Children's Committee 1980 The needs of the under-fives in the family. The Children's Committee, London
Clark J 1983 Evaluating health visiting practice. Health Visitor 56: 205–208
Clark J 1985 Delivering the goods. Nursing Times Community Outlook 81, 2: 23–28
Dingwall R 1977 The social organisation of health visitor training. Croom Helm, London

Dobby J 1984 Research into health visiting effectiveness (letter). Health Visitor 57: 292–293
Godber P 1981 Confidentiality of case records. Health Visitor 54:193
Goodwin S 1983a Caring for the carers. Part 2: Coping with stress. Health Visitor 56: 46–48
Goodwin S 1983b Open secrets. Nursing Mirror 156, 26:22
Green A, Macfarlane A 1985 Parent-held child health record cards—a comparison of types. Health Visitor 58: 14–15
Health Visitor 1980 Guide for health visitors on confidentiality. Health Visitor 53:30
Health Visitor 1983 Disclosing information to clients. Health Visitor 56:355
Hedley C, Grieve L, Hood J, Leyshom Y 1982 Using the need/problem orientated method of record-keeping. Health Visitor 55: 211–215
Hendy A 1983 The nursing process and health visiting. Health Visitor 56: 197–200

Irving D 1985 How to identify the needy. Health and Social Services Journal XCV: 18–19

Lambert C, Miers M, Edwards J, Farrow S 1985 Centralised records—who benefits? A discussion of issues raised by research into pre school developmental screening. Health Visitor 58: 11–13

Luker K 1982 Evaluating health visiting practice. Royal College of Nursing, London

Luker K 1985 Evaluating health visiting practice. In: Luker K, Orr J (eds) Health visiting. Blackwell Scientific Publications, Oxford

Marsden M 1985 Implementing the health visiting process. Health Visitor 58: 166–167

Messenger M 1982 The breastfeeding book. Century Publications Co Ltd, London

Nicholl A 1983 Community child health services—for better or for worse? Health Visitor 56: 241–243

Nicholl A 1984 The value of selective pre-school medicals in an inner city area. Public Health, London 98: 68–72

Nursing Times 1984 How more data can alter priorities. Nursing Times 80, 46:7

O'Connor P J, Willis M 1985 Clerical help for health visitors. Health Visitor 58: 261–262

Orr J 1980 Health visiting in focus. Royal College of Nursing, London

Orr J 1985 Health visiting and the community. In: Luker K, Orr J (eds) Health visiting. Blackwell Scientific Publications, Oxford

Owen C M 1980 Child health record booklet. Midwife Health Visitor and Community Nurse 16: 156–162

Pearson P 1984 Images of a health visitor. Nursing Mirror 159, 19: 21–23

Pearson P 1985 Parent-held records—what parents think. Health Visitor 58: 15–16

Powell J 1985 Keeping watch. Nursing Times Community Outlook 81, 2: 15–19

Robertson C A 1981 An evaluation of screening: an epidemiological approach. Measuring the effectiveness of health visitors. Health Visitor 54: 20–21

Robertson C A 1982 Becoming a health visitor—an obstacle course? Nursing Times 78, 36: 1508–1512

Robinson K 1983 Talking with clients. In: Clark J, Henderson J (eds) Community health. Churchill Livingstone, Edinburgh

Robinson K 1985 Knowledge and its relationship to health visiting. In: Luker K, Orr J (eds) Health visiting. Blackwell Scientific Publications, Oxford

Robinson K 1986 (personal communication)

Robinson J 1982 An evaluation of health visiting. Council for the Education and Training of Health Visitors, London

Rogers J 1982 Introducing the health visiting process. Health Visitor 55: 204–209

Royal College of Nursing 1980 Guidelines on confidentiality in nursing. Royal College of Nursing, London

Saffin K 1985 Card carriers. Nursing Times 81, 13: 24–26

Stanton A 1984 A question of help. Nursing Mirror Community Forum 158, 21: i–iii

Steering Group on Health Services Information (1984) Fifth Report to the Secretary of State. Chairman Mrs E Körner. Department of Health and Social Security, HMSO, London

UKCC 1984 Code of Professional Conduct for the Nurse Midwife and Health Visitor. 2nd edn. United Kingdom Central Council for Nursing, Midwifery and Health Visiting, London. paragraph 9

Whincup M 1981 The duties of a health visitor. Nursing Times 77: 567–568

Wilson M, Cowan J 1982 Putting the health visiting process into practice. Health Visitor 55: 209–211

In Chapter 9, we look at health visiting and handicap, mainly through the perspective of the prevention model, describing in passing important ideas from the Warnock Committee Report. We conclude with two examples of health visiting families who have a handicapped child, one example using the prevention framework and the other the family health needs format.

9

Families with a handicapped child

THE PREVENTION MODEL AND SOME WARNOCK IDEAS

The role of the health visitor is considered in this chapter by using the prevention framework, that is:
— preventing the occurrence of handicap and of later problems if disability is already present. This mainly involves health education and anticipatory guidance
— preventing the development of problems by discovering handicap early, or discovering other aspects of handicap where disabilities are already known to exist. These are important in order to enable timely care to be given
— rehabilitation and containment of the problem and support for the family. This is aimed at prevention of deterioration in the case of established handicap. It involves appropriate support through the emotional crisis and giving information on practical help.

Several ideas from a 1978 governmental report are very relevant to this work. Table 9.1 shows an outline of the prevention framework in this context and indicates where these ideas are particularly useful.

Warnock Report

Some important concepts for health visitors were contained in the Warnock Committee

161

Table 9.1 Health visiting and handicap: prevention framework

Aims	Some activities	Warnock ideas
To prevent occurrence of handicap or later problems	*Health education*: Public: for greater understanding Parents: anticipatory guidance Genetic counselling/abortion Pre- and antenatal care Immunisation: e.g. rubella, polio	Wider concept Partnership with parents
To prevent development through early diagnosis and care	*Surveillance, screening and referral*: Find hearing, vision, neurological problems; refer for assessment Listen to parental fears: act on them Monitor for multiple problems; assess functioning Clear records, share reports with parents:	Early discovery and education and partnership with parents
To prevent deterioration through rehabilitation and containment	*Practical and emotional help*: Support in stress: bereavement; marital tensions; morale boosting Practical advice and information Guidance on services and agencies Tell about voluntary organisations Catalyst for emergent groups Liaison with other professionals	Named Person and partnership with parents

Report. The government published a brief guide (Warnock, 1978) as well as the report itself, a sure sign that it was intended that the ideas in it should be read about and acted upon! Perhaps the four most important ideas for our work were those concerning, firstly, a wider concept of handicap, secondly, early discovery and education, thirdly, parents as partners and, lastly, the notion of a 'named person'.

1. The report proposed that special educational need, not medical disability, should determine the kind of schooling child was given. It pointed out that, taking a wider look at handicap, it could be seen that some 20% of children would need special help at some time in their school career.

It was envisaged that a range of educational provision should be available, including that enabling attendance at normal school backed up by appropriate health services. It was hoped that a more positive approach to handicap would emerge.

2. **and** 3. Early discovery of handicap, early education and the health visitor's part in these were discussed. The Court Report (1976) surveillance recommendations were endorsed, as was the need for parents to be involved in their children's assessment.

The report stressed that there should be a partnership between parents and professionals and that parents need advice, information and practical help in their important role as the main educators of their children.

4. Research undertaken for the Report (Warnock Report, 1978) showed that a very high proportion of parents found it difficult to obtain the advice they needed. It was therefore proposed that a designated Named Person should provide the main point of contact for families where a handicapping condition has been discovered.

As it was found that health visitors were in general the most, sometimes the only, helpful professionals in the early years, they were recommended as the Named Person up to school age. It was suggested that multiprofessional assessment might show another worker in frequent contact with the family to be more appropriate as the Named Person. He/She would, therefore, be designated to this role. Also, arrangements were proposed which would enable parents to ask to be put in touch with another professional, should their designated Named Person prove to be unsatisfactory.

A guide and advocate needed

A designated Named Person is very much needed. Many studies have shown that families caring for handicapped relatives tend not to receive full advice on services and entitlements to which they have a right. Sam Ayer's (1984) three-year study of 132 mothers caring for their severely mentally handicapped children led him to conclude that the current policy of 'community care' meant, in reality, 'institutional care in the community'. Despite the rhetoric, supportive facilities were so poor for these families looking after their own children that 'community care' could not be referring to family care.

Many of the families in Dr Ayer's study did not know about basic services available to help reinforce their efforts to care for their children themselves. High proportions did not know, for example, about a nappy service, home adaptations and the home help service. He said few acute crises are generated by these families' chronic problems of long-term management. It seems social workers do not tend to see them as 'appropriate' or 'deserving' cases. Dr Ayer drew up a checklist, outlined in Box 9.1, which, he suggested, parents and those seeking the welfare of these families could use to evaluate the provision of services locally.

Box 9.1 Community care for families: checklist (From Ayer, 1984)

Services providing reinforcement to help parents to care for their own mentally handicapped children

---

A full range of support from specialist services
Home visits, at least two monthly, by specialist social worker and/or community mental handicap nurse
Regular reports from these visits made available to parents
Short-term relief, counselling, classes etc.
Full information given to parents on statutory services
Priority placement on housing list for these families
Parents' workshops
Full laundry service
Special equipment available
Day care in school holidays

Where there are enough specialist social workers and/or community mental handicap nurses to provide frequent, regular visiting, then the health visitor is unlikely to be nominated the Named Person. These services do not yet seem to be widely available, leaving the health visitor in the main, to speak for and support parents of both physically and mentally handicapped children.

INCREASING AWARENESS

There are two sides to preventing the occurrence of difficulties. One is aimed at preventing the handicap ever happening and the other aims at trying to prevent problems arising out of known disability. We look first at the former and lead on into the latter.

PREVENTING HANDICAP

Aspects of everyday health visiting to do with increasing people's awareness of health needs, play a part in helping prevent handicap, for example in newborn babies. Enabling people to understand the value of vaccination and immunisation, particularly the vaccination against rubella, and public knowledge about the value of, for example, pre-conceptual and antenatal care regarding nutrition, smoking and alcohol, all help to produce healthy, normal babies. Other vaccinations, such as those against measles or polio, help prevent handicap occurring in otherwise healthy people as a consequence of those diseases.

Genetic counselling

A health visitor might tell parents about services that can help prevent handicap. For example, genetic counselling can help prospective parents understand the degree of risk attached to giving birth to a baby with an inherited genetic disorder. People who have a baby with, for example, multiple handicap may, after assessment and diagnosis of the baby's condition, be able to receive guidance about risks regarding future pregnancies. Cousins marrying or parents over 35 years may seek information. It has been suggested that genetic disorders occur in about one in twenty babies born alive (Winter, 1984).

PREVENTING LATER PROBLEMS

Through counselling

A service has been described in which a specialist health visitor was employed to follow up genetic clinic consultation with home visits (Harris & Weetman, 1982). This was done, for example, where it was felt that extra explanations would help people to better understand the risks. It was also given where people were thought to have great anxiety, or where blame seemed to be attributed to a particular member of the family.

Counselling was also undertaken, where necessary, to help parents overcome the problems of bereavement associated with having passed on a damaging gene to their child: the depression, the feelings of guilt and hostility. Follow-up visits were also made for counselling women who have an abortion following amniocentesis. This aspect of the service helps prevent the occurrence of later chronic emotional problems, which could affect the family.

Increased public understanding

Parents can feel shunned by society. Occasionally there may be a chance for health visitors who give talks to women's groups and others to help increase public awareness. They may be able to help engender the wider concept of handicap which enables greater acceptance and equal chance for children with these special needs. In this way, potential problems which many parents suffer over the social stigma attached to having a handicapped child in the family, could to some extent be avoided. The attainment of good public understanding and a caring attitude is

a huge task and health visitors may be able to play some small part in it.

Anticipatory guidance: in general . . . .

The health needs of handicapped children are the same as other children, except for the special requirements associated with their handicap. The families, therefore, may wish to discuss various aspects of, for example, nutrition, hygiene, safety, immunisation, dental care and illness recognition in the same way as families with normal children described in earlier chapters.

Stimulation and play with the baby or young child is one of the subjects that may be discussed between parents and their health visitor. This is classified in this chapter as part of a supportive programme aiming at containment and rehabilitation (see page 173). However, attention has been drawn here to a special consideration within these stimulation programmes.

. . . . and on the attachment process

Studying Down's syndrome children with their mothers, Berger and Cunningham (1983) felt that care has to be taken to prevent a problem occurring over the attachment and bonding between baby and mother. This is not so easy for babies with a difficulty that involves sensory impairment, such as movement disability, mental handicap or blindness. These can present something of an obstacle to the socially important and enjoyable two-way interactions in which parent and baby smile, vocalise, touch and gaze at each other (see Ch. 4, page 60). Furthermore, misinterpretations and interactive failures may lead to negative feelings and avoidance, on both sides, of further attempts towards emotional involvement.

Although slow to begin, Down's babies generally smile and maintain eye contact by about three months. In their small study, Berger and Cunningham found that after that age mothers of Down's babies played with and talked to their babies more often.

However, they did not tend to leave time for their babies to respond, thereby reducing the potential for social interaction. In comparison, mothers with normal babies conducted more two-sided communications.

After experimenting with various interactive approaches, it was found that parents imitating their baby's behaviour most increased the baby's responsiveness and improved parent—baby interaction. Berger and Cunningham concluded that it should be explained to parents that
— although mostly a few weeks delayed, smiling, eye contact and cooing invariably appear
— Down's babies need more time to cope with and to respond to stimulation
— their baby's gaze and eye contact show readiness to interact
— imitating their baby is one possible way of improving their social interaction with their baby.
In this way it is hoped that parents' increased awareness can help prevent the occurrence of problems with their emotional relationship with their baby on which so much depends.

In this section, examples have been given of health visiting work aimed at preventing the occurrence of handicap and of later problems. A wide range of 'normal' health visiting is relevant. It may also be possible to help public understanding of the 'wider concept of handicap'. In helping parents cope with their special needs, perhaps for genetic counselling or regarding bonding and attachment, another Warnock concept is employed by working in 'partnership with parents' to enable the best possible results and prevent the occurrence of later problems.

ON THE LOOK-OUT

The second and third of the Warnock ideas mentioned at the beginning of this chapter feature very strongly in secondary prevention: working in 'partnership with parents' in order to try to achieve 'early discovery and early education' for any incipient potentially handicapping problem. Screening and surveillance procedures and modes of discovery, keeping in touch with the District Child Development Team and good clear records and reports, are all part of this aspect of the work.

DISCOVERY

Only a very small number of handicaps are discovered at birth. For example, only 7 of the 82 handicapped children selected for the Child Study Sample of four-year olds by Chazan et al (1980) were discovered then. These were cases of Down's syndrome and spina bifida. A further 3 children with handicaps were discovered in the following few weeks. In some cases an episode such as an epileptic fit, meningitis or heart failure dramatically heralded the problem.

In most cases, however, a child's handicap reveals itself more slowly. Often the disability is apparent a long time before it becomes a handicap. Chazan et al said parents or professionals notice some aspect of functioning or behaviour which is unusual or absent. When, over time, it does not resolve itself, they become concerned about the implications. Often some triggering event crystallises the parents' or the professional's apprehensions and they decide to seek further advice and assessment. Chazan et al (1980, p. 40) gave an example of a mother who expects her child to say a word by 15 months. As the months go by and no word is spoken she becomes increasingly uneasy until a precipitating factor, such as a neighbour's comment on the child's speechlessness, causes her anxiety level to reach such a peak that she turns to some professional for advice.

Centile charts perform a very useful role in providing the necessary precipitating factor. They are drawn with demarcation lines which show quite clearly at what point a referral for further assessment should be made. Screening and surveillance of babies and young children were looked at in Chapters 5 and 6. We have looked at the importance of following up at home families who find it difficult or prefer not to attend screening clinics in order to discover problems as early as possible. Again centile charts are highly desirable because one can tell at a glance to what extent they have been completed. An additional consideration, once a handicap has been discovered, is the possibility, in some cases the probability, for example of deafness in Down's syndrome, of multiple handicap. The presence of further defects has always to be borne in mind.

Quite a range of handicap, including a high proportion of severely handicapped or disturbed children, was included in the Chazan et al (1980, p. 8) study sample. They investigated who discovered the handicap. 35 of the 82 in this sample had been discovered by professionals and 29 by parents who had then sought advice. In 2 instances, the mothers had been unable to persuade professionals of their children's problem, being dismissed as 'over-fussy' or 'over-anxious'. This highlights yet again the need to listen carefully to parents' views and anxieties. Quite a proportion of the mothers in this study were not fully aware of their child's problem. Many of these were from deprived and difficult circumstances. The 'partnership with parents' does not seem to have been put fully into effect.

An inverse proportion of facilities

A factor well known in health visiting was also highlighted (Chazan et al, 1980, pp. 25–26). The health visitors tended to have around the same sized caseload per head of population. However, some had as many as three times more children with problems than their colleagues working in another district. Added to this, the districts in which there were more problems had fewer facilities available, such as nurseries and playgroups. The researchers pointed out that this meant the health visitors were less able to share the care of these children with other workers and, inevitably, these families were receiving a lower standard of care.

It seems that in some cases, post-war housing policies had led to a very large number of children with problems being concentrated in a comparatively small area. This situation is reminiscent of Sue Phillips' (1986) problem. She was permitted, indeed encouraged, to spend time and effort acting as a 'catalyst', helping to create a much needed family centre which included day care and play facilities. This response to community need was successful, both in itself and from a health visiting point of view. Sue Phillips remarked, however, that in a health authority in which a daily quota of visits must be completed, there would not have been time for this sort of work. The community's needs would remain unmet.

ASSESSMENT OF FUNCTIONING

This screening and surveillance aspect of health visiting is much more than just discovering potential problems and handing them on for assessment, diagnosis and treatment. Discovery of handicap has significant implications for the family and the child. The question arises as to how to attain the best possible functioning for the child, how the handicap affects functioning and, from that, what special needs the family and child may have. Chazan et al's Screening Schedule Two, outlined in Table 9.2, can be a useful tool in thinking, with the parents, about the overall situation they currently face. The Schedule looks at five main behavioural areas, each aspect of which carries ratings on a five point scale ranging from normal functioning to severe handicap.

This sort of assessment, combined with problem oriented and detailed planning similar to that demonstrated by Barber and Kratz (1980), could provide a very useful basis from which to set the problems and planning in perspective. Barber and Kratz showed in a case study how the situation facing a family with a severely handicapped baby could be set out in the SOAP format. Immediate problems concerning the management and develop-

Table 9.2 Scheme for measuring functioning

Behaviour	Aspect
Sensory-motor	Locomotion
	Use of hands
	Vision
	Hearing
	Hand/eye coordination
Self-help	Feeding
	Toileting
	Dressing
	Competence around the house
Language	Expressive language
	Speech articulation
	Receptive language
	Listening to stories
Modes of activity	Level of activity
	Restlessness
	Constructiveness/destructiveness
Social, emotional and behavioural adjustment	Cooperation with adults
	Dependence
	Aggression
	Withdrawal
	Reactions to stress of deviant behaviour

From Chazan et al (1980, Appendix A)

ment of the baby, physical, emotional and social concerns regarding the mother, emotional problems for the father and problems the parents shared, were listed. Incipient environmental problems associated with long-term care, the baby's death and subsequent offspring, were covered separately. The functioning of the family and the child is inevitably a dynamic and changing process and therefore needs frequent review.

District child development team

The need for multiprofessional involvement and regular review was emphasised in the Court Report (1976). It recommended the setting up of more District Handicap Teams. Dr Christie (1986) has outlined the work of District child development teams, which in some areas provide the clinical and operational functions recommended for the District Handicap Team. These were:
— investigation and assessment
— to arrange for coordinated treatment

— to provide professional advice for parents and professionals involved in the care of the family
— a source of information on handicap and services available
— a training role.

Catriona Rouf (1983) argued that parents should be active participants of the care group, that they be told what is wrong with their baby and be involved in planning the care. She feels professional secrecy places an extra burden on the parents, leaving them feeling that they are without emotional or practical support.

Records and reports

Health visitors who do not attend the child development centre sessions may well need to write reports for the team. Sharing the information in the report or planning the contents of it with the parents, can make a contribution towards their involvement and their understanding of their baby. Parents now have a right to have a copy of any advice, information and evidence used in the Education Authority's Statement of Special Educational Needs (Health Visitors Association, 1985). Health visitors' records, including those of assessment and referral, are likely, therefore, to be available to the parents as of right.

Inform education authorities

The implications of the Education Act, 1981, concerning the rights of parents over information about the special educational needs of their child, their rights to assessment when their child is under two years and the Health Authority's statutory obligation to inform the Education Authority when the child is over two, are described by Dr Macfarlane (1985). He explained the parents' rights to participate fully at all stages of the subsequent assessment procedure and about their right to appeal if they do not agree with the final statement by the Education Authority.

In this section we have taken a wide look at aspects of screening and surveillance in the health visiting care of families with a young handicapped baby or child.

PRACTICAL AND EMOTIONAL SUPPORT

The Warnock concept of 'parents as partners' has been highlighted in the earlier two sections: it is just as important with regard to helping parents attain the best possible life for their child with these special needs and for the family as a whole, despite the handicap. The parents need to have someone to whom they can turn, a 'Named Person', to help them find and sort out information about available services and agencies which will enable containment and rehabilitation of the problems they face. They need that person, too, to act in liaison with these agencies, and also to care and give support with bereavement counselling, morale boosting and optimism in order to overcome emotional problems.

EMOTIONAL SUPPORT

Knowing how it feels

It is impossible for professional workers who have not, themselves, had a handicapped child to truly understand what it feels like. Some idea of the emotions involved can, however, be gleaned from books written by people who do know. There are, for example, two books about having given birth to a Down's syndrome baby. One tells of parents who decided they did not wish to take their baby home (Milne, 1982). The other described the circumstances and the parents' feelings surrounding the nine months their baby lived. The good times as well as the grief and the shock were described (Boston, 1981).

Personal experience provided a very sound basis from which Helen Featherstone (1980) was able to write about the anger, fear, loneliness, guilt and self-doubt which people can feel. She described too how these emotions and the burdens of physically coping can impose strains on the marriage. The emotions associated with visiting a severely handicapped son in hospital and the importance of the staff's attitude and approach were outlined in a short article by J E Dean (1982).

The bereavement process

Informing the parents

The experience of being told about their child's handicap is one which lasts in the parents' memory. It has been recommended that they should be told:
— the simple facts
— as soon as possible
— together
— in a quiet room
— by the consultant
— with a specialist health visitor in attendance.
The health visitor is then able to provide continuity, enabling further explanations and questions to be answered as necessary and providing the link with community services (Gath, 1985).

Know thyself

We have already looked in Chapter 7 at some aspects of bereavement counselling including the feelings of inadequacy that people can have when trying to help those who are grieving and the need for personal adjustment on attitudes towards death. Ann Fillmore (1981) has described how some professionals find it difficult to come to terms with their own grief and, consequently, are unable to advise their patients appropriately. Being inadequately aware of their own, and not facing up to their patients' natural reactions of sorrow, guilt, anger and need for acceptance of their own mortality, can lead them into using evasive tactics. This might result in, for example, a doctor refusing to allow parents to be informed about the terminality of their child's condition. This, in turn, can lead to emotional difficulties in the family which the health visitor will have to find some ingenious way of sorting out.

Giving support

Ann Gath (1985) and Yvonne Heavyside (1985) have discussed the stages of grief with regard to families with a handicapped baby. Yvonne Heavyside quoted a model of the various phases of the bereavement process, which maps out the way these phases manifest themselves and the way that the parents need, and can be given, help as each stage is reached. She also pointed out that it is important for nurses to:

— touch and handle the baby
— say something nice about the baby
— boost parents' morale regarding their ability to handle their baby
— respect parents wishes if they do not wish to discuss their feelings
— answer questions simply
— admit it if they do not know any answer and find out who does
— encourage hopefulness and optimism
— encourage assertiveness in the parents.

Most parents are likely to have to insist on their rights at some point on behalf of their child. The way that parents are able to cope, as with other critical life experiences such as the birth of a first child or adjusting to unemployment, is influenced by their emotional background and personality. Some people are more vulnerable than others. What has been shown, however, is that the optimism associated with early intervention programmes in which parents are involved, working with a trained home visitor to stimulate their baby, is emotionally beneficial. These programmes have a morale boosting effect (Gath, 1985) and can do much to alleviate depression, common amongst these mothers (Burden, 1980).

Studies of marriage breakdown related to having a handicapped child seem to indicate that it may be the early emotional trauma rather than the 'wear and tear' of looking after a difficult child that cause the marital tensions and later breakdown (Gath, 1985). It is also possible that parents of Down's syndrome babies fare better, on average, than parents of other sorts of severely educationally subnormal children (Gath, 1985) and tend to make a good

emotional adjustment (Murdoch & Ogston, 1984). The research is inconclusive at the moment, but is providing some indicators.

Morale boosting and reassurance using video

In North Devon, five videos were produced for parents of handicapped children at the various stages of their child's development and their emotional adjustment (Walker, 1984). The videos are concerned with:
— reassuring parents that help is at hand
— the child's right to lead as normal a life as possible
— the effects of stress on marriage and the siblings
— special needs in the child's development and education
— what will happen when the parents are too old to cope.

Support literature is left with the parents which reinforces the reassuring information in the video. The videos had first to be tested and then were to be made available to other health authorities at a nominal cost. The problems raised in these programmes are all touching on areas about which parents may have many questions and which they may wish to discuss with their health visitor. Having someone who is prepared to listen and let them think through their worries and feelings can help dispel anxieties, help them work through the grieving process and prevent pathological consequences.

Emotional support cannot really be separated from practical support which, in itself, offers optimism through involvement, explanations and concrete assistance. For the parents to feel cared for, any help offered needs to be given in response to what the parents themselves see as important.

PRACTICAL INFORMATION AND ASSISTANCE

Finding out

Parents become the experts on their handicapped child, but not without help. If the health visitor does not have a good knowledge of the condition and of the services and aids that pertain to the particular family needs encountered, then it is important to take steps to find out about them. The proportion of handicaps within any given caseload is very small. In addition to this, even within a given diagnosis, the nature of each individual child's circumstances can be very different. Generalist health visitors, therefore, cannot be expected to be fully informed on any particular handicapping condition that they might meet, nor, of course, the many variations within it.

The need then, is to find people and agencies who can give guidance. Perhaps the first people to turn to should be the

— specialist health visitor, if there is one
— consultant paediatrician or other specialist in charge of the case, for up-to-date and accurate information
— medical librarian, for appropriate literature
— health visiting nurse manager, for moral support!

Agencies that may be able to give some help are organisations such as the National Children's Bureau, the Voluntary Council for Handicapped Children and library services such as 'Help for Health' (see Ch. 2, p. 18). Robert Gann (1986) gives some good leads in his book about resources available for self-care. He has a section which gives information about the wide range of health care directories and journals which publish information on the statutory and voluntary services available. He provides a brief synopsis of the contents of each directory and source mentioned.

There are another two books that show families with special needs and their health visitors how to find help. One is the Mental Health Foundation's wide-ranging directory of around 10 000 self-help and community support agencies throughout the British Isles (Webb, 1985). These organisations are classified and listed according to the sort of problems that people may have. By using the key coding at the foot of each page a great deal of information can be learned about local

groups and agencies. The other book is the Disability Rights Handbook (The Disability Alliance, 1985), which is revised every year to produce up-to-date, comprehensive guidance on the rights, benefits and services available to disabled people.

It is worth searching round, too, for books written for parental guidance. There are, for example, the constructive and positively written books that help parents of Down's syndrome children. There is one that helps parents have a better understanding of the implications of their child's condition for themselves and their child (Cunningham, 1982), and others that help them give their child a helping hand (Cunningham & Sloper, 1978; Brinkworth & Collins, 1973).

There are also books available for parents who have children with other sorts of handicap. For example, there are two based on a behavioural approach: one group oriented, concentrating on communication with the child (Newson & Hipgrave, 1982), and the other providing more of a step-by-step guide to everyday problems (Carr, 1980).

In Griffiths and Russell's (1985) book, there are explanations of broad classifications of problems such as

— disorders of motor development
— visual handicap
— communication disorders
— special learning difficulties
— mental handicap
— multiple handicap

as well as explanations of assessment and 'parents as partners', which parents might find informative.

Taking another perspective, Diana Millard's (1984) book gives brief explanations of conditions such as

— cleft palate
— dislocation of the hips
— talipes
— cerebral palsy
— limb deficiency
— muscular dystrophy
— epilepsy
— diabetes
— cystic fibrosis

and describes practical ideas for coping with the everyday life of a handicapped child. In this book, recommended reading lists are provided for the child, for the parents and for the professional helper. Most of the books for parents have lists of useful addresses, providing, too, of course, useful guidance for professionals as well as the parents.

One book written for professionals working with developmentally handicapped children makes an excellent reference book for health visitors. Zelle and Coyner (1983) have provided a wealth of information on assessment and intervention for these children's first two years of life. Dipping into the appropriate sections may enable a better background understanding of the philosophy and the aims and purpose of the work.

Rights to information

Parents now have a statutory right to know about voluntary organisations that are able to give them advice and assistance (Macfarlane, 1985). The Named Person will need to make sure this information is given. A widely available introductory booklet is the Voluntary Council for Handicapped Children's (Russell, 1976), which lists some of the organisations that can help, and gives a brief overview of services available. Many Community Health Councils now produce a booklet which describes local facilities and organisations such as the one produced by Southampton and South West Hampshire Community Health Council (1979). Health visitors may also find it useful to have available the latest DHSS pamphlets that explain the rights to attendance allowances from the age of 2 (Roberts, 1983) and mobility allowances on reaching the age of 5 years.

Rights regarding assessment and education under the 1981 Education Act are explained in booklets written for the Advisory Centre for Education (Newell, 1983; Newell & Potts, 1984). They provide parents with a guide to various aspects of the Act, give tips, for example, on how to request assessment and appeal against decisions, suggest how letters might be written and, generally, help parents to be assertive and attain the services that they feel are most appropriate for their child.

Informal support

Groups

One in every three self-help groups is started with close cooperation with professionals (Robinson, 1978). Health visitors can quite often assume a catalytic role. Also, there is a need for some background support: this is hardly surprising as there are several inherent difficulties. Judy Wilson (1982) pointed out that they are generally organised and run by people who have problems in common with the members. This can present problems to the group because a leader with obligations to care for an ill child may, for example, suddenly have to cancel an evening with the group.

In many cases, members have not been 'joiners' before and may suffer, somewhat, from lack of experience in running a group. Added to this, the group is used as a stepping stone back to normal life, so that people are liable to leave when their situation has improved rather than stay on as lifelong members. Judy Wilson's research led her to feel that support for groups being set up is very important.

Research in general shows that around half of the parents with disabled children belong to a group. Cooke & Lawton (1984), however, found that considerably fewer than half of the 400 families with 10-year-old handicapped children they studied belonged to such a group. They pointed out that this finding matches a tendency found in another study of decline in membership after the child reaches six years of age. Parents who were members seem to have found them helpful. This was, however, mostly for the emotional support and practical advice they could give. Very few had received financial or practical help.

Friends and family

It is interesting to note that informal support

from friends, neighbours and family was found *not* to help on a day-to-day basis, but might help at a time of crisis. Babysitting was a problem for parents with severely handicapped children. It seems relatives and friends can be 'non-plussed' by the complexity of the problems involved, making parents unwilling to leave them. In effect, the informal support was found to be no greater for the families with severely than for those with mildly disabled children.

Cooke and Lawton found, too, that it was the mothers who bore the main burden of responsibility. Fathers were found to give help, where it was given, with child care and minding rather than with housework. There was a tendency for them to help even less where the child was severely handicapped. Baldwin and Glendinning (1983) also found women bore the brunt. The care of the handicapped children lessened their chances of returning to work which would have provided social and psychological benefits away from 'the daily grind'. Also these mothers were less able to subsidise the family income and help compensate for the increased costs associated with the care of a severely handicapped child.

Fellow feeling

Some people find that it is very reassuring to meet another family with a child with special needs similar to theirs. It can lessen the feeling of isolation and make it possible to find someone who is able to listen with empathy, without necessarily having to join and attend a group.

Health visitors are sometimes able to put people with unusual and obscure complaints in touch with each other through an information column in the Health Visitor journal. Dunning et al (1986) are concerned that the variation in disorders and in the way they affect people, might lead to a mismatch between people and cause distress. They suggest that health visitors contact their Regional Genetic Counselling Centre to enquire about families with similar problems who would be willing to be put in touch with

their family. Whether or not people do, in fact, need to be protected from meeting a variation of their problem, the genetic counselling service does provide a useful link.

Providing services and advice

The Named Person, or the person acting as such, should ensure that parents are offered all services to which they are entitled and any relevant advice. The aim is to help them increase the functioning of their child and the family as a whole to the best possible extent, in order to live as normal a life for them all as can be attained. This means, for example, helping parents find out about mobility aids and entitlements (Tarling, 1985; Nursing, 1985; Stevens, 1985), offering them respite care—before a crisis occurs, and, perhaps, working out with them their child's current functional needs so that appropriate services and advice can be offered. Sadly, many families have been found to have been inadequately advised and provided for (Ayer, 1984; Chazan et al, 1980, p. 101; Disabled Living Foundation, 1979, p. 43–55). Bathing, dressing, mobility and feeding are but a few of the problems that may be encountered and require habilitation.

Assignment of responsibility

A study by Gillian Parker (1984a) of the provision of incontinence services for handicapped children showed that the adequacy of the provision of services varied with the organisational structure of the community health services. In the districts in which the health visitor or the health visitor and subsequently the school nurse, had sole responsibility for the service, the service was properly provided. Where responsibility was divided between various people, it was much poorer.

Another factor was whether the service was offered spontaneously by the nurse or health visitor, as people hesitate to ask. Lack of knowledge of the service was the main reason for non-take up of the service. Gillian Parker (1984b) also found that advice tended to be inadequate on what steps parents could take towards improved continence for their child. Many did not realise, until their child started school, that an improvement could have been possible before. She thought that the Portage type of programmes would alert health visitors to just what could be achieved.

Pre-school training

Health visitors seem to enjoy being involved in Portage and other pre-school training programmes aimed at improving the child's abilities (Mansell, 1981; Cunningham et al, 1982; Cameron, 1982). Also, the programmes seem to engender positive feelings in the mothers taking part (Sloper et al, 1983). Sloper et al were a little apprehensive lest the mothers become dependent upon the visiting therapist and afraid to do what they feel is intuitively right. Another fact that emerged was that in some cases parents seemed to feel that the more effort they put into the programme, the more their child would improve. The fallacy of this was mentioned earlier in the chapter, in discussion about the need to aim for good interactional processes (see pp. 164–165). Sloper et al felt that perhaps more emphasis should have been put on explaining the interaction of maturational, environmental and inherent factors on the potential for development, and on teaching the underlying philosophy. This approach would aim at helping the parents understand, not only what to do, but more importantly why they are doing it. An overview of the sort of work undertaken in Portage schemes and the way it is planned, has been provided by Cameron et al (1984) whilst replying to what they felt were 14 criticisms of the system.

LIAISON

There may be many people involved in the care of a family with a handicapped child, particularly in the first year or so. There may be, for example, many visits to clinics, hospital and various agencies. The travelling can be costly and the experiences mentally exhausting. There is a great deal to be gained from liaison between the various people involved in this care, in order to successfully establish a coordinated service aimed at minimising, as far as possible, the confusion and trauma for parents.

It is best if the health visitor meets and knows, by name, the main people involved with the family. It might be possible to get to know several, for example, at a meeting of the District child development team. There may be, for example, a community physiotherapist (Sutcliffe, 1980), a social worker or community mental handicap nurse (Simon, 1981; Williams, 1980) alongside whom the health visitor might be working. Perhaps the most important professional to contact, preferably in the first instance in person, is the local specialist most involved with the family. This cooperation can provide two-way benefits: on one side, up-to-date and accurate information about diagnosis and treatment; and on the other, feedback for the specialist (assuming the family's permission is given) on how the family members are coping and what problems they are meeting.

Specialist or generalist?

Having researched the subject, the Disabled Living Foundation (1979, p. 63) found it could not prove the case either for or against specialist health visitors. However, it felt that overloaded generalist health visitors coping with a caseload of, perhaps, 7000 people would not have time to give adequate attention to families with a severely handicapped child. If they did give that time, then other work would have to be skimped.

Some of the arguments in favour, on the one hand of a generalist health visitor and on the other, of a specialist, are shown in Box 9.2. These families with a handicapped child face many problems. Some of them are outlined in a family health needs model in Boxes 9.3 and 9.4. Whoever looks after them, they need time and attention. Melinda Firth (1982) has made suggestions as to how

Box 9.2 Generalist or specialist? Arguments in favour of both

	Generalist health visitor	Specialist health visitor
EARLY DAYS	Useful in the early days, when there is non-acceptance of handicap, by parents. HV visits everyone, therefore acceptable: not stigmatising	Prolonged and repeated visits in initial period: parents need intensive help then, to prevent later problems.
	Can monitor children not yet officially diagnosed, only suspected	Assuming service adequately funded, more free to provide service
	Involved very soon after birth, where diagnosis immediate: probably met antenatally; already known where condition discovered later	Particularly useful in inner city work, where crises more common and normal HV overstretched
LIAISON	Better liaison with primary health care team, for example over parental need for counselling, information and support	May be better able to coordinate, cooperate with and alert other services on a broader front, for example physiotherapy, psychotherapy, special aids, adaptations and voluntary organisations
	In contact with 'normal' families living locally, who may offer moral support and invite to 'normal' mothers and baby group, etc	May be able to work more closely with District Child Development Centre Team
EXPERTISE	Avoids 'expertosis' as HV and parent learn together—parent in control, with HV helping to find out sources of information and appropriate help	Learns from previous experience and special training: can build up special skills and knowledge
	Can maintain contact with other professionals involved—an advantage if HV able to attend relevant Child Development Centre sessions, with parents there, decision-making	Can share knowledge with and train other HVs
		Especially useful where problems complex

generalist health visitors might be able to give an improved service to these families, for example, through training, information and reduced caseloads. Generally, health visitors with a specialist post tend to favour that approach (Disabled Living Foundation, 1979; Twinn, 1981). Cunningham et al (1982) said that where a highly motivated generalist health visitor continued to call when a specialist health visitor was visiting to help with training, this combination gave the most satisfactory service.

Whichever way, be it specialist, generalist or both, if the area carries a high level of problems and a low level of staffing, then the service is going to be spread too thinly to be effective. In this situation, health visitors need to keep their managers informed and up to date, not only on what they are able to achieve, but also on what they cannot.

This chapter has considered the work of the health visitor regarding families who have a handicapped child. Using the prevention model as a framework, we looked firstly at health education aimed at preventing the occurrence of handicap and, when it has occurred, at preventing the occurrence of later problems. Secondly, there was screening and surveillance aimed at early diagnosis and care to prevent the development of incipient problems. The third aspect was practical and emotional help aimed at rehabilitation and containment of the problems in the case of known disability or difficulty. The relevance of some of the concepts of the Warnock Report were included. Two examples follow, the first uses the family health needs framework from Box 9.4 and 9.5 and the second, the prevention format.

EXAMPLES OF WORK WITH FAMILIES WITH HANDICAPPED CHILDREN

The first example uses the family health needs framework (see Box 9.5) in outlining a health visitor's thinking on the way to visit a family recently informed of their child's diagnosis.

Box 9.3 A family with a handicapped baby: health needs of parents

Environmental	Mental/emotional	Social aspects
Adequate housing e.g. for safety and mobility	**Emotional** *support*	*Overcome potential isolation*: Meet other person (s) with similar problem e.g. local self-help group or National organisations or through special introduction
Financial support: (extra costs of handicapped child and one parent less able to work)	Parents *told together* about handicap and follow-up at home (by GP?) and given chance to hear again what forgotten from initial interview	*Time as normal family*: Home help service Babysitting (volunteer) Ability to have normal holidays—respite care
Knowledge of *benefits and entitlements*–when attendance and mobility allowances become due and extra sources such as Rowntree Family Fund	Feel people prepared to *listen, and care*; encouragement to express anger, grief, resentment, guilt (these feelings likely to result in marital tensions)	*Overcome feeling of social stigma* Acceptance by relatives and friends
Encouragement to claim these entitlements	*Regular visits*: professional awareness of crisis periods e.g. when anticipated attainments are not achieved	*Develop own interests* Especially the mother, perhaps opportunity to return to work
Knowledge of aids and equipment e.g. clothing, bedding, laundry, fares, adaptations	*Chance to talk* about worries about future	Encouragement to be *forceful*: In order to gain entitlements and supportive services
Physical	**Knowledge** of condition and equipment, also training available, medical needs, including likelihood of surgery, etc.	
Overcome tiredness—extra time and effort taken by care of baby, hospital appointments, etc.—home help?	Help with sorting out confusion of advice	
Knowledge about hoists and mobility and other aids, to help with *physical management*	*Preparatory knowledge* about dressing, feeding, sleeping, toilet training etc.	
Genetic counselling re further children, if relevant	*Confidence* to follow own initiative on care of baby/child	

Box 9.4 A family with a handicapped baby or child: some health needs of the children

Physical	Mental/emotional	Social aspects
Handicapped baby/child		
Play and fun:	*Loving home*: to be accepted and without overprotection	*Normal absences from parents* Acceptable babysitter Play and fun and satisfactory relationship with siblings, other children, grandparents, other relatives
Programme of exercises and/or activities appropriate to developmental attainments—stimulating but not overwhelming	Attachment—allowed enough time to respond and take part in two-way interaction: time to respond to stimuli	
Access to toys e.g. from Toy Library	*Overcome effects of separation* e.g. hospitalisation and respite care	Arrangements to be made for later access to playgroup or nursery class, if required
Regular developmental assessment and hearing, vision, communication, and measurements of head, length/height, and weight	Play and fun and sleep, general behaviour, etc–approach as appropriate	*Notification* to Education Authority
Special care according to need: e.g. Down's—skin, chest, extra vitamin supplement		*Approach*: 'potential ability' not disability; special needs not 'handicap'
Safety relevant to developmental attainment level		
	Siblings	
	Attention of parents (and professionals)	*Access to normal family life* with parents–outings, holidays
	Discussion with parents regarding family tensions (due to anger, frustration and grief associated with adjustment to handicap)	Respite from extra household duties (especially caring older sister)
		May feel social stigma re handicap: needs acceptance by friends and ability to bring them home

Box 9.5 Example one; the Firth family

Environmental	Mental/emotional	Social aspects
Parents Financial support: knowledge of benefits and entitlements Encouragement to claim the entitlements (high costs + mother less able to work)	Emotional support: parents told: follow up by Dr Green and regular visits by HV Encouragement to express anger, grief, resentment and guilt (feelings likely to result in marital tensions) and to talk about worries about future	Overcome potential isolation: meet other people with similar problem, perhaps through Cystic Fibrosis Research Trust Overcome feeling of social stigma re coughing and smelly stools: acceptance by relatives and friends: support group may help with ideas
Physical Genetic conselling re further children, if relevant, and for emotional support		
Children: Paul Continued assessment, especially of measurements of height and weight, to monitor rate of disease Special care re physiotherapy, diet and supplements.? chemotherapy	Loving home: to be accepted and as others, without overprotection Overcome effects of separation through hospitalisaton	Arrangements for nursery, if required Approach: 'potential ability', not disability Notification to Education Authority
	Anne Attention of parents, to minimise jealousy over extra attention to brother	Access to normal family life with parents—outings and holidays Meet other families with CF through Cystic Fibrosis Research Trust

The second, outlined using the 'prevention' approach (see Box 9.6), is about some aspects of work with a family with a Down's syndrome child.

EXAMPLE ONE: THE FIRTH FAMILY

On her way to visit the Firth family, Heather Vaughan (HV) thought about some of the special needs that the family now had. Their 4-year-old daughter, Anne, who now attended playgroup, was in full health. However, their 2-year-old son, Paul, had just been confirmed as a case of early cystic fibrosis.

Fortunately, the District used centile charts for weight, height and head measurements, and so the gradual move towards the 3rd centile (in spite of a good appetite) was easy to monitor. Frequent pungent smelling stools and then some chest infections caused HV to refer the matter to the GP before the measurements dropped below the 3rd centile. It would be necessary to continue the monitoring of Paul's growth. This was now likely

to be mainly undertaken during, what would probably be, frequent visits to the hospital.

Paul would now be on a special fat-restricted, high calorie and protein diet with enzyme and vitamin supplements, physiotherapy and, possibly, antibiotics. His parents had a great deal of learning and work ahead of them. The health visitor intended to tell Mrs Firth about the Cystic Fibrosis Research Trust if she did not already know of it. The secretary of the local branch had been very helpful when HV had phoned. She had described the sort of information and emotional support the Trust was able to give. Ms Vaughan intended to tell the Firths what had been said and how they could contact the Trust if they should wish to.

In due course, HV would check that the Firths were aware of the benefits and allowances to which they might be entitled, and she would encourage them to take them up. However, just at the moment it was the need to listen, should Mrs Firth wish to talk about how she felt, that was likely to take greatest priority at the visit. At the most recent meeting of the primary health care team, talking about emotional adjustment Dr Green had said that the parents had been told

Box 9.6 Example two: the Edwards family

Aims	Some activities
To prevent occurrence of handicap or later problems	*Health education*: Public: joint discussion at local Women's Institute—Mrs Edwards, HV and GP Parents: anticipatory guidance as for all children, but especially on stimulation and on two-way communication for bonding Information about genetic counselling service; amniocentesis and abortion discussed
To prevent development through early diagnosis and care	*Surveillance, screening and referral*: Monitored for multiple problems; listened to parental fears and acted upon them; assessed especially for vision and hearing—teaching parents how (GP: heart, respiratory and endocrine disease) Assessed developmental progress and functioning Records and reports shared with parent—information for education authority
To prevent deterioration through rehabilitation and containment	*Practical and emotional help*: Support: active listening in bereavement phases, morale boosting, too Practical advice and information, e.g. financial entitlements and nappy service Information about voluntary organisation able to give advice and support: Down's Children's Association—accompanied mother to clinic Help due to special training in Portage scheme Contact with District Child Development team

the diagnosis by the consultant. Dr Green had known the date of the appointment and had visited the mother at home the next day in order to answer her queries and to show his concern.

The health visitor had a copy of 'Help starts here' in her pocket, but she would gauge the extent to which Mrs Firth was accepting the handicap before she produced it. It might be better to give it at the following visit. She knew Dr Green had not mentioned genetic counselling. That service would probably be able to provide

good emotional support. This was another point HV would mention either at this meeting or the next one, perhaps the following week.

There would be the matter of notifying the education Authority and, perhaps, arranging for a special nursery place, depending on the extent of any special needs. In order to be helpful to the mother, it would be important for HV to know just how much Paul's handicap was likely to affect his functioning and how, over time, he was, in fact, progressing. She had already made an appointment to see the consultant and expected to be in touch by telephone from time to time.

The health visitor could not help hoping that the couple would contact the Trust. She felt it was likely to be the best source of guidance, for example over jealousy by Anne and other problems associated with the great amount of attention that Paul would be getting. From the telephone conversation HV thought, too, that their approach would be optimistic and positive. She arrived on the doorstep a little apprehensive, partly in case some of the anger inevitably associated with bereavement processes would be directed at herself, and partly in case she misread some of Mrs Firth's feelings and wishes at this very difficult time.

EXAMPLE TWO: THE EDWARDS FAMILY

Honor Vincent (HV) had enjoyed seeing Amanda Edwards playing amongst the children at the playgroup she had just been visiting. It seemed she was presenting the staff with no particular problems. A Down's syndrome child, she was progressing well and clearly benefited from the stimulus provided by the other children.

After the early stages of grief over the handicap her mother had gone 'all out' for acceptance by the community. Mrs Edwards had been very keen to arrange a panel discussion session at the local Women's Institute on handicap and had asked HV and the GP to join her. It had been quite a success. They had talked in depth about the early days, the inevitable bereavement, grief for the loss of the expected normal child, and Hilda Edwards had been embarrassingly glowing about the professional support at that time. The Cunningham books had been found particularly reassuring and encouraging. Mrs Edwards had described how she had tried to encourage her daughter to do things, but only at her own rate, and to concentrate on two-way communication between them as they played.

The Women's Institute session was rather symbolic, in a way, of the fact that the HV, GP and mother had worked together as a team. For example, explaining about genetic counselling had been shared between HV and the GP. The mother had taken an active part with HV in monitoring for possible defects, in particular, hearing, vision and developmental assessment. Dr Smith had regularly checked for heart and endocrine disorder and, fortunately, there had been none. Hilda Edwards had been worried about hearing, and the yearly visits to the audiometry clinic had paid off: significant deafness had been discovered at this most recent visit and arrangements were under way for a grommet operation in the near future.

When they had been assessing Amanda's progress, HV had always shown Hilda Edwards the records as she wrote them up. She also showed the mother reports, such as the ones for the Education Department, so she should be informed on exactly what was being said and could contribute her opinion. There was no doubt that she had become the expert on her own child and that the help from the Down's Children's Association had played a significant part in that. Also, the emotional support from the

local branch had been invaluable. A mother with an older Down's syndrome child had accompanied Hilda Edwards to the clinic to see her through the embarrassment she had felt in those early days, and a very good friendship had developed. They now frequently baby-sat for each other.

Amanda had been somewhat slow in becoming continent, so the Edwards had decided to take up the nappy service. However, toilet training was now being so successful they had just cancelled the supplies.

When she had visited the family soon after the birth of the baby, HV had felt remarkably ignorant and useless from a practical point of view, with nothing but a textbook knowledge of Down's syndrome. Fortunately, she had been able to attend a Portage scheme course and it had been fun working with the mother on it. They had both attended the District Handicap Team clinic sessions when Amanda was assessed. Liaison and teamwork had worked very well, both at this level and, of course, with the primary health care team.

Mrs Vincent wondered, as she walked back to her car, whether arrangements would be made, as the Edwards wished, for Amanda to attend their local school. She hoped so. Anyway, they knew how to appeal against any decision they felt unjust.

USEFUL ADDRESS

National Children's Bureau
8 Wakeley Street
London ECIV 7QE
Tel 01 278 9441

REFERENCES

Ayer S 1984 Handicapped children in the community. Nursing Times 80, 37: 66–69

Baldwin S, Gendinning C 1983 Employment, women and their disabled children. In: Finch J, Groves D (eds) A Labour of Love: Women, Work and Caring. Routledge & Kegan Paul, London

Barber J H, Kratz C R 1980 Towards Team Care. Churchill Livingstone, Edinburgh: p 93–99

Berger J, Cunningham C 1983 Early interactions between infants with Down's syndrome and their parents. Health Visitor 56: 58–60

Boston S 1981 Will, My Son. The life and death of a mongol child. Pluto Press, London

Brinkworth R, Collins J E 1973 Improving babies with Down's syndrome and introducing them to school. National Society for Mentally Handicapped Children, Belfast

Burden R L 1980 Measuring the effects of stress on the mothers of handicapped infants: must depression always follow? Child: care, health and development 6: 111–125

Cameron R J (ed) 1982 Working Together. Portage in the UK. NFER-Nelson, Windsor

Cameron R, Chambers G, Martin S 1984 What is wrong with Portage? Health Visitor 57: 142–144

Carr J 1980 Helping your handicapped child. A step-by-step guide to everyday problems. Penguin, London

Chazan M, Laing A F, Bailey S M, Jones G 1980 Some of our children. The early education of children with special needs. Open Books, London

Christie P N 1986 Management of the handicapped child. Midwife Health Visitor and Community Nurse 22: 67–69

Cooke K, Lawton D 1984 Informal support for the carers

of disabled children. Child: care, health and development 10: 67–79

Court Report 1976 Report of the Committee on Child Health Services, Fit for the future. Cmnd 6684. HMSO, London

Cunningham C 1982 Down's syndrome. An introduction for parents. Souvenir Press, London

Cunningham C C, Aumonier M E, Sloper P 1982 Health visitor support for families with Down's syndrome infants. Child: care, health and development 8: 1–19

Cunningham C, Sloper P 1978 Helping your handicapped baby. Souvenir Press, London

Dean J E 1982 Communication between professionals and parents of handicapped children. Nursing Times 78:1371

The Disability Alliance 1985 Disability rights handbook for 1985. The Disability Alliance's guide to benefits and services for all people with disabilities. The Disability Alliance, London

Disabled Living Foundation 1979 The specialised health visitor for the handicapped baby, young child and school child. A report. Disabled Living Foundation, London

Dunning J A, Mueller R F, Smithells R W 1986 Information wanted (letter). Health Visitor 59:29

Featherstone H 1980 A difference in the family. Life with a disabled child. Harper and Row, London

Fillmore A 1981 The dying child and professional withdrawal. Health Visitor 54: 328–330

Firth M 1982 How good is professional support following a diagnosis of mental handicap? Health Visitor 55: 215–220

Gann R 1986 Health information handbook: resources for self care. Gower Press, Aldershot

Gath A 1985 Parental reactions to loss and disappointment: the diagnosis of Down's syndrome. Developmental Medicine & Child Neurology 27: 392–400

Griffiths M, Russell P 1985 Working together with handicapped children. Souvenir Press, London

Harris R, Weetman M 1982 Genetic counselling and the work of a medical genetics centre. Health Visitor 55: 343–345

Health Visitors Association 1985 The health visitor's role in child health surveillance. A policy statement. Health Visitors Association, London

Heavyside Y 1985 Handicapped babies and their families. Midwife Health Visitor & Community Nurse 21: 388–392

Macfarlane J A 1985 The Education Act 1981. British Medical Journal 290: 1848–1849

Mansell C A 1981 Portage—not just another course. Nursing Times 77: 1807–1808

Millard D M 1984 Daily living with a handicapped child. Croom Helm, London, p 12–15; 39–47; 55–60

Milne P 1982 John David. The child that changed their lives. A novel. Virago Press Ltd, London

Murdoch J C, Ogston S A 1984 Down's syndrome children and parental psychological upset. Journal of the Royal College of General Practitioners 34: 87–90

Newell P 1983 ACE special education handbook—the new law on children with special needs. Advisory Centre for Education, London

Newell P, Potts P 1984 Under-5s with special needs. Pre-school children: the new law and integration. Advisory Centre for Education, London

Newson E, Hipgrave T 1982 Getting through to your handicapped child. A handbook for parents, foster-parents, teachers and anyone caring for handicapped children. Cambridge University Press, Cambridge

Nursing 1985 Civil and government benefits for the disabled. Nursing 2, 33: 966–967

Parker G 1984a Incontinence services for the disabled child. Part 1: the provision of aids and equipment. Health Visitor 57: 44–45

Parker G 1984b Incontinence services for the disabled child. Part 2: the provision of information and advice. Health Visitor 57: 86–88

Phillips S 1986 A centre for change. Nursing Times Community Outlook 82, 7: 15–17

Roberts G S 1983 The attendance allowance. Nursing Times 79, 28: 54–55

Robinson D 1978 Self-help in relation to health care. Midwife Health Visitor and Community Nurse 14: 265–267

Rouf C 1983 Parents care too. Health and Social Services Journal XCIII:415

Russell P 1976 Help starts here. For parents of children with special needs. National Children's Bureau for the Voluntary Council for Handicapped Children, London

Simon G B 1981 Local services for mentally handicapped people: the community team, the community unit and the role and function of the community nurse, social worker and some other members of the CMHT. British Institute of Mental Handicap, Kidderminster

Sloper P, Cunningham C C, Arnljotsdottir M 1983 Parental reactions to early intervention with their Down's syndrome infants. Child: care, health and development 9: 357–376

Southampton and South West Hampshire Community Health Council 1979 Information booklet for parents with mentally handicapped children. Southampton and South West Hampshire Community Health Council, Southampton

Stevens T 1985 Aids centres and the Disabled Living Foundation. Nursing 2, 33: 968–971

Sutcliffe B J 1980 Physiotherapy in the community. Midwife Health Visitor and Community Nurse 16: 166–170

Tarling C 1985 Assessing the mobility needs of the dependent person. Nursing 2, 32: 947–950

Twinn S 1981 The specialist health visitor for handicapped children: luxury or necessity? Health Visitor 54: 478–479

Walker E 1984 Sharing the video. Health and Social Services Journal XCIV: 350–351

Warnock M 1978 Meeting special educational needs: a brief guide to the report of the Committee of Enquiry into education of handicapped children and young people. HMSO, London

Warnock Report 1978 Report of the Committee of Enquiry into the education of handicapped children and young people. Cmnd 7212. HMSO, London, p 76–78

Webb P 1985 Someone to talk to directory 1985. A directory of self help and community support agencies in the UK and Republic of Ireland. Mental Health Foundation, London

Williams R 1980 A community service for mentally handicapped children. Nursing Times 76: 2011–2012

Wilson J 1982 Stepping stone to normal life. Health and Social Services Journal XCII:1253

Winter R M 1984 Who needs genetic counselling? Update 28: 1159–1163

Zelle R S, Coyner A B 1983 Developmentally disabled infants and toddlers: assessment and intervention. F A Davis Company, Philadelphia

In this chapter we look at some of the special problems encountered by families who have, during the past few decades, come to live in Britain. These problems might include health factors associated with environmental and social difficulties, a language barrier and cultural differences. In order to be able to help effectively, health visitors need to get to know about and to understand these families' particular viewpoint.

Knowledge and understanding

Family health needs
   Environmental factors
   Physical health
   Mental/emotional factors
   Social aspects of health

Examples of work with families who have immigrated

10

Families who have immigrated

KNOWLEDGE AND UNDERSTANDING

First we consider the importance of health visitor knowledge and understanding of the particular customs and beliefs of the families they visit. We then use the family health needs format to look at some problems that may be encountered by families who have immigrated fairly recently and at the problem of sickle cell anaemia. In this model, seen in Box 10.1, matters are categorised into environmental factors such as accommodation and income, physical health and mental factors and, lastly, social factors such as the extended family and self-help groups.

The same but more so

Health visiting families who have come from abroad is, in essence, no different from that described in the rest of this book. The aims of the work and the range of matters discussed are just the same. The difference lies in the increased potential for communication difficulties and for health visitor ignorance of cultural factors. For example, a fundamental aim in health visiting is to tailor the preventive health care to suit the particular individual or family. This is obviously more difficult if the health visitor does not know about the family's cultural background and/or religion, or, for example, what it feels like to be a black person in a predominantly white population. It is never easy to

Box 10.1 Family health needs framework showing health related factors described in this chapter

Environmental factors	Physical health	Mental/emotional health	Social aspects of health
Common problems — poor housing in inner city areas — low status, low paid occupation — work long hours, often at night — imported traditional food expensive *Very different* from home environment: — weather — traffic — socialisation patterns — city instead of rural — traditional clothing — food — colour prejudice	*Health education* 1. For feeding and other practices to improve perinatal morbidity and mortality rates 2. Nutrition, vitamins and exposure to sunlight to prevent rickets in children and osteomalacia in women 3. Lead in imported medicaments and cosmetics: danger re surma—updated health visitor tests for lead *Screening and support* re ethnic minority group related disease e.g. sickle cell disease—need screening for family members and counselling, as well as care services	*Knowledge* Language problems—a barrier to use of health and welfare services Health visitor could: Use — phonetic translation — Henley hints — flash cards Learn — Asian language Checklist — suitability of local health services Work with — linkworker (if available) — opinion leaders *Mental health* Potential for misunderstanding in cross-cultural interpretation of behaviour Strains of adjustment e.g. anxiety, guilt and shame on being obliged to break religious Laws (e.g. by examination by male Dr)	*Religious practices* Health visitors need to: — understand these in outline — expect variation — respect views Recording religion (and ethnic origin) — sensitive issue — can help health care priority and resource allocation decisions *Support from*: — family — friends — childminding *Self-help groups*: — for support — as pressure group — source of information on needs of ethnic minorities

know exactly what is in the mind of a client, but it is significantly more difficult where life experiences and language form a barrier.

The potential for stereotyping provides another example. This is always a possible trap, but perhaps, is more likely if the health visitor knows only a limited amount about the relevant religion and customs and makes assumptions about the family's beliefs and behaviour (Hunkins, 1983). These problems of communication and understanding, where they exist, are of course felt by client and worker alike.

The provision of practical care can also be more difficult. For example, it is not easy to help women overcome social isolation where there are few other women in the locality of the same or similar cultural background. The obstacles associated with being able to offer acceptable and relevant health education

where the family has relatively uncommon cultural beliefs and little has been written on the matter, provide another example.

To some extent, cross-cultural problems affect anyone who moves to a new environment, for example, from city to rural life or from 'the North' to 'the South' in Britain. However, the degree of adjustment and the challenges are significantly greater when moving between countries, particularly where the way of life is so different.

Guidance for health visitors

In these past few years, there have been series of articles which have given health workers an outline of the cultural beliefs and customs and some of the specific health problems of the main minority groups now in Britain (Schofield, 1981a, 1981b, 1981c; Henley & Clayton,

1982a, 1982b, 1982c, 1982d, 1982e, 1982f; Mayor, 1984a, 1984b; Black, 1986, 1985a, 1985b, 1985c, 1985d, 1985e, 1985f, 1985g). A number of health visitors have followed up their researches by visiting the country of origin of the people for whom they care (Pearson, 1982a, 1982b, 1982c; Rudge, 1983; Rhodes, 1985a, 1985b).

Organisations such as the Commission for Racial Equality, the King's Fund Centre and the Health Education Council are able to provide reading lists of books, articles, reports and pamphlets. Their addresses will be found at the end of the chapter.

Learning about life-style and religious beliefs is one thing. Getting to know about people's feelings is another. Brent Community Health Council (1981) provided a perspective of black people's relationship with the health service which many health workers might not have considered. Racism, stereotyping, and being used as cheap labour were among the matters described, and the booklet shows clearly how people can feel. Melba Wilson (1983) pointed out that there is not a 'black community' as some people imply, and that black people are as diverse as any other. Being seen as 'a problem' or being given an identity merely as 'immigrant' can be very hurtful. There are now many indigenous black people. They are bringing to society a new dynamic influence and this needs recognition.

Racial awareness courses should be part of the educational programme (Clark, 1985; Stevenson, 1985). These can help health visitors review their own assumptions about 'normal behaviour' and take a more empathetic and understanding approach in the study of other cultures. Health visitor students who are themselves members of minority groups could help with these learning processes (Stevenson, 1985) and if conversant with the language and culture, they might have an important role to play (Inter Departmental Consultative Group, 1984, pp. 8, 15; Clark, 1985). The handbook by Mares et al (1985) explores many of these key issues, as well as being a very useful resource and reference manual.

Health visiting nurse managers need to know to what extent their staff have the knowledge relevant to the people they visit. Twenty health visitors working in a multi-cultural inner-city area were questioned about their knowledge of Asian cultures in a small study by While and Godfrey (1984). In the main, the health visitors demonstrated a significant lack of knowledge and had not had post-registration training in this field. This ties in with June Clark's experience of the scarcity of appropriate courses.

It sounds as if 'do-it-yourself' is the solution until courses become available. Health visitors could ask the leaders and workers from local ethnic minority self-help groups to come and speak to them and, perhaps, lead discussions. There is so much to discover. However, if there is the will to learn about people's beliefs and customs, then a way can be found: and it is important that these customs should be understood in the context of the way they have been adapted, both to suit society as it is encountered and to contend with racism.

FAMILY HEALTH NEEDS

ENVIRONMENTAL FACTORS

Many immigrants to Britain find themselves obliged to settle in the very poor parts of cities and towns and to take badly paid jobs—two factors that increase the likelihood of poor health. Previous generations living in these areas also suffered from similar ill-health. For example, in the past there was a tendency for many children in central Glasgow to get rickets, just as there is now in their Asian counterparts (Dunnigan et al, 1985). Elizabeth Watson (1984) found poor housing and environmental factors increasingly significant over time regarding the health of disadvantaged mothers and infants.

In Batley where Hazel Rhodes (1985a, 1985b) worked, she found that unemployment was twice as high amongst the Asian community as amongst the indigenous community. Asian men tended to have the more poorly paid, lower status jobs, but worked very long hours and night shifts to increase their income. Although on similar incomes, 90% of the Asians owned their own homes, whereas less than 45% of the indigenous people did so. Overcrowding was commonplace for the Asian families. Three-quarters of their population had more than one person per room, compared with just over one tenth of the indigenous population, perhaps reflecting the Asians' need to band together and buy to overcome the difficulties of finding rented accommodation. These families are coping remarkably well in very difficult circumstances.

Several families had come from one area of the Gujerat and had settled into a relatively homogeneous community which had Asian shops readily available. This 'cornershop environment' meant the families were able to help each other. It also meant that for the women there was little contact with British culture and customs and that they could manage quite well without speaking English. There was also very little incentive for the men to learn any more than they needed to communicate at work.

These people came from a well-organised village and from relatively wealthy, prominent and property-owning families. Family members have a mutual obligation to help care for each other. They are unused to welfare provision by the government. A great deal of the women's and children's time there is spent in the fresh air, which enables socialisation between the women and safe play and exploration for the children. Life in their Yorkshire mill town is very different.

Many other people from abroad experience a similar change in their circumstances. For example, they have a lowered status, the climate is not so good and traffic can be very dangerous. 'Natural' ways of meeting and chatting with neighbours are not available, and it is not safe to let the children run free to play and explore their environment in the way that the parents themselves were brought up. They meet colour prejudice and/or racism.

Clothing which is an important part of the cultural heritage of some families is not always suitable, for example silks worn in winter. Traditional food, especially if imported, can be very expensive. The climate, the inner-city environment and the social structure of the British system are not supportive of the traditional patterns of behaviour of people, not only from India and Pakistan, but also from, for example, Vietnam, the West Indies, Africa and many parts of the Mediterranean. Not all are lucky enough to join a sub-community based on their own culture. Some people can be very isolated at the same time as they are trying to adjust to the new environment.

Health visitors are in a unique position because they call on families routinely, without the families having to request it. In this way, information can be given about the voluntary and statutory services available to help people cope with their difficulties. Advice and suggestions to promote good health and prevent ill-health form an integral part of this service.

PHYSICAL HEALTH

Examples are given here of the way that help can be provided, such as health education using an interpreter which seems to have helped to reduce the perinatal mortality rate. Two other examples are facilitating screening and providing counselling for families with a specific condition such as sickle cell disease, and giving advice on the acquisition of vitamin D in campaigns to eradicate rickets. Responding to specific difficulties, such as the possibility of lead in surma (an imported eye cosmetic popular in some cultures), helping to identify whether lead is present in it and warning of the potential for harm, provides the last example.

Health education with interpreters

Health visiting services have been shown to be effective and to help improve perinatal mortality rates for Bengali families in an inner London area. Elizabeth Watson (1984) studied the health of 100 women and small babies there and their use of the services by the time the baby was eight weeks old. 28 of the families were Bengali, 49 were from the indigenous population and the rest were a heterogenous group from ethnic minorities which she classified as 'English speaking immigrants'. With one exception, this latter group spoke English well and were able to communicate easily with the health service workers.

The children across all the groups had reported high levels of morbidity and admission to hospital in the early weeks of life. All the mothers used the services. The perinatal mortality rate had previously been higher for Bengalis than for the indigenous population. With preventive health service efforts, it had dropped to the same rate. However, subsequent interviews, when the babies were aged 8 months and 14 months, revealed an increasingly adverse influence of social conditions on the health of disadvantaged mothers and babies. The Bengalis in the study were distinctly appreciative of the health visitors' care, particularly over artificial feeding practices and the use of an interpreter. They had all learned to use the sterilisation units correctly.

It was suggested that it would be better to stress the value of breastfeeding than to concentrate on artificial feeding techniques (Watson, 1984). However, before becoming too zealous on this issue, it would be wise to ask the mothers more about their reasons for their choice. Lack of privacy in these young mothers' overcrowded homes and the lack of traditionally available family support may be important factors in their decisions on how to feed their baby (Mayor, 1984b).

Some of the specific health problems of children of parents from Asia (Black, 1985d), from the Mediterranean and around the Aegean Sea (1985e), from the West Indies and Africa (1985f) and from Vietnam or of Chinese descent (1985g) have been outlined by John Black. He drew attention to congenital abnormalities associated with a particular ethnic group, such as sickle cell disease in families of African descent or beta thalassaemia amongst Asian and Mediterranean families. He said that, if properly treated, these diseases tend to cause less distress and disability than, for example, cystic fibrosis, the commonest of the genetically determined recessive conditions in Europeans (Black, 1985a).

Sickle cell anaemia

It is surprising that neonatal screening for phenylketonuria, present in 1 in 7000–10 000 live births in the white races, is thought important enough to be fully available, whereas screening for sickle cell anaemia, which affects at least 1 in 400 of the West Indian community (Black, 1985a), is still limited in its availability. It is important that the presence of sickle cell disease, in whatever form, is known both to the families and the professionals who care for their health. This is necessary so that the appropriate interpretation in illness can be made and anticipatory action taken (Black, 1985f; Konotey-Ahulu, 1985; Prashar et al, 1985; Serjeant, 1985; Anionwu & Hall, 1983; Gray, 1982; Anionwu, 1982).

Both the Sickle Cell Society (Health Visitor, 1982) and the Organisation for Sickle Cell Anaemia Research (OSCAR), whose new addresses will be found at the end of the chapter, can provide information about the disease and counselling. Anne Gray points out that there is a great deal of professional ignorance about the disease. She says that 'at risk' antenatal patients should be screened as routine and that specially trained health visitors should visit the homes of affected women to provide counselling and to arrange for other members of the family to be screened if they wish it. Health visitors should check on what facilities are available for this in their locality.

Rickets

Rickets is sometimes a problem amongst Asian children. Important factors are:
— inadequate exposure to sunlight

— strict vegetarian diet
— household cows' milk used for infant feeding
— inadequate maternal intake of vitamin D during pregnancy (Black, 1985d).

In a pilot study some Muslim, Sikh and Hindu women who were pregnant were interviewed by Val Box (1983) to find out the effectiveness of dietary advice and/or of information about exposure to sunlight in the prevention of rickets. She had an experimental group and a control group. Women who were counselled on diet were able to remember only about half of the advice. At such an interview there is a limit on what can be remembered, and all that group forgot they had been told about exposure to sunlight. Surprisingly, blood samples showed that the control group, who were not given special advice on food, had increased their levels of vitamin D to a greater extent than the experimental group. It was speculated that this was due to greater exposure to sunlight.

With the exception of very strict vegans, Val Box concluded that, as an Asian diet provides about the same amount of vitamin D as that of the indigenous population, health visitor education should be concentrated on exposure to sunlight and vitamin D supplementation. Dr Black (1985d) warned about the potential problem of overdosing for children given standard vitamin drops as well as foods fortified with vitamin D.

A campaign to reduce rickets in Glasgow was monitored by Dunnigan et al (1985). Low dose supplements were found to be so successful that the campaign had been extended to women at risk of osteomalacia. In another study, vitamin D given to pregnant women was shown to correlate with their babies having improved length and weight as compared with the babies from the control group who had no supplement. This was especially so when the babies were 9 and 12 months old (Brooke et al, 1981). An annual dose, either by injection or by mouth, was found to provide very good serum levels of the vitamin (Stephens et al, 1981).

Lead in cosmetics

Lead is sometimes used in medicines and cosmetics in the Third World. There has been considerable concern about lead sulphide in surma, an eye cosmetic popular amongst Asians (Aslam & Healy, 1982). Although it is illegal to import it, in actuality it is posted in as a gift or brought back from a holiday. The original surma was much safer and was made from matter such as soot or vegetable dyes. It may be applied to babies' eyes several times a day from about two weeks onwards. Children may rub their eyes and then suck their fingers and consequently swallow lead.

The problem is to find a way of discovering the presence, or otherwise, of lead in surma. Currently there is no completely satisfactory, non-hazardous test for use by the mother in the home. Drs Healy and Aslam (1984) have suggested tests which need particular chemicals and could be undertaken in the home by a health visitor in less than five minutes. Where the presence of lead was indicated, confirmation would be needed by qualified personnel. Aslam and Healy have found that samples of surma coming into the country in hand luggage from Mecca and Medina invariably contain lead. They advocate education about the dangers of surma as, whatever is tested, new supplies are likely to be arriving. Posters and pamphlets entitled 'Surma, the gift that can be dangerous' are available from the Department of Trade and Industry Consumer Safety Unit (address at end of chapter).

This section has given some examples of ways health visitors may be involved in preventing illness and promoting good health for families who have immigrated. The example of sickle cell disease might more properly be classified under the previous chapter on preventive health care regarding handicap as nowadays it is of concern to significant numbers of people whose parents immigrated decades ago.

MENTAL/EMOTIONAL FACTORS

There are basic health needs (a) for knowledge about health promotion and prevention of ill-health and (b) for stability and security to enable and promote good mental health. Language difficulties can prevent understanding and full use of health services. Moving to a new country inevitably brings with it stresses and strains.

Knowledge

The language barrier

It is important that health visitors find a way to overcome language problems. The service is bound to be inadequate for families who face this difficulty. In effect, they are debarred from the basic choice of whether or not to use it. An increasing number of foreign language health education pamphlets, leaflets, tape-slides, films and videos are becoming available (Health Education Council, 1986; Chauhan, 1980), but these do not solve all the communication problems. The best solution would be the employment of health visitors who speak the relevant language, but that is currently a rare occurrence.

A booklet for health visitors and midwives which will translate, phonetically, key questions and statements in a common Asian language, is being produced by Redbridge Health Education Service. Training in its use is planned and it seems likely to make a very positive contribution. Many other schemes are being tried out (Wandsworth Council for Community Relations, 1978). June Clark (1985) suggested that there would be great benefits if health visitors went to classes to learn their clients' language. Even partial understanding would help overcome many problems.

Where no language classes are available, there might be a community leader or a family prepared to give some lessons. If health visitors were told how to say it, they might be able to write down the words phonetically for some of their favourite foreign language health education leaflets. Gradually the families visited could teach the proper pronounciation and there could be distinct advantages in this exchange of learning. It might help to provide a less formal atmosphere and would be especially useful in families where the women have not been taught to read.

Where the dialogue has to be in English with people whose knowledge of the language is limited, it may be much improved by using Alix Henley's (1982) hints on how to make it easier to get across the meaning. It is a question of a careful choice of words and a well thought-out approach. A list of her suggestions was reproduced in Community Outlook (1981). Another way of improving communication and helping people to understand could be the use of flash cards. Barbara Rudge (1983) saw these used in health education projects in India and felt they might also be helpful here.

Many useful ideas were put forward in two workshops organised by Training in Health and Race and the Centre for Ethnic Minorities Health Studies. The booklet that was subsequently published described how initiatives were being taken to improve the uptake of antenatal services. It included a checklist of basic points about the accessibility and relevance of maternity services for recent immigrants, especially those who cannot speak English (Appendix II). Health visitors should be aware of the extent to which their local services measure up and should plan to help their clientele overcome obstacles (Pearson, 1985).

Cross-cultural understanding and acceptance

In many places interpreters are available, but the service tends to have its limitations. For example, like the health visitor the interpreter may come from a significantly different class (normally higher) and cultural background: this results in reinforcement of the 'deference barrier' associated with contact with officialdom. Also these communications tend to be hospital- rather than client-centred and the service is not always easily available (Mays & Levick, 1985).

An advocacy scheme was set up in Hackney in 1980. Five women were employed on a wide-ranging basis. For example, as well as interpreting they not only helped people learn about their rights and spoke on their behalf, but also helped health workers to understand the problems and perceptions of non-English speaking women. These workers were specially selected on account of their language skills, their warm and compassionate personalities, and the fact that they had children themselves and came from the local community. The success of the scheme was easily demonstrated in the increased antenatal attendance, improved haemoglobin levels and baby birth weight for non-English speaking mothers (Winkler & Yung, 1981; Watson, 1984; Cornwell & Gordon, 1984).

This idea of employing workers from the community has spread. A DHSS report recommended a major new initiative in maternity services to take account of the problems of communication and cultural differences that discouraged Asian mothers. The Asian Mother and Baby Campaign was subsequently launched and now some ninety 'linkworkers' have been employed on a nationwide basis in areas with a large Asian population. Training videos are available (Alibhai, 1984).

The workers act as a bridge between the Asian communities and the health service, and work in partnership with the health professionals to help full communication in both directions between client and health professional. The project is to be evaluated and will assess health statistics, the subjective views of the people involved and changes in professional practice (Alibhai, 1984; Hadley, 1986).

The way that innovatory ideas are accepted or otherwise in a community are complex. Philip Rack (1982, pp. 191–192, 237–240) explained the mechanisms and pre-requisites for change. He demonstrated the value of opinion leaders, for example the influence of the senior Asian women (especially the

mother-in-law), in matters of pregnancy, childbirth and childrearing and of the Hakim or Vaid in general health issues. Linkworkers should be able to help health professionals understand these factors from a local and very practical point of view.

Mental health

Stresses and strains

Probably the best description and explanation for health visitors of mental illness in the context of cultural variation is that provided by Philip Rack (1982). He describes the feelings that immigrants can have during the processes of adjustment and the expected behaviour in various cultural groups, and gives thought-provoking examples of misunderstanding and misdiagnosis.

Health visitors attend seminars and seek advice from a unit especially set up in Islington in order to give psychotherapy and counselling, by people familiar with a variety of cultural backgrounds and languages (Francis, 1984). The cultural shock as a result of the unpleasant experiences associated with moving to Britain can manifest itself in various states of mental illness (Black, 1985a).

Hazel Rhodes (1985b) was able to compare the differences in the pace and way of life of Asian women whom she knew in Batley with their relatives whom she met in Alipor. In India they had servants and were freer from stress. In addition to the stresses and strains associated with employment and accommodation, the differences of culture can be very hurtful. She explained how the health of women and children is seen in Alipor as a family matter. The honour and status of the family is called into question if family difficulties and problems are made public. Zohra Ali Zubair (1984) described the deep anxiety, guilt and shame that women can feel when they are seen (and internally examined) by a male doctor, that is a man other than their husband.

Health visitors need to do their best to understand the problems of adjustment and to overcome language difficulties, as far as they can, in order that an appropriate and compassionate service is given which enables recently immigrated people to maintain a good level of health.

SOCIAL ASPECTS OF HEALTH

Respect for religious beliefs, social isolation and loss of family support, the need for child-minding and the importance of self-help groups are examples of social matters that are pertinent, of course, to all health visiting care groups, but are particularly so for people who have recently immigrated.

Religious beliefs

It is important for health visitors to be sensitive and aware of the religious customs and spiritual beliefs of the people they care for, so that they can take these factors into account in their discussions and suggestions. A well-researched outline of the customs of a wide range of religions has been drawn up by Chris Sampson (1982). Within any given religion there is, of course, a great deal of variation and, as Sampson points out, an intermingling of ideas between the different philosophies.

It is important to be mindful of the particular views of any given family. Individuals may vary significantly in their degree of orthodoxy, or they may choose to put a different interpretation on certain matters within their religion. For example, Mary Peel (1983) pointed out that some members of a Moslem community may believe that birth control is forbidden by their religion, whilst others point out that Moslem scholars 'have regarded all safe legitimate contraceptives to be permitted'.

As with all families, it is worth making a note on the records of a family's religion if this is known and important to them, so that their beliefs can be respected. Recording this is less likely to be seen as a potential source of prejudice and discrimination than making a note of ethnic origin. Many modern health visiting records have a space for both of these

features and health visitors have to think very carefully about their use. For example, the 1981 Census did not include a question on race or ethnic origin as it was felt it would not be acceptable (Population Trends, 1982). A statement of racial origin put on health visiting records gives no indication of how long it is since the person or the family members immigrated and about the degree of adjustment—nor whether they were born and educated in Britain! Religion gives more directly useful information. However, it is probably best to ask the family members how they feel about their religion being noted on the records.

Health visitors and their clients are more likely to be happy that health visitor records should include sensitive matters such as religion and/or ethnic origin if it is quite evident that the purpose is to provide equality of opportunity and/or to monitor the active implementation of such a policy. If they can see that the information is used, and used in a completely non-name-linked statistical and analytical manner, to plan and create local health and support services appropriate to the particular needs of the client groups—and to quote recent examples—then that would be evidence enough. Where it is just a matter of labelling and with no apparent benefit, they are less likely to concur.

Family factors

The degree of family support and community companionship available varies significantly for individual immigrants. In Batley, many of the older generation of the family were still in Alipor (Rhodes, 1985a), though families lived close together as an extended family. The family circle may be able to cope with child-minding whilst the mother is at work or attending a clinic. In the study in Tower Hamlets, Bengali women were found to take their babies with them, as did 60% of the 'English speaking immigrants'. 'Indigenous mothers' were far more likely to rely on their mothers or other relatives to look after their child when they went out (Watson, 1984).

The Bengali men tended to undertake a much wider range of help at home than the other men in that study, but were less likely to take time off work so they could be available when the new baby and the mother came home. Catherine Watson (1984) showed how domestic responsibilities and being unable to go out alone at night can limit the chances for non-English speaking women to learn the language. It seems, however, that the project workers in Hackney were helping some of the women to enroll in classes. Individual circumstances and opportunities can vary greatly.

Child-minding

There is some concern about the provision of day care for under-fives, particularly those of Asian and Afro-Caribbean descent. It is pointed out that research projects indicate that mothers from immigrant backgrounds are far more likely to work full time than non-migrant mothers. They are also more likely to have problems in finding and keeping a place with a child-minder. It was suggested that health visitors could be in a good position to recruit child-minders from amongst the Asian and Afro-Caribbean communities (Inter Departmental Consultative Group, 1984, pp. 12–14, 20; Clark, 1985).

Ideas for new initiatives for day care and schemes which help overcome racial disadvantage as well as sources of funding for such projects have been described by the Inter Departmental Consultative Group (1984) for Provision for Under-Fives. Ealing Council, the GLC and DHSS have got together on a project which is run by the Family Welfare Association. There are many activities, for example: play sessions are available; health visitors are there to advise on child care; a social worker gives advice on welfare services; and counselling sessions and classes are held in English conversation (Community Care, 1985).

Self-help groups

There has been a 'mushrooming' of self-help groups amongst the ethnic minorities in recent years. Many of the groups are health related, especially with regard to antenatal, child and adolescent health care and improved care for diseases which are specific to certain ethnic minorities. Melba Wilson (1983) found that many groups were founded in response to inadequacies, particularly a lack of understanding, in the health services. She quoted a DHSS circular which suggested that district health authorities should consult with representative organisations from ethnic minorities in order to form appropriate policies and allocate resources for health care.

However, it seems that dialogue between the health service hierarchy and the voluntary community groups is still a long way off. Health visitors, working with linkworkers where appropriate or possible, may be able to help bridge that gap. They will, however, need their managers' support if the messages from the groups are going to influence the 'health service hierarchy' and achieve a more appropriate service. In this chapter we have looked at the implications for health visiting with regard to some of the issues associated, in one case rather tenuously, with immigration. After an introduction about the need for adequate health visitor education and understanding, a family health needs framework was used to separate out and consider some of the environmental, physical, mental and social matters affecting health.

EXAMPLES OF WORK WITH FAMILIES WHO HAVE IMMIGRATED

The first example describes an antenatal visit to a Hindu household by a health visitor and a linkworker. The second is about background support given to a self-help group seeking sickle cell screening services in their area. The examples are outlined in family health needs formats in Boxes 10.2 and 10.3.

EXAMPLE ONE: AN ANTENATAL VISIT TO THE PATEL FAMILY

Hermione Verrall (HV) and Mrs Sharma, a linkworker, were visiting the Patels because Lalita

Box 10.2 Example one: an antenatal visit to the Patel family

Environmental factors	Physical health	Mental/emotional health	Social aspects of health
Common problems — poor housing in inner city areas — low status, low paid occupation — work long hours, often at night for first and second sons — third son unemployed: Claiming supplementary benefit: entitlements in pregnancy explained *Very different from home environment:* — weather — traffic — socialisation patterns — city instead of rural	*Health education* 1. Value of vitamins and exposure to sunlight in prevention of rickets in children and osteomalacia in women Normal diet taken Explained about free vitamins and milk 2. Lead in imported medicaments and cosmetics: Family sought HV tests for cosmetics One item referred to Pharmacy Dept (*Plans* to — discuss immunisations — explain infant surveillance scheme)	*Knowledge* Language difficulties but minimised through work with linkworker Use of pictorial scheme to provide reminder of explanation *Mental health* Strains of adjustment: women seem well adjusted. Husband reported as anxious about unemployment	*Religious practices and traditional customs* Linkworker able to explain individual preferences and views of family members *Support from:* — family — friends

Kumari Patel, the 19-year-old wife of the third son in a Hindu household, was pregnant. The family lived in a deprived inner city area where there was a small Hindu community.

The family were delighted to find that Mrs Sharma had come with the health visitor. Their teamwork was building up a good reputation. They were introduced to Lalita Kumari's husband who was at that time unemployed. He took no part in the subsequent discussions and left the three women of the household to converse with their visitors. One was Lalita Kumari's mother-in-law who had come to live some years previously with her oldest son on the death of her husband. The wife of the oldest son was also present.

With Mrs Sharma's help, HV conversed with all three women, seeking, in particular, the opinion of the mother-in-law, as it was likely to be held in high regard within the household. The women had heard of the lead-testing service the health visitor carried with her, and they brought three cosmetics for her to test. Two passed the tests and one needed to be checked by the pharmacists and arrangements were made for this.

Diet was discussed. The Patels explained how they had found good substitute foods for those that were normally unattainable in Britain. A local shop made some traditional foods available. The value of exposure to sunlight was described as well as how to get hold of vitamin D.

Mrs Sharma explained that having heard the good news about Lalita Kumari's pregnancy through a neighbour, she had brought the health visitor to help explain the value of early attendance at an antenatal clinic and to answer any questions they might have, for example about welfare benefits. First she explained that the health authority had decided to start a midwives clinic for Muslim and Hindu women in early pregnancy. Antenatal classes were discussed and, as her husband did not wish to attend, Lalita Kumari asked if her sister- or mother-in-law might come too. This was agreed and they opted to come to the series of classes in the local health centre, specially arranged for non-English speaking families. Mrs Sharma promised to be there.

The conversation then moved on to the free services (including milk and vitamins) available, as the couple were at the time on supplementary benefits. Whilst HV was explaining she filled in a pictorial chart to provide them with a reminder, as none of the women had been taught to read.

Another visit was arranged for two months later, when HV promised to discuss immunisations and the local infant surveillance scheme if they wished it.

As they walked towards the car, Mrs Sharma and HV talked about the success of the midwives' early pregnancy clinic where the women were able to have their own family with them at the examination—conducted by a woman. In due course, the success of the clinic and evidence of the number of women wishing to be examined by women for religious reasons, led to the appointment of a part-time female obstetrician.

EXAMPLE TWO: 'THE GROUP' AND SCREENING FOR SICKLE CELL ANAEMIA

As she happened to be passing by at the right time, Henrietta Varley (HV) decided to look in on 'The Group', a health education based self-help association of young mothers in an inner city area of London. This group had grown out of a series of antenatal/postnatal classes in which many of the young women (or their husbands) had been at school together. HV slipped quietly in and sat in a chair on the edge of the circle where some twenty mothers were in hot debate over what constituted 'normal discipline' in the context of 'child abuse'.

Adele Brown, a mother whom HV knew quite well, caught her eye and indicated she would like a word outside. Mrs Brown came quickly to the point and explained that her sister's only child had recently died with sickle cell anaemia. It had not been diagnosed in the early stages of the illness and inappropriate treatment had been given (Konotey-Ahulu, 1985). 'The Group' had taken the matter very much to heart and had decided to do something positive about it by pressing for sickle cell screening services in their district. Had HV any ideas?

The health visitor asked what approaches had been considered and was told that they had thought of a petition to the district general manager. Mrs Brown's brother-in-law had sent a letter of complaint to the health authority about the tardy diagnosis, due mainly to inadequate screening services. They thought that that might help, but felt intuitively that a sickle cell awareness campaign would need to be launched, in order to get enough interest for the necessary allocation of funds for the service.

It seems that the group had no information on just how many people it might affect in their own area and in the district. However, as there were a large number of families of West Indian origin, it was likely to be a significant number. HV suggested that they tried to find accurate figures as far as they could, perhaps by using local population figures from OPCS small area statistics (Population Trends, 1982). She also suggested that they contact the Sickle Cell Society and invite someone to come and offer them guidance.

Mrs Varley undertook to ask her nurse manager whether health visitor records might give reliable information about the number of babies of Afro-Caribbean descent born locally. She said she would write a proposal for the Community Unit general manager and would be able to follow it up when he came on his next 'ground roots' visit which was scheduled in two months' time. It occurred to HV that it would be a good idea to look at the current District Plan to see if a screening service was planned and what priority it had been assigned.

Having asked how Mrs Brown's sister was, HV heard that her health visitor had been very supportive through the illness and since the death. Family and friends were helping the couple

Box 10.3 Example two 'The group' and screening for sickle cell anaemia

Environmental factors	Physical health health	Mental/emotional health	Social aspects of health
Common problems — poor housing in inner city areas — low status, low paid occupations — poor facilities *But*—some parts of community very cohesive	*Health education* Self-help group discusses many aspects of physical health *Screening and support* re ethnic minority group related disease—sickle cell disease—need for screening facilities for forewarning of presence or possibility of disease	*Knowledge* Self-help group discusses many aspects of mental and emotional health Seeking to find information: will contact Sickle Cell Society *Mental health* Care for couple through bereavement period	*Self-help group* Provides focus for socialisation and mutual support Can act as pressure group Source of information on needs of ethnic minorities *Support for Mrs Brown's relatives* — family — friends — group members — HV in early days

to adjust. They had been very pleased that 'The Group' had decided to take up the issue. HV left the premises feeling very glad she had called in.

It was another six months before the screening was given top priority and it was in full swing a year after that.

USEFUL ADDRESSES

Commission for Racial Equality,
Information Department,
Elliot House,
10–12 Allington Street,
London SWIE 5EH
Tel 01 828 7022

Consumer Safety Unit,
Department of Trade and Industry,
Millbank Tower,
Millbank,
London SWIP 4QU

Health Education Council,
78 New Oxford Street,
London WCIA IAH
Tel 01 631 0930

King's Fund Centre,
126 Albert Street
London NWI 7NF
Tel 01 267 6111

Organisation for sickle cell anaemia research (OSCAR),
22 Pellatt Grove,
Wood Green,
London N22
Tel 01 889 3300/4844

Redbridge Health Education Service,
Ilford Chambers,
11 Chapel Road,
Ilford Essex,
IGI 2QS
Tel 01 533 0813

Sickle Cell Society,
Green Lodge,
Barretts Green Road,
Park Royal,
London NW10 7AP
Tel 01 961 7795/8346

REFERENCES

Alibhai Y 1984 Forging a new partnership. Nursing Times 80, 37: 19–20

Anionwu E 1982 Sickle cell disease. Health Visitor 55: 336–341

Anionwu E, Hall J 1983 A handbook on sickle cell disease: a guide for families. Sickle Cell Society, London

Aslam M, Healy M 1982 Present and future trends in the health care of British-Asian children. Nursing Times 78, 32: 1353–1354

Black J 1986 The new paediatrics: child health in ethnic minorities. British Medical Journal, London (**This is a reprint of the seven articles below**)

Black J 1985a The difficulties of living in Britain. British Medical Journal 290: 615–617

Black J 1985b Contact with the health services. British Medical Journal 290: 689–690

Black J 1985c Asian families I: cultures. British Medical Journal 290: 762–764

Black J 1985d Asian families II: conditions that may be found in the children. British Medical Journal 290: 830–833

Black J 1985e Families from the Mediterranean and Aegean. British Medical Journal 290: 923–925

Black J 1985f Afro-Caribbean and African families. British Medical Journal 290: 984–988

Black J 1985g Chinese and Vietnamese families. British Medical Journal 290: 1063–1065

Box V 1983 Rickets: what should the health education message be? Health Visitor 56: 131–134

Brent Community Health Council 1981 Black people and the health service. Brent Community Health Council, London

Brooke O G, Butters F, Wood C 1981 Intrauterine vitamin D and postnatal growth in Asian infants. British Medical Journal 283:1024

Chauhan V 1980 Community information (Asian languages) directory. Commission for Racial Equality and Citizens Advice Bureau, London

Clark J 1985 Understanding the under-fives. Nursing Times Community Outlook 81, 11:8

Community Care 1985 Shanti Niketan opens its doors. Community Care 547:7

Community Outlook 1981 Chat sheet. Nursing Times Community Outlook 77, 28: 239–241

Cornwell J, Gordon P (eds) 1984 An experiment in advocacy. The Hackney multi-ethnic women's health project. Report of a conference organised by the King's Fund in collaberation with City and Hackney Community Health Council. King's Fund Centre, London

Dunnigan M G, Glekin B M, Henderson J B, McIntosh W B, Sumner D, Sutherland G R 1985 Prevention of rickets in Asian children: assessment of the Glasgow campaign. British Medical Journal 291: 239–242

Francis W 1984 Out of the textbooks and into the consulting room. Community Care 535: 19–20

Gray A 1982 Sickle cell disease. Nursing Times 78, 31: 1324–1325

Hadley A 1986 Mothers' advocate. Nursing Times 82, 6: 16–17

Health Education Council 1986 Health education for ethnic minorities. Resource list prepared by the Health Education Council, 2nd ed. Health Education Council, London

Health Visitor 1982 The Sickle Cell Society. Health Visitor 55:341

Healy M A, Aslam M 1984 Identification of lead in Asian cosmetics—a test for use by health visitors. Public Health, London 98: 361–366

Henley A 1982 Asian patients in hospital and at home. Oxford University Press, Oxford

Henley A, Clayton J 1982a Cultural patterns. Health and Social Services Journal XCII: 833–834

Henley A, Clayton J 1982b What's in a name? Health and Social Services Journal XCII: 855–857

Henley A, Clayton J 1982c Catering for all tastes. Health and Social Services Journal XCII: 888–889

Henley A, Clayton J 1982d Religion of the Muslims. Health and Social Services Journal XCII: 918–919

Henley A, Clayton J 1982e Five signs of Sikhism. Health and Social Services Journal XCII: 943–945Henley A, Clayton J 1982f Illness and the life cycle. Health and Social Services Journal XCII: 972–974

Hunkins S V 1983 West Indians' sexual attitudes (letter). Health Visitor 56: 7

Inter Departmental Consultative Group 1984 Services for under fives from ethnic minority communities. Report of a subgroup on provision of services for under fives from ethnic minority communities. Department of Health and Social Security, London

Konotey-Ahulu F 1985 Ethnic minorities and sickle cell disease (letter). British Medical Journal 290: 1214

Mares P, Henley A, Baxter C 1985 Health care in multi-racial Britain. Health Education Council and National Extension College, Cambridge

Mayor V 1984a The family, bereavement and dietary beliefs. Nursing Times 80, 23: 40–42

Mayor V 1984b Pregnancy, childbirth and child care. Nursing Times 80, 24: 57–58

Mays N, Levick P 1985 When maternal instinct isn't enough. Health and Social Services Journal XCV: 870–871

Pearson M 1985 Racial equality and good practice maternity care. A report of two workshops held in Bradford organised by Training in Health and Race and the Centre for Ethnic Minorities Health Studies. Health Education Council and National Extension College for Training in Health and Race, London

Pearson R 1982a Understanding the Vietnamese in Britain. Part I: background and family life. Health Visitor 55: 426–430

Pearson R 1982b Understanding the Vietnamese in Britain. Part II: marriage, death and religion. Health Visitor 55: 477–483

Pearson R 1982c Understanding the Vietnamese in Britain. Part III: health beliefs, birth and child care. Health Visitor 55: 533–540

Peel M 1983 Islam and family planning (letter). Health Visitor 56:436

Population Trends 1982 Editorial. Sources of statistics on ethnic minorities. Population Trends 28, Summer: 1–8

Prashar U, Anionwu E, Brozovic M 1985 Sickle cell anaemia—who cares? A survey of screening and counselling facilities in England. The Runnymede Trust, London

Rack P 1982 Race, culture and mental disorder. Tavistock Publications, London

Rhodes H 1985a From Alipor to Batley. Nursing Times Community Outlook 81, 24: 39–44

Rhodes H 1985b From Batley to Alipor. Nursing Times Community Outlook 81, 28: 8–14

Rudge B 1983 Health education, Indian style. Health Visitor 56: 373–376

Sampson C 1982 The neglected ethic. Religious and cultural factors in the care of patients. McGraw-Hill, Maidenhead

Schofield J 1981a Behind the veil: the mental health of Asian women in Britain. 1. Life in Asia. Health Visitor 54: 138–141

Schofield J 1981b Behind the veil: the mental health of Asian women in Britain. 2. Migration and life in Britain. Health Visitor 54: 183–186

Schofield J 1981c Behind the veil: the mental health of Asian women in Britain. 3. Preventing stress—the role of the health visitor. Health Visitor 54: 248–251

Serjeant G R 1985 Sickle cell disease. Oxford University Press, Oxford

Stephens W P, Klimiuk P S, Berry J L, Mawer E B 1981 Annual high-dose vitamin D prophylaxis in Asian immigrants. Lancet II: 1199–1201

Stevenson O 1985 Education for community care. British Medical Journal 290: 1966–1968

Wandsworth Council for Community Relations 1978 Asians and the health service. A directory of measures implemented by Area Health Authorities to meet the needs of the Asian community. Commission for Racial Equality, London

Watson C 1984 The vital link. Nursing Times 80, 30: 18–19

Watson E 1984 Health of infants and use of health services by mothers of different ethnic groups in East London. Community Medicine 6: 127–135

While A E, Godfrey M 1984 Health visitor knowledge of Asian cultures. Health Visitor 57: 297–298

Wilson M 1983 Networking for health. Health and Social Services Journal XCIII: 565–567

Winkler F, Yung J 1981 Advising Asian mothers. Health and Social Services Journal XCI: 1244–1245

Zohra Ali Zubair 1984 Preface. In: Cornwell J, Gordon P (eds) 1984 An experiment in advocacy. The Hackney multi-ethnic women's health project. King's Fund Centre, London

This chapter considers some of the ways health visitors can help to prevent the occurrence, development or deterioration of situations involving child abuse and looks at some of the difficulties for health visitors in this field of their work.

Small but important

Preventing child abuse

Identification and selection

When problems arise

11
Child abuse

SMALL BUT IMPORTANT

The framework

Child abuse should be studied in the context of cross-cultural family and societal violence. Here it is possible to take only a limited look at the topic. We use the prevention model (see Table 11.1) as a framework for outlining some of the aims of health visitors with regard to child abuse and neglect, that is their attempts to:

— prevent the occurrence of such problems, for example by improving people's understanding of the basic needs and development of babies and children and of the factors associated with child abuse, in order to engender good bonding and good parent—child relationships and interaction.

— prevent the development of child abuse and neglect where strains and tensions are becoming too great, for example by trying to identify the most vulnerable people, and ensuring a 'life-line' (someone to talk to in a crisis) and that help such as a day nursery place is available, to help relieve the stress in the household.

— prevent deterioration of the situation in cases in which child abuse has or seems to have occurred: for example, by keeping in touch with the family if their child is taken into care and helping them cope with their child's behavioural problems on return to the family.

Table 11.1 Prevention model of health visiting aims regarding child abuse

Aim	Through	Examples
To prevent occurrence of child abusing situation	Teaching	Parenthood courses — in school — antenatally Child abuse discussions, e.g. incest
	Normal supportive services	Tell about groups and agencies
To prevent development of stress & tensions leading to child abuse	1. Identifying those vulnerable 2. Enabling extra support for them	In liaison with midwives Observations of health visitors Tell of self-help groups, e.g. OPUS Health visitor special initiatives More frequent visiting
To prevent deterioration where child abuse seems to have occurred	Child-centred decisions with nurse management support	Use social and clinical evidence Full and contemporaneous records Multi-profession decision & action Evidence in court where necessary Continued support for parents if child removed

Keeping up to date

Child abuse has always been a feature of society (Radbill, 1980; Korbin, 1980; Borkowski et al, 1983). Attitudes towards it have changed over the past twenty years since interpretation of X-rays alerted doctors to patterns of physical violence towards children. More recently, concern has also focused on child neglect and emotional and sexual abuse.

A feeling that something could and should be done about child abuse has been developing rapidly. In recent years, there has been a great outpouring of literature intended to help guide health and welfare workers. Early literature was mainly devoted to alerting people to the problem and to encouraging them to take action. Suggestions on how to discover the people most prone to this problem have been proliferating. Now a number of research projects are being undertaken, leading to increasingly perspicacious commentary. For example, Nigel Parton (1985) has brought together a great deal of the available data and has drawn attention to the need for clearer definitions of child abuse and for a more wide-ranging and supportive solution to the problem.

Ideas will change as informed understanding of the subject improves. It is therefore important that health visitors have plenty of opportunities to keep up to date by going on courses, by reading and through mutual support groups and nurse manager help (see Ch. 2, pp. 18–19). However, it is becoming more difficult to attend courses now that resources are being cut back (Thorneley, 1986). For this reason, the nurse managers' role in facilitating and enabling the best possible practice becomes very important.

A small part of health visitors' work . . . .

Helping parents overcome the strains and tensions of child care is an integral part of most health visitors' everyday work. Child abuse pertains to a very small part of this and lies at one extreme of the range of need for care and support (see Fig. 11.1).

The government does not collect statistics on child abuse. Normally the numbers quoted, such as 7000 children physically abused by their parents in England and Wales in 1984, are derived from an extrapolation of figures from National Society for the Prevention of Cruelty to Children (NSPCC) teams who have access to statistics which cover less than 10% of the country. The figures quoted can therefore provide only an indicator (Laurance, 1985). The numbers of reported cases of child abuse and neglect have been increasing over recent years. However, it may well be due to a greater readiness to report the problem.

Where more firm figures are available, it can be seen that serious and acknowledged child

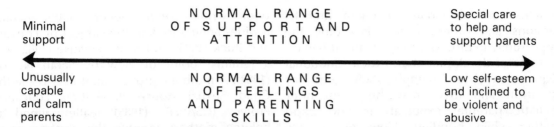

Fig. 11.1 Continuum showing range of child care supportive work. Above the continuum shows the extent of health visiting involvement, below shows parents' feelings and skills.

abuse and neglect represent only a very small proportion, if any, of most health visitors' work. For example, there are very few children involved in care proceedings, a matter of about 4 children per 10 000 each year (Dingwall, 1983). Also, only a small number of pre-school deaths caused by 'violence or accident' are due to child abuse. In Ontario, for example, they amounted to around 4 to 8% of the deaths (Greenland, 1986). In comparison, accidents in the street or in the home account for extremely high numbers of death and disability.

.... with high anxiety levels

Health visitors tend to find child abuse a particularly stressful aspect of their work. There has been a great deal of media attention focused on this problem, both in defence of parents where a child is thought to have been taken into care unnecessarily, and at the other extreme where a child has been harmed having been returned to his parents.

However, this was not mentioned in Valerie Weeks' (1982) study of the ways in which non-accidental injury caused professional anxiety. Health visitors who had been involved with actual or suspected cases reported most concern over their ongoing relationship with the family. Next came worries that their suspicion of child abuse might be unfounded and concern about legal proceedings. There was anxiety about insufficient training and information about procedures for dealing with cases, inadequate nurse manager support and problems with caseload size. There were

several other worries, including those associated with borderline cases and children's behavioural difficulties on being returned to their parents after having been 'in care'.

As child abuse is such a worrying topic and also one about which much has been written, this chapter concludes with a list of helpful books and papers not included amongst the other references.

PREVENTING CHILD ABUSE

Both education and support have a part to play in promoting good child care. For example, learning about a child's development and basic needs may help engender good bonding and parenting skills. It can be useful to people to know about the services available to help parents under stress. Better understanding by the general public and more open discussion about taboo subjects such as child sexual abuse, may help prevent its occurrence. Support, for example in the form of having someone to turn to and trust, may help parents talk through their problems, lower stress levels and help avoid abuse of the child.

Health education

Both learning about child care in general and about child abuse in particular, may help to prevent the occurrence of child abuse. Some health visitors become involved in giving or advising on preparation for parenthood courses in schools and in teaching in antenatal sessions and other groups. Providing the opportunity to discuss and learn about babies' patterns of development and their emotional requirements, for example their need for attention and love, may help engender realistic parental expectations and good mother—child bonding. However, as we discussed in Chapter 3 (see pp. 45–46), there are no glib solutions to preparation for parenthood. It is difficult for people to visualise it in advance.

There are advantages if lessons in school also include discussions about child abuse. An understanding of the factors associated with this problem and knowledge of the facilities and services available, may help families with tensions and worries to recognise the need to seek timely advice and help. It might also lessen fears about seeking that support. A concise and very useful overview of child abuse has been written for the non-professional by Dana Ackley (1977). Molly Meacher (1982, p. 3) has sketched out a neat synopsis of current ideas on the nature, size and causes of the problem.

These same articles would also be useful as a general introduction for women's groups and other organisations. Some of the articles and books referred to in the next two sections of this chapter may be found useful in stimulating debate and discussion on general child abuse. It is a very wide subject. Child sexual abuse is provided here as an example.

Child sexual abuse

As in other aspects of child abuse, there is much to debate. Identifying the problem and finding effective and acceptable measures to deal with it are even more difficult than, for example, with physical abuse. Public and professional awareness of incest, for example, are said to be at a level roughly equivalent to that for physical abuse 15 years ago (Vizard, 1985).

Groups wishing to discuss this topic should be encouraged to read a variety of books and articles, in order to get a range of views. Three books written for the general public include a wide-ranging look at the subject by Forward and Buck (1981) and Jean Renvoise (1982) and a feminist point of view by Sarah Nelson (1982). A mothers' group might like to see the Child Sexual Abuse Prevention Education Project (CSAPEP) (1985) leaflet aimed at helping mothers identify the occurrence of sexual abuse in their own family. Pamela Holmes (1986b) described a book specially designed to help children know how to cope with improper approaches. There has been a proliferation of this type of literature in America. Commenting on this, Nicholas Tucker (1985) described some unfortunate side-effects of what he saw as an over-reaction to the problem. He said that in America there were examples of over-zealous accusations of incestuous behaviour, for example, in custody proceedings in the divorce courts.

Group discussion of this topic is very likely to lead to questioning about local facilities and ways officialdom copes with the problem. Health visitors need to be sure they know exactly what the policy in their locality is on the management of child sexual abuse and how liaison between the relevant professionals is put into action (Vizard, 1985; Renvoise, 1982, pp. 166–216; Nelson, 1982, pp. 77–78; Forward & Buck, 1981, pp. 138–139). They need to know this both for their practice and in order to provide such a group with a clear picture of how cases are handled. It would also be useful to have made personal or telephone contact with the agencies willing to give adults and children confidential help (Pownall, 1985; CSAPEP & Driver, 1985), in order to be able to give an accurate account of the range and style of services available.

It has been suggested that 10% of adult Britons were sexually abused as children (Elliot, 1985). Widespread knowledge about confidential and supportive services for the sexually abused may do much more than encourage reporting of early cases. It could help discourage its occurrence in the first place, once potential, particularly incestuous, abusers were less certain they could rely on hiding behind a veil of secrecy.

General health visitor support

Supportive work is one of the basic mainstays of a health visitor's work. It involves, for example, telling mothers about local groups and schemes which offer help to young families. This was mentioned in Chapter 4 (pp. 66–67). In Chapter 5 (pp. 91–93), helping people with loneliness, depression and stressful problems, such as having a persistently crying baby, were described. In some cases, this everyday work will help defuse and avert problems that might otherwise have led to child abuse. Support services more specific to child abuse are described in the next section.

In this section we have taken a brief look at some of the ways health visitors may be able to help prevent the occurrence of child abuse. Education, both on babies' emotional needs and on child abuse itself, was discussed, as was the preventive value of everyday support work in health visiting. Child sexual abuse was given as an example of the value of open debate on the subject.

IDENTIFICATION AND SELECTION

In this section we look at the means currently available to try to discover the people most vulnerable to the stresses and strains that can lead to their abusing their children. In essence the aim is to prevent the development of child abuse in families who have these difficulties, by providing them with the degree of extra care and support that seem to be required.

A form of screening?

The process of identification and selection of vulnerable people might loosely be considered screening. However, the process does not lead to the discovery of immediately verifiable early cases of child abuse, nor does it discover a pre-symptomatic phase which, if it received no attention, would inevitably result in child abuse. Many, or possibly, most of the selected families will have no major problem. The purpose is to draw health visitors' attention to those most likely to be 'at risk'. These schemes provide a rather crude tool for selection. They need to be used with circumspection and to be given a great deal of thought about what is really being picked out.

Many health visitors are concerned about 'labelling' and the development of disparaging attitudes towards families selected by this type of scheme. This matter was touched on in Chapter 3 (page 46). However, where health visitors are clearly able to provide the selected families with extra time and support, a feature incorporated, for example, in the Portsmouth scheme (Powell, 1985), or where facilities such as preferential day nursery places for families under stress are readily available, then concern will be less. The advantage of being able to channel help where it is most needed is likely to be seen to outweigh the disadvantages of the system.

What and how extensive is the problem?

Some basic questions are:
— Exactly what is child abuse?
— How widespread is it?
— Who does it and why?
— Where is the borderline between physical child abuse and 'normal discipline'?
— To what extent is early discovery and support and/or therapy successful?

Answering these questions is difficult and in some cases impossible, basically because there is not and will not be a fully agreed definition of child abuse. Welfare professionals use the phrase to cover an enormous variety and range of notions and aspects of the problem. Agreed definitions, such as that for physical abuse quoted in governmental documents (Department of Health and Social Security, 11986, p. i), are generally stated in such broad terms that they could, if taken literally, include an enormous number of families. Another problem is that researchers using different definitions have necessarily come to a variety of conclusions so that studies cannot be compared and many questions inevitably remain inadequately answered (Parton, 1985, pp. 133–146). Either way, as ideas on child abuse are culturally defined and socially determined (Meacher, 1983, p. 3), definitions and ways of thinking about it are certain to continue to change over time.

A variety of basic approaches to the study of child abuse have been described by Nigel Parton (1985, p. 154–172) amongst them a national survey of family violence in the United States by Straus, Gelles and Steinmetz. Straus et al found that child abuse, far from being rare, was part of the normal pattern of a large number of children's lives. The lower the income level, the higher the rate and degree of violence tended to be. They found that amongst the poorest families, stress did not increase the likelihood of violence—high stress levels are part of normal life for them.

Many studies find a correlation between low socio-economic levels and child abuse. Professor Greenland's (1986) study of 100 child abuse and neglect deaths in Canada also found this tendency. As far as he could discover, only 6 out of 100 came from the white collar or professional classes. It is worth noting in passing that in a significant number of the cases (9) the suspected perpetrators were baby-sitters and not the parents.

An attempt was made by Elmer (Parton, 1985, pp. 166–167) to study the long-term consequences of child abuse by following up 17 children, abused under one year of age, eight years after they were originally examined, and comparing them with two other groups of children, matched for age, race, sex and socio-economic status. The children in one of the control groups had suffered accidents under one year of age; those in the other control group had had no record of either similar accidents or child abuse. To their astonishment the researchers found that *all* the children appeared fearful, anxious and depressed and demonstrated social and developmental problems. Subsequent work led them to feel that research into child abuse was discovering more about lower-class children in general, rather than specifically about abused children. There is an obvious need for further research using fully matched control groups.

Identifying those in need of support

A basic premiss of Kempe and Kempe (1978, p. 22) was that

abusive parents come from all walks of life.

Although this may be so, it looks, from the research quoted above, as if they are unevenly spread across the social classes. There seems also to be an element of uneven selection and classification slanted towards lower class parents (Dingwall et al, 1983, p. 101).

The Kempes wrote the most influential of the early treatises on the subject. They described a cycle of abuse in which poorly-parented children grew up to become parents who cared badly for their children and so on through generations. In their work they had discovered four factors implicit in child abusing families shown in Table 11.2, some aspects of which they said could be sensed from parental reaction to the newborn baby. These are listed in Box 11.1. A list of Lynch and Roberts' (1977) significant factors which they said could be gleaned from the midwifery notes will be found in Box 11.2 . More recently, attention has been turning towards identifying parents during pregnancy too, in order to promote good bonding after delivery (Ounsted et al, 1982).

Table 11.2 Four factors implicit in child abusing families (from Kempe & Kempe, 1978, p. 24–38)

Factor	Features
Potential for abuse—acquired over the years	Lack of mothering imprint Isolated—cannot trust or use others Spouse passive—he/she cannot give Unrealistic expectations of the child
Child appears different to parents	For example, hyperactive, retarded, suffers from a defect, appears similar to disliked person
Crisis or series of crises	Cannot cause, but precipitates abuse
Life-link lacking	No one to turn to in a crisis and to tell about feelings and problems

Box 11.1 Parents' reactions in labour and delivery rooms (from Kempe & Kempe, 1978, p. 81)

Factors sensed	Reaction to new baby	Worrying signs
Potential for abuse	What mother said	Passive response to baby
How parents perceive child	How she looked	React to him with hostility
Degree of tension	What she did	Seem disappointed over baby's sex
	How father reacted	Do not look baby in the eye
	Midwife's anecdotal information	Parents not loving towards each other

Box 11.2 A method for predicting bonding failure in the maternity hospital (from Lynch & Roberts, 1977)

Five factors from midwifery notes
Mother under twenty for first baby
Referral to maternity hospital social worker
Baby admitted to special care unit
Emotional disturbance recorded
Recorded concern over mother's inability to cope

Table 11.3 Health visitors' measure of mother–child interaction (from Dean et al, 1978)

Percentage of mothers	Coded	Description of situation by health visitor (coded later)
68	No concern	No stated environmental, behavioural or interactional difficulties
21	Mild concern	Any one word concerning environment or behaviour
7	Moderate concern	Prolonged separation Non-supporting situation Unrealistically high expectations of baby History of psychiatric illness—either parent History of prolonged marital discord
3	Great concern	Type of interaction between mother and baby (e.g. eye contact, physical contact) Presence of physically neglectful situation History of unstable/violent background—either parent
		(where description qualified, qualification discounted in coding)

Research in Aberdeen took another approach. Dean et al (1978) studied health visitors' assessment of mother—child interaction to see if the more vulnerable families could be discovered this way. They found that health visitors could sense when families were having emotional difficulties, but tended to discount these and to concentrate on the more physical 'mothering skills'. They felt that if health visitors had the courage of their own convictions, they could identify the families most likely to be in need of extra help. In the event, two thirds of the children in the family situations coded as causing the health visitor moderate or great concern (see Table 11.3), later suffered accident, injury or failure to thrive.

Spurred on by this sort of research, health visitors started to set up pilot schemes which attempted to checklist factors which would find the families most in need of help (Woods, 1981; Waterhouse, 1981; Fort, 1986). One example is Claire Johnson's (1985) scheme in Rochdale, in which 22 factors were selected. Special weighting was given to items shown by earlier research to be important. The scoring system chosen seemed to be successful in making it possible to identify the vast majority of parents who would need help.

Around two thirds of the families selected through this scheme had one or more episodes of suspected or actual non-accidental injury, neglect, failure to thrive or emotional deprivation during the year of the study. It follows that a third did not. They all had a yellow sticker on their file. There is a clear advantage to new or 'stand-in' health visitors if there is a systematic method of drawing attention to the families most likely to be suffering significant problems. However, there is also the disadvantage associated with the ethical problem of 'labelling' a family and, perhaps, not telling them they have been classified in this way.

This type of scheme is useful from a planning point of view, making it possible to estimate the number of 'at risk' families in a caseload. It can help indicate the relative need for supportive services and levels of staff in and between areas. There is little value in pinpointing the families most likely to be at risk if there is no hope of offering them extra support.

Support services

There are self-help groups specially set up to help families finding it difficult to cope with stress and the tensions of parenthood. Anne Ashley (1980) described the history of the voluntary associations providing anonymous telephone counselling services and their subsequent proliferation. Some are able to provide group meetings too.

The work of the self-help groups in the Organisation for Parents Under Stress (OPUS) has been studied by the Mental Health Foundation (Meacher, 1982). A large number of people who had joined a group had benefited significantly. They were better able to talk about their problems and had changed their patterns of caring for their children.

Many of the volunteers had themselves experienced abuse as children. Many had had worries about their relationship with at least one of their children, which enabled them to empathise with the people they were trying to help. A 24-hour support service was felt to be important.

Few of the callers to OPUS suffered from unemployment or housing problems. Most were able to afford their own phone. Health visitors should remember that the families likely to feel most stressed, the low paid and the unemployed, are the least likely to use these self-help groups. They will need appropriate services organised locally.

Health visitors set up a walk-in unit in Hertfordshire (Butler, 1983). In that area, a great deal of time was spent in professional discussions about children 'at risk', and the unit was proposed as a way of providing a practical solution to some of the difficulties faced. It was a flexible facility, providing a place where:
— children could be left in safe hands for a short time
— mothers could
  — meet other mothers
  — discuss problems with the health visitor
  — join in activities with the children
— health visitors could observe
  — child behaviour
  — mother—child interaction.

The health visitors found it very helpful to be able to give the mothers reassurance and advice based on these observations, another example of the interlinking of health education and support in our work.

The success of the unit has led to a decision to amalgamate with a local play group to form a family centre. Several unemployed fathers have already shown an interest in it. It will be able to provide health education and support on a full family basis, increasing understanding and reducing stress, thereby helping to prevent child abuse and other problems.

In this section we have looked at schemes for identifying families thought to be 'at risk', with a view to providing them with extra care and attention, and at examples of special supportive services. The health visitor's aim is to help minimise the degree of tensions, misunderstanding and other difficulties and so prevent the development of situations leading to child abuse.

WHEN PROBLEMS ARISE

The main thrust in this aspect of health visiting is in trying to prevent a crisis situation. However, we now turn to what happens when a crisis does occur. The decisions about what should be done are inevitably difficult and need to be child-centred and based on both medical and social factors. Support from nurse managers and inter-professional decision-making and action are very important factors.

Who is the client?

For some families the strains and tensions become too great and, to some degree, child abuse occurs. Where this has or seems to have happened, decisions have to be taken in order help the family and to try to prevent further deterioration of the situation.

Deterioration for whom? Normally in health visiting each member of the family is considered a client. However, particularly in matters pertaining to child abuse, the child is seen as the primary client. Where parental interests conflict with those of their child, the child's welfare takes precedence.

What is normal and what is abuse?

The decision at one end of the scale might be, for example, to suggest a place for the child at the day nursery to ease family tensions by giving the parents and child a break from each other.

At the other extreme, it might be to encourage the parents to make immediate contact with the social services department and seek help or even for the health visitor to do so. The former decision would be based on the assumption that the problem was currently within reasonably normal limits but might get worse, the latter on the assumption that the situation seemed to be significantly more dangerous. Where is the borderline and how do we decide which conduct amounts to normal family behaviour and which to child abuse?

It is easy to classify as abuse a situation in which a parent or carer is clearly vindictive and cruel or has killed a child. However, most cases involve grey areas and therefore are not so clear-cut. There are guidelines but in essence the decision has to be based on a value judgement. It is interesting to note that a small study found the relative seriousness of various theoretical incidents of child mistreatment were categorised by health visitors and social workers in a remarkably similar way (Fox & Dingwall, 1985).

EARLY DECISIONS

Warning signs . . . . .

Sometimes non-accidental injuries come to the notice of health visitors because parents confide in them. In some cases, they are initially based on suspicions. This can be because:
— the child has bruises which show a particular pattern
— there is an inadequate explanation of the injuries, such as inconsistencies in the account
— there has been a delay in seeking care, perhaps the mother treated the injury and it was seen with another injury.
Additional warning signs can be apprehension by the child and disturbed parental behaviour (Ross et al, 1977) and the child being stunted in height and/or weight.

. . . . . and caution

There are traps for the unwary. Misunderstanding or, for example, inadequate knowledge of traditions amongst ethnic minorities can lead to misdiagnosis of child abuse (Chan, 1985; Black, 1986). Inexperience in differentiating between non-accidental injury and accidental injury or failure to recognise certain medical conditions can lead to similar problems (O'Doherty, 1982; Oates, 1984).

Health visitors find themselves 'gatekeepers' to the system in which people become labelled as 'abusers' (Gelles, 1975). They are faced with inherent anxieties associated with attempting to decide the relative risks of physical injury, for example against the less immediately visible risks of emotional injury due to separation from the family (Moore, 1985).

A wide range of factors

Dingwall et al (1981, p. 21–22) found health visitors identified more cases than social workers confirmed because the former:
— combined social and clinical evidence

— were more particularly concerned with children, rather than the family as a unit
— were more concerned with the short term, i.e. the pre-school years
— had greater concern for current symptoms than possible causes of the problem.

Both of the professions (and the parents) used 'justifications' and 'excuses', for example the particular cultural or economic circumstances of the family, to absolve parents to some extent. Assessments were made under a 'rule of optimism' in which, where possible, staff think the best of people.

This approach provides a solution to the problem of the tension in our society between its special regard for the privacy of the family and yet the need to inspect if children are to be protected. In exchange for free access, health and welfare services promise parents that they will think the best of whatever they find. This rule then, breaks down where parents resist inspection by these child protection agencies or where the family's circumstances have ceased to be private and have become public knowledge (Dingwall, 1983). Dingwall et al (1983, p. 101) suggest that this:

. . . . . would seem to filter moral character in such a way as to hold back some, upper-, middle-, and 'respectable' working-class parents, members of ethnic minorities and mentally incompetent parents while leaving the 'rough' indigenous working class as the group proportionately most vulnerable to compulsory measures.

Reports on how the system has failed (Department of Health and Social Security, 1982, p. 69) show that, amongst many others, these two factors are important, for example

many allegations of abuse by members of the public turn out to be well-founded. . . . . The child or children must be seen.

Professor Greenland's (1986) study of child abuse and neglect deaths showed, as has other research, the importance of continuous assessment of the progress of the child and the need to respond to warnings by neighbours and concerned relatives. An outline of the factors he showed to be key issues in

Box 11.3 Some of the factors associated with deaths due to child abuse and neglect (from Greenland, 1986)

Child
Young baby, especially under one year
Already sustained broken bones/fractured skull
At or below third centile for weight and height
Severe behaviour disorder, difficult to rear
May express help-seeking behaviour

Parents
Already known to child protection agency
Underlying social and emotional stresses
Lack system of social, family or professional support
History of:
    criminal assaultive behaviour
    abuse of drugs and alcohol

Professionals
Inexperienced and unskilled professionals, such as medical/social workers
Poor interdisciplinary action and communication
Fail to respond to:
    warnings by neighbours and relatives
    help-seeking behaviour of parents

helping to identify high risk situations are listed in Box 11.3.

More than half the victims in Professor Greenland's study died during their first year of life, a quarter died in their second year and fewer than 5% after the age of five. About half the victims were at or below the third centile for height or weight, and about the same number were already known to the child protection agency. Well over half had had previous injuries treated by a physician.

GUIDANCE

By nurse managers

It is clear that there are many factors to be considered in the decisions to be made. Health visitors, particularly the less experienced, need to have direct contact with and support from nurse managers in order to enable
— case discussion
— help with action planning
— preparation for case conferences
— preparation for court
— help to resolve allied emotional difficulties from the earliest stages in this type of work

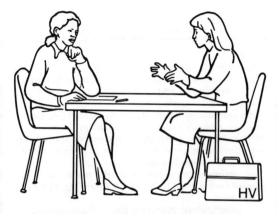

DIRECT CONTACT AND SUPPORT

Fig. 11.2 Direct contact with and support from the health visitor nurse manager.

Box 11.4 Outline of an example of non-accidental injury to children procedures manual

> **Procedure for nursing staff**
>
> Aim: identification and regular surveillance to prevent occurrence of injury
>
> 1. *Where injuries*, established or suspected:
>   *Immediate action*
>   'Place of Safety' if necessary to prevent further injury
>   *Ensure*:
>   a. Seen by doctor
>   b. Inform Principal Area Officer, Social Services (PAO)
>   c. Inform Nursing Manager(NM)
>   d. Plus written report to NM for PAO
>
> 2. *Where suspicion* but no immediate medical problem:
>   a. Discuss with GP
>   b. Inform NM
>   c. Inform PAO
>   d. Written report to Social Services
>
> 3. (i)   Case conference:
>   Convened by PAO—can be requested by others
>   (ii) Previously notified cases:
>   NM keeps file—submit regular report
>   (iii) Legal services:
>   Inform NM where legal involvement

(see Fig. 11.2). The local authority procedures manual on non-accidental injury to children is likely to encourage this (Department of Health and Social Security, 1986). An example of procedures for nursing staff is outlined in Box 11.4.

The Jasmine Beckford case highlighted the fact that although health visitors are responsible for their own actions, it is necessary for nurse management to provide support (Nursing Times, 1985; Jay, 1985). The health visitors in the Lucie Gates case were found in two reports to have acted conscientiously, but their managers were condemned for failing to provide adequate advice, support and supervision. It seems that the nurse managers failed to assess the problems and had not provided policies for nurses involved in child abuse cases. Neither of the nursing officers nor the senior nursing officer in the case had health visitor qualifications or experience (Nursing Times, 1982). Nurse managers without a health visitor background need to read widely about child abuse, and themselves need support until they have become experienced in this aspect of their work.

A graphic account has been given by Jane Schofield (1983) of the stress associated with setting up a good relationship with a couple and then moving away from her usual non-judgemental approach on account of child mistreatment. Both parents were drug addicts.

The mother, in particular, seemed very receptive to health visiting and talked about improving the children's welfare. However, the children's condition went from bad to worse while the parents lives were dominated by the search for drugs, and the decision had to be made to protect the children. Miss Schofield said how lonely she felt and recounted the emotional confusion associated both with the decision to take the children into care and the experience in court. Later, an accidental fire at the flat when the parents were 'high' killed the father and nearly the mother too. This provided proof that it had been the right decision, but it had been and still was painful. She felt she had learned the hard way.

A six month trial in which a specialist nursing officer dealt only with child abuse was found to be particularly successful. The health visitors appreciated the accessibility at all times, the crisis support which helped to alleviate anxiety and the help with preparation for case conferences (Bailey et al, 1984). The trial was a small one but it increased enthusiasm for a specialist post amongst the health visitors taking part.

On violence to staff

One of the issues over which health visitors need particular support is associated with the degree of risk they run working in the homes of families in which violence is relatively commonplace. Guidance has been given at health visitor meetings on how to look out for signs of approaching violence (Health Visitor, 1983d; 1986) and guidelines are outlined in Box 11.5. It seems that the arrival of the health visitor can become the 'trigger event' in a situation of rising tension. The health visitor can become a scapegoat and finish up as a 'lightning conductor' for the violence. The mere presence of professional people and the extra anxieties associated with the visit, can cause them to become the object of aggression.

Robert Dingwall (1984) suggested that economic stringencies have led to an increase in this danger for community nurses. He also said that, in a way, there has been a conspiracy of silence on the issue, perhaps to prevent exacerbating the problem by attracting public attention to it. In his research, however, he found that some employers were clearly not taking the problem seriously, even after an incident had taken place. He felt that an over-emphasis on training can lead to the misguided assumption that violence can be blamed on the failure of a nurse to use the proper techniques. This he felt diverts attention away from the need for an appropriate managerial response to the basic problem.

Box 11.5

Some signs of potential aggression and violence (from Health Visitor, 1983d; 1986)

Flushed face
Trembling hands
Sweating
Raised voice
Expression of anger/hate/excessive criticism
Excitable
Pacing around
Kicks furniture
Stands up to tower over visitor

Box 11.6 Outline of HVA guidance on staff safety (From Health Visitor Association, 1984, pp. 4–6)

Policies to:
— identify hazardous areas/times of day
— outline authority's actions to minimise hazards, e.g. working in pairs, visiting on priority occasions, at certain times
— provide guidance on reporting hazards/incidents
  — management discover scale of problem
  — to inform visiting staff of need for special care
— respect health visitor's opinion of advisibility of revisit by same health visitor
  — ensure safety if revisit to take place
— state procedures to be taken following an incident
  — immediately attending any GP/occupational health
  — report matter to police
  — complete report to line manager & health & safety rep
  — authority support of prosecutions

Precautions, where relevant:
— not visiting alone after dark
— visiting: on priority occasions; notifying colleague at end of visit; with colleague outside house; in pairs; with nurse manager; doorstep only; see only at clinic
— clinic work: with minimum levels of staff where isolated; security precautions
— use of special alarm equipment—value debatable

Training should:
— centre on health visitors most at risk
— ensure familiarity with authority's safety policy and procedures available to help avoid violence
— teach how to identify potentially violent situation; simple techniques to prevent/avoid physical aggression

---

Some student health visitors are given self-defence training during their course, others gain what information they can from books such as Pat Butler's (1982) *Self-defence for women* or Kaleghi Quinn's (1983) *Stand your ground*. It is most important to try to keep the situation as calm as possible to avoid having to use a physically defensive strategy and getting trapped, and to have a clear idea of possible exit routes (Health Visitor, 1983d). An outline of the Health Visitors Association's (1984) health and safety guidance on staff safety will be found in Box 11.6. It is to be hoped that it is being widely discussed and instituted at field level.

On records

Nurse managers should aim to enable their health visitors to make up their notes contemporaneously, that is as near in time as possible to the visit, and certainly on the same day or within 24 hours. This is for accuracy and in case the evidence they contained should ever be needed in court (Godber, 1981). An audio-typing service is an obvious advantage.

Advice from tutors on recording information is no longer likely to be against making a permanent note of 'discrediting information', which is what Dingwall (1977) had found in his research in the early 1970s. If there is any suspicion of abuse, factual and pertinent evidence of what has been said, seen or done, both by the health visitor and/or family members, must be recorded.

Box 11.7 Important items to record where child abuse is suspected

---

What has been *seen* by health visitor:
— traumata such as burns, cuts, bruising, noting location and appearance
— height and weight on percentile chart, noting changes in serial observation
— developmental attainments, if possible on a bar chart or step-ladder centile chart, noting changes in serial observation
— parent—child interaction, noting reactions to each other's intiatives e.g. by touching, visual contact

What has been *said* by parent(s) recounting:
— their viewpoint and explanations of the situation
— health history, particularly evidence of organic reasons for failure to thrive
— developmental milestones, e.g. aware of and responsive to bath, ability to sit unsupported, speech development (at appropriate ages)
— family history, e.g. alcohol, drugs and history of violence

What has been *done* by health visitor:
— appointments made with family, e.g. to visit GP or clinic and for further visits by health visitor
— co-professionals contacted, e.g. GP, social worker, NSPCC
— meetings attended
— dates
   — of home visits
   — notes left for family when not found at home
   — family seen but no access to child
— contact with nurse manager re problem, e.g. not able to see family and/or child

---

June Helberg (1983) described factors that need to be assessed and documented, some of which are incorporated into the list of important items for recording in Box 11.7

Borderline cases

It is difficult for health visitors to reach decisions when they come across what they feel are borderline cases. It is best if they can share their problem anonymously with a sympathetic co-professional who is a good listener, perhaps a social worker, another health visitor, a GP or their nurse manager. A 'hypothetical case' presented in such a way that the family could not be identified, means the health visitor can speak freely and will 'label' no one. The process of explaining the pro and cons that make the case so borderline might trigger a decision one way or the other: either, for example, that there is no real problem, or that the suspicion seems justified and should be taken a step further and formally reported.

FORMAL PROCEEDINGS

The main purpose of setting in motion the formal procedures (see Box 11.4) is to protect the child through coordinated help to the family. Three agencies have a statutory investigatory role in the protection of children: the Social Services Departments, the NSPCC and, on occasions, the police. Health visitors have no statutory powers and are unable to undertake the prolonged and frequent visiting necessary for crisis management. The time it takes up would prejudice the preventive work for the rest of their caseload.

Reporting the problem to the social services department puts the process into action. Where there seems to be great and immediate danger, the child is taken to a place of safety such as a specially selected foster home. In all cases, a case conference will be called, and the urgency with which this is done will be determined by the apparent degree of risk to the child. If at the case conference the problem is confirmed, the child's name will be entered on to the Child Concern/Abuse Register and a plan of action for care and support of the family proposed.

Hazards

There has been considerable criticism of the system, for example that it can be protectionist and over-used (Buckle, 1979; Thomas, 1980). The case conference has been described as a blunt and expensive instrument, conducted like a secret trial, convened in haste and leading to ill-thought-out, ill-informed conclusions with a resultant lack of trust between social and health workers (Barrie, 1979; Moore, 1986). Communication between health visitors and social workers has been described as far too one-sided (Musanandara, 1984).

A governmental draft guide to inter-agency cooperation has made many suggestions which, if followed, should help overcome many of these difficulties. It should also help clarify where the responsibility lies for maintaining regular contact with and coordinating the work of the various agencies involved. These and other key matters, such as coordinating and ensuring a comprehensive review of the case at least six monthly, are clearly stated as the duty of a designated social worker from either the social services department or the NSPCC (Department of Health and Social Security, 1986).

It has been suggested that in certain rare circumstances a health visitor (or other nurse) might be nominated 'prime worker' to work with a 'case coordinator', a level 3 social worker, dealing with all the administrative arrangements which are the responsibility of the 'key worker' (see Fig. 11.3). Relevant circumstances might be if the health visitor were the only worker acceptable to a family with, for example, problems of emotional

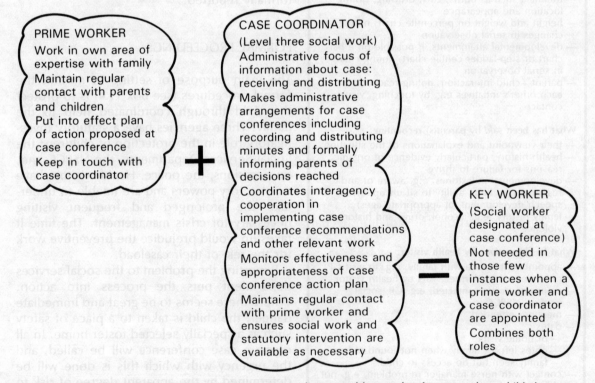

PRIME WORKER
Work in own area of expertise with family
Maintain regular contact with parents and children
Put into effect plan of action proposed at case conference
Keep in touch with case coordinator

+

CASE COORDINATOR
(Level three social work)
Administrative focus of information about case: receiving and distributing
Makes administrative arrangements for case conferences including recording and distributing minutes and formally informing parents of decisions reached
Coordinates interagency cooperation in implementing case conference recommendations and other relevant work
Monitors effectiveness and appropriateness of case conference action plan
Maintains regular contact with prime worker and ensures social work and statutory intervention are available as necessary

=

KEY WORKER
(Social worker designated at case conference)
Not needed in those few instances when a prime worker and case coordinator are appointed
Combines both roles

Fig. 11.3 Outline of functions of prime worker, case coordinator and key worker for cases where child abuse and neglect exists or is suspected.

abuse and neglect. This arrangement could only be made if there were agreement between the line manager and the health visitor, who would be given relief from some other caseload work (Health Visitor, 1983a, 1983b; Fawcett-Henesy, 1986).

Continued contact

In line with the policy of providing extra help for families with greater problems, staffing levels permitting, a family with child abuse and neglect difficulties would be given an increased level of visiting. This would be for surveillance of child development and nutrition, health education and some emotional support for the parents. Very occasionally, health visitors become more involved (Cannon & Walker, 1985).

When the child has been removed into care, it is important that the health visiting service is still provided. From one point of view, the child still needs to be monitored and foster parents can be very grateful for support and advice (Health Visitor, 1983c). From another point of view, it is important both to support the parents and to help them talk through the situation, and to remain in touch in readiness for the child's return.

Health visitors would expect to write a report on the case or to attend every case conference. This would occur at least every six months. If health visitors can be as open as possible with the parents about, for example, the content of their reports, it gives the parents a chance both to discuss the criteria and the issues involved and to make appropriate moves to sort out the situation (Department of Health and Social Security, 1986, p. 18). Some will want to contact parents' organisations such as PAIN, Parents Against INjustice (Holmes, 1986a; Whitehouse, 1986), or the Family Rights Group for specific help and support (addresses at the end of the chapter). Parents Aid (1987) provides a useful booklet for parents with children in care or likely to be so.

A few health visitors are obliged to go to court and give evidence about their work with the family. Under these circumstances there is particular advantage if they have been open and truthful about their aims and opinions on how the family has been progressing, so the parents learn nothing new in court. It is obviously an extremely painful experience for the parents, and is generally unnerving and distressing for the health visitor too. Peter Godber (1980a, 1980b, 1980c, 1981) has written lucidly and reassuringly on court procedure, and the Court Training Services offer pertinent advice on all the key aspects.

We have just taken a brief look at health visitors' work aimed at preventing a worsening of the situation when child abuse is discovered or suspected. Earlier in the chapter there were examples of the way health visitors aim, through education, to prevent the occurrence of child abuse and, through selection and support, to prevent development of stresses and strains which can result in child abuse. The discussion has also provided yet another example of the use of the prevention framework proposed in this book.

EXAMPLES OF WORK IN THE FIELD OF CHILD ABUSE

The first example is of work with an exasperated young mother with an attention-seeking three-year old and a 'difficult to rear' baby. The second is of caseload-wide work aimed at preventing the occurrence and development of stresses and strains that can lead to child abuse. Outlines will be found in Tables 11.4 and 11.5.

EXAMPLE ONE: THE WALKER FAMILY

Mrs Hester Vines (HV) had completed her health visitor training six months previously and had taken up a post in a small town. Mrs Walker, whom she had first met antenatally, had a three-year-old son, Paul, and a small baby.

A questionnaire was completed for the local computerised baby surveillance system at the third visit, when the baby girl was four weeks

Table 11.4 Example one: the Walker family

Aim	Through	Examples
To prevent occurrence of child abusing situation	Teaching	Discussions at visits: babies' need for fondling and attention; tensions and child abuse
	Normal supportive services	Told about groups and agencies at birth visit, not followed up
To prevent development of stress & tensions leading to child abuse	1. Identifying those vulnerable 2. Enabling extra support for them	Computerised system indicated high risk baby More frequent visiting Discussion about difficulties; FIS and other entitlements
To prevent deterioration where child abuse seems to have occurred	Child-centred decisions with nurse management support	Use social and clinical evidence: naked weight and appearance; family history and social support Full, shared and contemporaneous records Multi-profession decision & action

old. The result was that she was classified as 'high risk' (Powell, 1985). It was at the seventh home visit when the baby was twelve weeks old that Mrs Walker had confided that the previous week, in a moment of extreme anger, she had found herself shaking the baby. She had checked herself and felt she had not harmed her, but was terribly distressed because she felt she might yet do that. The health visitor explained that she was obliged to tell her nurse manager of such cases when they arose. Mrs Walker acceded to that and added that she felt she needed help.

The matter was discussed at length, with HV encouraging Mrs Walker to express her feelings about the problem. It seems that Mr Walker never helped in the house or with the children; he was not violent, but was rather withdrawn. He was employed by a firm of contract cleaners and the family claimed family income supplement and allied entitlements. They had no family or friends

locally and Mrs Walker had not made any contact with any local mothers' groups. She had had a very autocratic upbringing with some violence.

Baby Mary was the sort who was not very responsive to fondling: wriggling and struggling whenever she was held. She frequently posseted after meals, cried a great deal when left alone, for example in her pram, and was likened to 'Aunt Susan, who is always wingeing'. Paul, having been a 'good baby' was now attention seeking, and it was one of his apparently contrived 'accidents' that had triggered the frustration which was eventually vented on the baby.

In due course, the baby's developmental tests were noted on the step-ladder centile charts and HV, as normal, weighed her naked, plotting the result on a percentile graph, both measures continuing well within normal limits. There were no signs of bruises, burns or wheals.

Mrs Walker and HV discussed the idea of Paul attending a playgroup in the mornings and, if it were possible, getting a temporary place at a social services department day nursery two or three mornings a week. The health visitor explained she would need to tell the appropriate social worker about the problems Mrs Walker was having and that he/she might need to visit to assess for eligibility for these hard-to-come-by places. Mrs Walker said she was happy for that to be set in motion. They agreed too, that HV should contact the GP in order to ensure that an appointment be arranged for the baby to be checked over soon. A record of the visit was made before leaving the flat and HV arranged to return in two days' time.

Mrs Vines had phoned her nurse manager for an appointment and found Mrs Nora Major (NM) in her office that lunchtime as arranged. Just as Mrs Walker had found it helpful to pour out her heart to HV, HV was now grateful for NM's preparedness to listen sympathetically and to make practical suggestions. The health visitor reported that this family was not already on the Child Protection Register, and they discussed how the reports should be written. NM agreed that there would probably be playgroup and day nursery places for the children and asked if HV knew about the District 'Troublesome Baby Group' set up by some health visitors for such parents. They showed trigger films to stimulate discussion and found it had evolved into a good self-help group. She also asked if the GP knew about the problem, to which HV replied that he had undertaken to see the baby that morning.

In the event, the family was given the playgroup place for Paul and a two mornings a week nursery place for some months for Mary, which Mrs Walker found very therapeutic. She attended the 'Troublesome Baby Group' and found some good friends there. After a case conference, the family had been put on the Child Protection Register. Things went well and the name was removed at another case conference three months later. For some time after that, NM would enquire every few months how the family were progressing.

EXAMPLE TWO: STRATEGIES AIMED AT PREVENTING CHILD ABUSE

Miss Helen Voisey (HV) was reviewing schemes aiming to minimise the incidence of child abuse, both by working within her caseload and in the local community. Part of the caseload work involved trying to identify the people most vulnerable to this problem in order to offer extra support as it was needed, particularly through the

Table 11.5 Example two strategies aimed at preventing child abuse

Aim	Through	Examples
To prevent occurrence of child abusing situation	Teaching	Parenthood courses in school: liaison— school nurse & teachers Group discussions on child abuse
	Normal supportive services	Tell about groups and agencies Normal 'therapeutic listening'
To prevent development of stress & tensions leading to child abuse	1. Identifying those vulnerable	Combined sudden infant death & child abuse surveillance scheme
	2. Enabling extra support for them	Tell of telephone crisis contact self-help groups More frequent visiting
To prevent deterioration where child abuse seems to have occurred	Child-centred decisions with nurse management support	No recent experience of suspected or actual child abuse

first year of their baby's life. Work in the general locality involved trying to improve understanding about child care and matters associated with child abuse, to encourage open discussion, less apprehension about seeking help and greater knowledge of how to seek help, as well as better parent–child interaction.

In order to have some relevant support services, the West Seahaven District Health Authority had set aside some joint funding towards a family centre in the poorest part of town. The local authority social services day nurseries gave highest priority to cases involving actual or suspected child abuse.

It was a question of finding the families who most needed help. The previous year the health visitors had decided it would be a good idea to start an infant surveillance scheme similar to the one in Portsmouth in which both child abuse and sudden infant death factors were incorporated (Powell, 1985).

A working party had been set up and HV had been invited to join it. It had meant a great deal of hard work, looking up papers from the library and finding out how other authorities' schemes were working out. Now decisions were made and the scheme they had instituted was running smoothly.

Some 5% of HV's caseload were rated as 'high risk', and so far she had had none rated 'very high risk'. Very few needed the sort of supportive help that was required in the areas nearer the centre of town. Many of the women in her caseload were able to afford babysitters to give them a break, had mothers or sisters living nearby, or had joined a specially organised self-help babysitting circle. She had just introduced two new mothers to a newly developing group and had been invited to lead a discussion on child abuse at one of their monthly evening meetings. It seems they had heard about her talks at the women's groups of the local churches.

At a recent meeting of community health nurses and teachers at the local school there had been a great deal of interest in health educational aspects of child abuse. The school nurse, HV and the general studies teacher had spent a good deal of time discussing various aspects of the topic, and had swapped ideas and given each other leads on relevant articles and pamphlets. The other two had not known of the Ackley (1977) paper; HV heard about pamphlets specifically for children, about which some of 'her mothers' might like to know. The teacher had asked if HV knew a mother who would be prepared to come and bath her baby and to talk about what it really feels like to be a mother—the difficulties as well as the joys. One mother, an ex-teacher, had since offered to go.

It seemed to HV that working together with other professionals had helped improve all their contributions towards health education over child abuse. She had worked with the priests and vicars and was now working with the teachers and, as ever, with the school nurse. Working with other

health visitors had helped bring in a useful new infant surveillance scheme.

However, Miss Voisey concluded, child abuse could never be thought about or dealt with in isolation, but was necessarily an aspect of wider considerations. For example, in health education it is just one part of any discussion on parentcraft, in caseload work a relevant part of wider infant surveillance and, for the individual parent, part of and influenced by their social situation.

USEFUL ADDRESSES

Court Training Services,
79 Merton Hall Road,
Wimbledon,
London SW19 3TX
Tel 01 540 7487

Family Rights Group,
6–9 Manor Gardens,
Holloway Road,
London N7 6LA
Tel 01 272 4231/2
01 272 7308

PAIN, Parents Against Injustice,
Conifers,
2 Pledgeon Green, nr Henham,
Bishop's Stortford, Herts.
Tel 0279 850545

REFERENCES

Ackley D C 1977 A brief overview of child abuse. Social Casework 58: 21–24

Ashley A 1980 Voluntary self-help for parents under stress in Britain. Midwife Health Visitor and Community Nurse 16: 244–246

Bailey J, Ramm K, Warner U 1984 The nursing officer's role. Nursing Times Community Outlook 80,11: 102

Barrie H 1979 Personal opinion—on case conferences. Midwife Health Visitor and Community Nurse 15: 188–192

Black J A 1986 Misdiagnosis of child abuse in ethnic minorities. Midwife Health Visitor and Community Nurse 22: 48–53

Borkowski M, Murch M, Walker V 1983 Marital violence—the community response. Tavistock Publications, London

Buckle J 1979 NAI registers: a substitute for communication. Social Work Today 10, 30: 23

Butler A J 1983 A walk-in unit for pre-school children and their mothers. Health Visitor 56: 411–412

Butler P 1982 Self-defence for women. New English Library, London

Cannon D, Walker J 1985 Getting off the treadmill. Health Visitor 58: 192–193

Chan M C K 1985 Chinese and Vietnamese families (letter). British Medical Journal 290 1588

Child Sexual Abuse Preventive Education Project, Driver E 1985 Have your children been sexually abused? CSAPEP, c/o Hungerford House, Victoria Embankment, London WC2

Dean J G, MacQueen I A G, Mitchell R G, Kempe C H 1978 Health visitor's role in prediction of early childhood injuries and failure to thrive. Child Abuse and Neglect 2: 1–17

Department of Health and Social Security 1982 Child abuse. A study of inquiry reports 1973–1981. HMSO, London

Department of Health and Social Security 1986 Working together. A draft guide to arrangements for interagency cooperation for the protection of children. DHSS, London

Dingwall R 1977 The social organisation of health visitor training. Croom Helm, London, p. 108

Dingwall R 1983 Child abuse—the real questions. Nursing Times 79, 25: 67–68

Dingwall R 1984 Who is to blame, anyway? Nursing Times 80, 15: 42–43

Dingwall R, Eekelaar J, Murray T 1981 Care or control? Decision-making in the care of children thought to have been abused or neglected. A summary of the final report. Social Science Research Council Centre for Socio-Legal Studies, Wolfson College, Oxford

Dingwall R, Eekelaar J, Murray T 1983 The protection of children. State intervention and family life. Basil Blackwell, Oxford

Elliot M 1985 The child assault prevention programme. Health Visitor 58: 187–188

Fawcett-Henesy A 1986 Who is the key worker? Community Care 605: 20–21

Fort A 1986 The spider's web. The Health Service Journal 96: 558–559

Forward S, Buck C 1981 Betrayal of innocence: incest and its devastation. Pelican Books, Harmondsworth, Middlesex

Fox S, Dingwall R 1985 An exploratory study of variations in social workers' and health visitors' definitions of child mistreatment. British Journal of Social Work 15: 467–477

Gelles R J 1975 The social construction of child abuse. American Journal of Orthopsychiatry 45, 3: 363–371

Godber P 1980a The health visitor in court–1. Health Visitor 53: 83–84

Godber P 1980b The health visitor in court–2. Health Visitor 53: 162–164

Godber P 1980c The health visitor in court–3. Health Visitor 53: 206–209

Godber P 1981 Confidentiality of case records. Health Visitor 54: 193

Greenland C 1986 Preventing child abuse and neglect deaths: the identification and management of high risk cases. Health Visitor 59: 205–206

Health Visitor 1983a Child abuse: a step forward. Health Visitor 56: 41

Health Visitor 1983b Health visitor's role in child abuse clarified. Health Visitor 56: 43

Health Visitor 1983c Children in care: HVs should be more involved. Health Visitor 56: 115

Health Visitor 1983d Violence: coping strategies for HVs. Health Visitor 56: 442

Health Visitor 1986 Violence to health visitors: health authorities must have safety policies. Health Visitor 59: 27

Health Visitor Association 1984 Health and safety in the community—some guidance on safety policies from the Health Visitors' Association. Health Visitors' Association, London, p4–6

Helberg J L 1983 Documentation in child abuse. American Journal of Nursing 83, 2: 236–239

Holmes P 1986a Innocent parents. Nursing Times 82, 3: 16–18

Holmes P 1986b It's OK to say no. Nursing Times 82, 3: 18

Jay M 1985 The Jasmine Beckford case. Death of a child in care. The Listener 114, 2931: 6–7

Johnson C 1985 Identifying children at risk: a system for health visitors. Health Visitor 58: 195–196

Kempe R S, Kempe C H 1978 Child abuse. Fontana, London

Korbin J E 1980 The cross-cultural context of child abuse and neglect. In: Kempe C H, Helfer R E (eds) The battered child 3rd ed. University of Chicago Press, London

Laurance J 1985 Collating information to prevent child abuse. Primary Health Care 3, 11: 6

Lynch M A, Roberts J 1977 Predicting child abuse: signs of bonding failure in the maternity hospital. British Medical Journal I: 624–626

Meacher M A 1982 Self-help groups for parents under stress: a contribution to prevention? Mental Health Foundation, London

Moore J 1985 For the children's sake. Nursing Times 81, 42: 19–20

Moore J 1986 All in the family. Community Care 609: 22–23

Musnandara T 1984 Communication between workers: the key in cases of child abuse? Health Visitor 57: 233

Nelson S 1982 Incest: fact and myth. Stramullion Co-operative Ltd, Edinburgh

Nursing Times 1982 New team to look at Gates death. Nursing Times 78: 2010

Nursing Times 1985 The Beckford case has shown it is vital to have sufficient clinical managers to back up community staff. Nursing Times 81, 50: 3

Oates R K 1984 Overturning the diagnosis of child abuse. Archives of Disease in Childhood 59: 665–666

O'Doherty N 1982 The battered child. Recognition in primary care. Bailliere Tindall, London

Ounsted C, Roberts J C, Gordon M, Milligan B 1982 Fourth goal of perinatal medicine. British Medical Journal 284: 879–882

Parents Aid 1987 Guide for parents with children in care: 101 questions and answers. 4th ed. Parents Aid, 66 Chippingfield, Harlow, Essex CM17 0DJ

Parton N 1985 The politics of child abuse. Macmillan, London

Powell J 1985 Keeping watch. Nursing Times Community Outlook 81, 2: 15–19

Pownall M 1985 A family affair? Nursing Times 81, 43: 58–61

Quinn K 1983 Stand your ground: a woman's guide to self-preservation. Orbis, London

Radbill S X 1980 Children in a world of violence: a history of child abuse. In: Kempe C H, Helfer R E (eds) The battered child 3rd ed. University of Chicago Press, London

Renvoise J 1982 Incest: a family pattern. Routledge and Kegan Paul, London

Ross K R, Smith E S, Williams E O, Bradley S J, Wright J D 1977 Frozen awareness. A guide to diagnosis and management of non-accidental injury to children. Wolverhampton Area Review Committee, Wolverhampton

Schofield J 1983 Visiting can be stressful, too. Nursing Mirror 157, 13: 20–21

Thomas T 1980 Blinded by the light when the red button is pushed. Health and Social Services Journal LXXXX: 950–951

Thorneley N 1986 Child abuse lessons from the past (letter). Nursing Times 82, 2: 12

Tucker N 1985 A panic over child abuse. New Society 74: 96–98

Vizard E 1985 Facing the facts. Nursing Mirror 161, 17: 14–15

Waterhouse I 1981 A bar on abuse. Health and Social Services Journal XCI: 1302–1303

Weeks V 1982 Health visitors, stress and non-accidental injury to children. Health Visitor 55: 75

Whitehouse A 1986 The anguish of the parent. Community Care 597: 20–22

Woods J 1981 A practical approach to preventing child abuse. Health Visitor 54: 281–283

SUGGESTED FURTHER READING

Child sexual abuse

Johnson R A 1985 Incest Crisis Line. Health Visitor 58: 187

Mills J 1985 Breaking the last taboo. The Listener 114, 2933: 11–12

Trowell J 1985 Working with families where incest is actual or feared. Health Visitor 58: 189–191

Vizard E 1984 The sexual abuse of children. Health Visitor 57: 234–236

Vizard E 1984 The sexual abuse of children—part 2. Health Visitor 57: 279–280

Wild N J 1986 Sexual abuse of children in Leeds. British Medical Journal 292: 1113–1116

Decision-making and evidence

Hall J G, Mitchell B H 1978 Child abuse—procedure and evidence in Juvenile Courts. Barry Rose, Chichester

Vernon J, Fruin D 1986 In care. A study of social work decision making. National Children's Bureau, London

Emotional abuse

Gath A 1984 Emotional abuse. Maternal and Child Health 9: 229–232

Gath A 1985 Recognition and treatment of emotional abuse. Update 31: 445–452

Trowell J 1983 Emotional abuse of children. Health Visitor 56: 252–255

General

Carver V (ed) 1978 Child abuse, a study text. Open University Press, Milton Keynes

Jones D N 1982 Understanding child abuse. Hodder and Stoughton, London

Kempe C H, Helfer R E 1980 The battered child. 3rd edn. University of Chicago Press, London

Lee C M (ed) 1978 Child abuse, a reader and sourcebook. Open University Press, Milton Keynes

Renvoise J 1978 Web of violence. A study of family violence. Penguin Books, Harmondsworth

The law

Bailey J M 1980 The law and the community nurse. Nursing Department, Cumbria Area Health Authority, Caldcotes, Caldewgate, Carlisle CA2 5TT

Burr M 1982 The law and health visitors. Edsall, London

Department of Health and Social Security 1985 Review of child care law. Report to ministers of an interdepartmental working party. HMSO, London

Mother–infant bonding

Robson K M, Powell E 1982 Early maternal attachment. In: Brockington I F, Kumar R (eds) Motherhood and mental illness. Academic Press, London

Valman H B 1980 Mother-infant bonding. British Medical Journal 280: 308–310

In this last chapter, we look at some of the administrative changes that have affected health visiting in recent years, some of the challenges that face the profession and the need now for greater political awareness. Some of the current debates and recent initiatives are mentioned. Finally, our three basic models are considered in the light of a community-based health project, which is one of the new initiatives in health visiting.

Influences and challenges
  Recent issues
  Making the most of it

Ideas and initiatives

A future for the models

12

Health visiting— which way now?

INFLUENCES AND CHALLENGES

Administrative changes over recent years have meant that, despite high levels of agreement that prevention is better than cure, health visiting, alongside other community services, has had to fight for funds in competition with more prestigious and powerful medical lobbies. Naturally, there are fears that expenditure on community health services would not be adequate to enable proper care if the demands for limitless resources for high technology medicine prevail (DHSS, 1986, p(i)).

The purpose and the nature of health visiting is not always easily understood by people oriented to acute care. However, an increasing number of health visitors are writing and explaining about their work and about the results of new initiatives they have been undertaking. There are plenty of debates within the profession. One is on the relevance of community-based health projects, and the book concludes by showing how the three frameworks used in the earlier chapters are also relevant for this type of work.

RECENT ISSUES

The reorganisation of the health service in 1974 brought health visitors from the relative obscurity of the Medical Officers of Health Local Authority departments into mainstream nursing and funding through the NHS. They moved from a unit that clearly sympathised with and supported their preventive role, into the much larger arena of the Health Authorities, which were, until then, almost totally concerned with acute clinical care.

The Debate and 'identity'

There was an obvious need to be able to explain the health visitor's role in clear terms. In 1974, tutors were expressing concern about the definitions associated with the theoretical aspects of the course that described the practice of health visiting (Council for the Education and Training of Health Visitors, 1977). A wide ranging debate was set up by the Council for the Education and Training of Health Visitors (CETHV) (1977, 1980, 1982) in which many health visitors participated.

The self-questioning and the discussions of the CETHV's 'Investigation' coincided with a new phase in which more health visitors were prepared to write about their work and to try to find ways of evaluating it. Clear evidence of this trend can be seen in the significant improvement over recent years of the quality and content of the *Health Visitor* journal.

In the changing times of the mid-seventies, this rigorous professional self-examination naturally engendered some feelings of professional insecurity. On the other hand, it did mean that these practitioners were not just unthinkingly continuing traditional patterns of practice. They were aiming to take a critical look at what they were hoping to achieve and at the significance of various aspects of the work and to find ways of explaining it.

Not all health visitors have been thinking and acting so systematically. The Community Nursing Review Team for England (Cumberlege Committee) felt community nurses in general were too limited by their traditional roles and 'in a rut' (DHSS, 1986, p. 2–3; 11). They suggested that health visitors, district nurses and school nurses should work together in groups providing neighbourhood nursing services. It was proposed, for example, that the nurses should undertake work based on more systematically identified

health needs with improved nurse management closer to the consumer, that there should be more involvement by the consumer and good team-work by primary health care team members.

The team felt that better organised and locally planned collaborative ventures could be significantly more responsive to the needs of each particular neighbourhood and to the individuals within it. The proposals provide an exciting challenge and some very useful pointers for the next phase in the history of our work. The role and skills of the health visitor were certainly appreciated by the team, a matter taken up later in this chapter (pp. 222–223).

For the most part, the move into the larger arena has made the work of the health visitor more widely and better understood. Their particular nursing role has been accepted. Evidence of this can be seen, for example, in their being specifically named alongside nurses and midwives in the Act of Parliament that unified the various aspects of the nursing profession (DHSS, 1979).

Competing for resources

The fight for funds presents a different problem. Factors such as structural changes, the apparent need to demonstrate dramatic success and the influence of the acute care model of health, mean health visitors need to make particular efforts to explain locally about the purpose and value of their work.

Peter Townsend (1982) explained the evident contradiction between the government's declared intentions to strengthen community health services and the reality, instead, of ever increasing resources in the field of acute care. He described important factors underlying this. One is that recent structural changes have led to a weakening of the already subordinate position of community health and community care. For example, the appointment of more consultants and the centralisation of management structures have meant that the political voice for acute sickness hospitals has been strengthened.

The dominance of the idea of health in which the body is seen as a machine for which a medical engineering approach is appropriate is another factor. Some managers tend to think in terms of this medical model of 'health—illness' rather than the more complex social model of 'health—future health', which takes into account more the important non-medical factors such as the social and environmental influences on families. It is far more difficult for these people to speak for and explain about preventive health work such as health visiting. This has obvious implications for the allocation of funds for the service.

The Griffiths style of management has drawn another matter in to the equation. The general managers' three to five year appointment puts pressure on managers, as well as government, to demonstrate their 'success'. This factor also favours the dramatic, readily quantifiable aspects of health care. It can be observed in the chosen patterns of expenditure and in governmental statements about, for example, more consultants' posts, reductions in hospital waiting lists and the number of hospitals being built.

There is a further problem. Wide-ranging identification of morbidity rates in various areas of the District, the logical approach to proper preventive health care, is unlikely to be encouraged by some of the new managers for whom visible 'success' is important. Instead of being seen as a sensible base from which to make health care decisions, it can be perceived as a potential Pandora's box, liable to throw into public focus and debate evidence of many preventable problems which require attention. To deal with these would need a reallocation of funds which would have to be weaned away from the more powerful medical lobbies, a disincentive in itself. Also, there is no Dr Kildare type of dramatic appeal, the basis of good 'success' headlines, in work with people such as under-privileged young couples, the elderly, the handicapped and the unemployed.

It can be seen then that the system is loaded against prevention and community care at the moment. However, there are many people who wish to enhance the work. The managers likely to be most sympathetic to the public health needs are the new general managers for the community units. To a certain extent, they have become the successors to the Medical Officers of Health. They are unlikely to be trained in public health matters, but will probably learn fast. There is an urgent need to help them understand about the purpose and value of preventive health care and it is up to health visitors to explain. It is worth remembering that these managers, too, will need ways of demonstrating 'success'. Let us hope they are made aware of criteria for measurement, such as home accident rates, which are significantly more meaningful than, for example, the number of home visits undertaken by health visitors!

Now they are out in the larger arena, health visitors must become more politically aware. However, as Sheila Jack (Health Visitor, 1984) pointed out, attributes such as competitiveness and power necessary for politics can be quite opposite to the qualities required in the practice of health visiting and other forms of nursing. However, Miss Jack's own example shows what can be achieved (Dopson, 1986).

MAKING THE MOST OF IT

Given the current economic climate and the increased activities in favour of acute care, it does not look as if there will be a significant and widespread increase in preventive health nursing in the short term. We have yet to find out if staffing levels will keep up with, for example, the rising birth rate and pressures to provide preventive health care in preparation for the increasing numbers of very old elderly people. However, there have been plenty of examples in recent years of health visitors using their initiative and organising their time in the best way they can for the particular community they serve.

Freedom to initiate

The question arises as to whether health visitors are normally free to use their professional knowledge and understanding in order to undertake the sort of work *they* see as most important for their locality. Some Health Authorities do restrict their health visitors to certain types of activities, by excluding tasks such as health education in schools or work with the elderly. Others restrict their ability to be innovative by insisting, for example, on a certain number of home visits to be completed each week.

All too often, though, it seems that myths arise about Health Authority policies for health visiting. Judith Fitton (1983, 1984a, 1984b) surveyed the views of the community nursing leaders of 45 Northern England Health Authorities about preventive care of the elderly. The results of her work led her to feel that health visitor practice was constrained by 'phantom policies'. She speculated that there are both health visitors and nurse managers who see themselves governed by the sort of policy they would find convenient, that is a policy reflecting traditional priorities and/or their personal views. In reality it seems that 60% of the Authority policies in the study were 'laisser-faire'. In these Health Authorities, the nursing leaders felt that the health visitors themselves should decide their priorities and whom to visit. The health visitors were in fact at liberty to do what they thought best.

It has been pointed out by Sue Grierson (1983) that health visitors should not feel controlled by management and that they should be free to plan their work on the basis of their up-to-date practical experience and their detailed knowledge of their particular locality. She also suggested that health visitors should make sure that enough time is made available for discussions with their managers on what can be done to improve the service. The enabling role of management depends on this type of positive communication.

It is also important to understand managers' true position and intention. For example, the personal opinions of managers may, at first glance, mistakenly be taken to represent Authority policy. A health visitor was reported

as telling a meeting how she had planned to present her views at a local public enquiry. On being advised by management against taking this 'political action', she enquired further and found out that, in reality, she was perfectly free to make her own decision about the matter (Health Visitor, 1981). It was worth discovering what was meant by the advice. However, any repercussions there might have been affecting her later relationship with the manager through not taking the advice, were not reported.

Professional decisions and 'Griffiths' management

Issues of control and the extent to which health visitors are individually able to decide their approach, their priorities and their methods of practice, become more important as health visitors and other nurses come under the wing of the newly appointed general managers. As part of their explanations about their work, health visitors need to describe to these managers how important it is to be able to respond, for example, to street level nuances of which they become aware in the course of their work and, as described at various points in this book, to the particular needs of the families in their locality.

However, it seems likely that the ability to respond to the local situation will remain. Firstly, it would be logical for these new style managers to delegate the task of preventive health care to community nursing management. Secondly, a good manager will not knowingly quell initiative and stifle potentially useful innovation. Such a disaster is only likely if the manager is ill-informed or misinformed. It is up to the health visitors and other community nurses to ensure that the new managers are able to learn about the nature and purpose of their work. The brief given to the community nursing management can then incorporate that understanding.

This section has considered some implications of moving health visiting from the public health centred departments of the Local Authorities into the National Health Service. These include aspects of resource allocation and health visitors' ability to use their initiative and implement new, useful ideas.

IDEAS AND INITIATIVES

There have been many debates and discussions about what form initiatives should take and how best to use the scarce resource of health visiting. There is no shortage of people in medical and paramedical work who can see how health visiting could help in their particular speciality, for example, over alcoholism, drugs, pre-conceptual care, preventive health care for the middle aged and the problems of adolescence. There have been many interesting ideas put forward and many worthwhile projects undertaken. For example, an epidemiological approach has been suggested: some health visitors have been involved in widening community-based work and in inner city schemes. The debate as to whether health visitors should continue to maintain a generalist approach or should increasingly take on a more specialised remit, continues.

There can be no single solution or any one formula for all time. The best course will be if health visitors continue to debate and undertake new initiatives and also put great efforts into explaining what they are doing and why. This way, objectives, achievements and any underlying problems will be better understood, responsiveness to local requirement will receive appropriate attention and a thinking profession will be making a progressive contribution to health care.

An epidemiological approach

One of the recent debates was mainly initiated by Baroness MacFarlane (1982; Nursing Times, 1981). The wide variations in local need led her to suggest that health visitors should become the epidemiologist of the primary health care team. She questioned the value of 'attachment' to GPs and suggested that health

visitors might identify local health trends and health needs and find ways of improving them, perhaps on a 'patch' basis.

There is no lack of literature which is available to provide ideas and guidance on epidemiological concepts and practices (Richards, 1980; McCarthy, 1982; Farmer & Miller, 1983; Waters & Cliff, 1983; World Health Organisation, 1982). Jane Robinson (1983), however, proposed caution over the idea of health visitors becoming epidemiological missionaries and going out and seeking new health needs based on these kind of studies. Firstly, her research had made her very aware of the heartfelt needs amongst families at an individual level and she defended the traditional generalist approach in health visiting. Dr Robinson was also concerned about the 'spurious scientific respectability' implicitly endowed upon such small scale epidemiological studies, which would in fact be far too small to be able to produce statistically reliable conclusions.

The meaning of 'an epidemiological approach' was taken by Muir Gray (1983) to mean something rather broader. He saw it as a population-based approach as opposed to the more common approach in medicine which is concerned only with those individuals who happen to have made contact with the services. He said health visitors' interest in the wider population is a distinct attribute. Dr Gray emphasised that the challenge in health care is to attend to problems where there is currently nothing being done. He agreed about the importance of personal attention to individual families. However, he pointed out that health visitors' ability to focus attention on community-wide factors make them aware of those people with a need for preventive care but who tend to make contact with the health services too late.

There is a need to be able to continue to support and care for individual families and at the same time to continue to use the wider awareness of the community to make contact with the more vulnerable people, as far as this is possible. There are many ways in which these goals can be attempted.

Community-based initiatives

Group and individual talent in the community can be encouraged, often with the health visitor working in a 'catalystic' capacity. Work with groups has always been a normal part of the job, but particularly with regard to health education, such as in schools or at antenatal classes. Now, as Jean Orr (1982, 1983) has described, health visitors are finding a wide variety of ways of responding to personal and community health need. She regretted that, relatively, so few write about what they are doing.

One example of a new initiative in the community was when two health visitors worked in a women's health shop which provided one-to-one education and health promotion, as well as support for self-help groups (Robinson & Roberts, 1985). Another example is Tyler and Barnes' (1986) groups which were set up to offer support and education to patients suffering from long-term ill-effects due to stress. The health visitors described how they evaluated the results of their work with the groups and showed just how much can be saved in the costs of tranquillisers or anti-depressants through the significantly smaller cost per head of running these courses. The GPs were beginning to refer people to them *before* putting them on medication, an obvious compliment to the success of their work.

One health visitor was employed specifically to work with groups in the community and freed of the normal commitment to individual families. Vari Drennan (1984) described how she worked evenings and weekends to fit in with the groups' needs. The project was backed by a steering group, some members of which met the health visitor regularly, providing constructive support and helping to evaluate achievements. Mark McCarthy (1985) emphasised the value to project workers in the community, both of a steering group, which should include local people, the funding agency and the participants, and of a built-in evaluation to enable development of ideas as the project progressed.

An approach on a more individual level can also be successful. There have been some moves towards encouraging women in a locality to take some training and then provide help for a particular family or families. There is very little difference between client and helper in some of these schemes. The idea is a little reminiscent of a strategy mentioned in the introductory chapter, where the Manchester and Salford Ladies Sanitary Reform Association trained and employed 'respectable working women' to visit homes (Owen, 1983). It is possible they were more acceptable to and empathetic towards working class mothers than had been the earlier volunteer 'lady' visitors.

An excellent example of this approach is the scheme in Dublin which is under the auspices of the Child Development Project (1984). Here some women who have demonstrated a particular aptitude in bringing up their own children, have been trained as 'Child Development Aides' (CDA). They have then worked under the guidance of Irish health visitors, visiting and supporting first-time mothers. In due course, some of the mothers who were visited in this scheme, have themselves become CDAs. Other examples of this approach are those of the Lisson Grove Health Centre (Wood, 1985) and Newpin (Mills & Pound, 1986) schemes.

Ideas on community health initiatives can be found in Sue Dowling's (1983) *Health for a change* and Caroline Smith's (1982a) booklet describing some sixty schemes. Guidance on how to set up voluntary groups and promote health, where to look for help and how to apply for funds is also available (Smith, 1982b). The Department of the Environment 1970's research into self-help groups in inner city areas of London, showed there were fewer groups in these areas than elsewhere. This research enabled some useful advice to be given on how groups in inner cities might be encouraged (Knight & Hayes, 1981).

Inner city work

It is now well known that special attention is

needed in many inner city areas. Multiple problems including poor environmental conditions, families on low income, high levels of unemployment and mobile populations from a diversity of backgrounds and cultures, mean specially tailored solutions need to be devised.

Recent reports on primary health care in the London inner city areas were reviewed by Alison While (1982). Each had suggested more resources and improved staffing levels. She questioned whether this would prove to be the solution to the problems and suggested that a change of approach might be more important. She felt there was a need for more sensitivity to the acceptability of the services offered to inner city dwellers. The present 'middle class medical model' seemed inadequate and a more flexible approach was advocated.

A study by Downham et al (1980), which looked at the provision of child health services in Newcastle upon Tyne, showed that services were not concentrated in the parts of the city where they were most needed. Downham et al also felt that the most important factor is the *quality* of the services and that it is this that affects the extent to which they are used. However, they said that improving the quality of services is very difficult whilst they remain quantitatively inadequate.

The transfer of control from Area to District Health Authorities in 1982, should be making it easier to respond to particular local need and implement special projects. Elizabeth Watson (1984) described three inner city initiatives which aimed at improving the health of the local people. One at the Thomas Coram Research Unit set up experimental 'walk-in' clinics, which adopted a wide view of child health surveillance and included concern with the mothers' mental health. 20% of the children attending were found to have special problems. The mothers appreciated the broader approach and continued to attend as the children got older. This was in contrast to the normal, shorter pattern of clinic attendance in which the initial frequent visits with

a new baby tail off sharply, with few people returning to discuss the care of toddlers and young children.

Child health surveillance programmes were rejected in the Riverside project in Newcastle upon Tyne, in favour of giving parents common clinical information which research had shown was ill-understood. In this way, the project enabled parents to make their own decisions, to take responsibilty for their children's health and to motivate them to take the necessary action.

In a third example of inner city initiatives described by Elizabeth Watson, one in Nottingham, the number of routine examinations was reduced. The emphasis was changed towards dealing with the problems identified by parents, nursery teachers and others in contact with the child. Health visitors, of course, had a key role. It had been suggested that they should refer children to a named doctor. Dr Nicoll (1983) described how this more flexible system was both more efficient and effective in detecting new problems, by concentrating doctors' valuable skills where a problem is already suspected and by using other people's skills in recognising that some aspect needs further examination.

A birth scoring system for identifying 'at risk' babies was implemented in Nottingham. It showed that around 5% of the babies in the more affluent areas were classified as high risk, as opposed to 30% in some inner urban wards. Here the health visitors' workload was increased because, not only was there a large number of high scoring babies, but the birth rate was also higher. It had been decided to allocate new staff, as they became available, to these inner city wards and to maintain the level of health visitor services in the more affluent areas. The scheme would be dependent, though, on attracting staff to work in these inner city areas (Madeley & Latham, 1979).

One health visitor accepted the challenge of inner city work in a very positive way. Sue Phillips (1986) found herself working on a historically under-resourced housing estate, with high levels of social deprivation. The estate was on the edge of two Local Authorities, neither of whom was keen to accept responsibility for providing facilities. She decided that some part of her time must be spent campaigning for increased services, working as a 'catalyst' behind a community-based project to set up a family centre. This activity was undertaken in partnership with parents, local residents and local workers. She was allowed to work on her own initiative and received encouragement over the project from her managers.

The question was raised as to whether health visitors shoul be involved in 'political action' of this nature (Phillips, 1986). Health visitors, like other workers, face the problem that where change is sought, this is recognised as a form of political activity. However, deciding to take no action to change things and supporting the status quo, is also 'political action'. The difference is that the inactivity associated with tacit acceptance makes it less noticeable.

Acceptance of things as they are can have derogatory effects. When searching for possible failures in the child care services associated with infant deaths, Jepson et al (1983) concluded that health visitors should not work in grossly deprived areas for too long because they would eventually accept conditions that would be considered abnormal by an outsider. A health visitor busily engaged in background help aimed at improving the local situation is perhaps less likely to be so accepting and immune to the reality. Sue Phillips provides a good example of what *can* be done in the face of gross social deprivation and we shall return to her work in the next section.

A common dilemma facing health visitors working in inner city areas is associated with expectations that they will fill in the gaps created by the lack of social services and staff. Working in Southwark during the strike by social workers brought this fact into sharp focus for Jane Schofield (1984). She described how easy it is to respond to people's crisis situations and to slip into a social work role. Routine visiting suffers as a consequence, and the risk of missing important health problems

in other families is increased. It is important, she says, to be clear about what we are employed for, and that it may help to remember that other workers would not step over into our nursing role if there were a shortage. In essence, each Authority must be held responsible for its own obligations—and health visitors should undertake health visiting.

Specially assigned or generalist?

There is a debate within the profession on the extent to which specialisation or generalism should be encouraged (Barratt, 1985). Each has merits and there seems plenty of room in health visiting for both. Some fear a two-tier profession (Davidson, 1979), but this seems to be based on a misunderstanding of the term 'specialist'. What is actually meant is 'specifically employed' or 'specially assigned' to certain duties, for example, for the elderly, the handicapped (see Box 9.3), for diabetics (Nursing Times, 1983; Jackson, 1981) in the Child Development Project (1984) or, as we have seen above, for group work (Drennan, 1984). In the Cumberlege Report (DHSS, 1986) it was suggested that these specialist health visitors should be brought into neighbourhood nursing services, in order to work closely with district nurses, school nurses and health visitors.

On training, the Cumberlege Report suggested a broad-based health visitor type of course for all these community nurses, in which students would opt for a specialist module. This would, for example, be in maternal and child health, health education, nurse practitioner work or the elderly. It was a relief to find that the authors stated emphatically that they were in no way proposing the introduction of a generic nurse and that they were particularly 'seeking to preserve the type of skills possessed by the health visitor' (p. 44). An all-purpose public health nurse would find it impossible to be well enough educated across the necessary range of preventive *and* acute care. Added to that, acute care would inevitably be rated as higher priority and preventive health care work would be sure to suffer (While, 1986). It was the potential for working together in order to share knowledge and approaches for the benefit of the clientele, that lay behind the Report's proposals.

There are advantages in specialisation. Specially employed health visitors are less likely to be side-tracked by crisis work or other health visitors' clinic sessions, and are therefore free to devote themselves to their particular client group. This can be especially useful in areas of deprivation, but only if theirs is an additional post.

These health visitors are not 'special'. Their range of basic skills is just the same. However, their narrower remit makes it easier for them to acquire a better depth of knowledge for the group they look after. As was suggested in Chapter 9 (Table 9.4), other health visitors may find them useful to turn to if they are also caring for the same sort of client group.

The disadvantage of the narrow remit and homing in on one care group is that it militates against an awareness of and an involvement with the wider community beyond that particular group. Here the traditional broader remit of the generalist health visitor is invaluable. Having a theoretical remit which has concern for the community as a whole enables, encourages and improves the potential in health visiting. There are several key factors. For example:

1. Acceptability

The universality of the service increases its acceptability and minimises the possibility of stigma. Specialist health visiting has a higher level of acceptability, even if it is concerned with a low status group, on account of the general image of health visiting.

2. Creativity

The wider remit and freedom to choose from a variety of ways to provide preventive health care, both for traditional and for new client groups, enables use of initiative in, for example, setting up pilot schemes to discover better ways of working.

3. Access

Being able to take the service to any group of people without their having to come forward and request it, encourages a search for acceptable and effective ways of taking preventive health care to vulnerable families or groups who are currently under-utilising the services.

Both specialists and generalists make timely use of skills and knowledge aimed at increasing people's independence in their health care. Both are versatile enough to be able to support individual and group work, whichever seems most appropriate. It seems very likely that the evolution of health visiting will see them both living in a symbiotic relationship for many years yet.

In this section we have looked at suggestions and projects which show some of the current influences on the way health visiting is moving forward. An epidemiological- or population-based approach, work with groups and individuals from the local community and some inner city work, have been described.

A FUTURE FOR THE MODELS?

There remains the question as to whether the ideas and models described in earlier chapters are likely to be relevant to future health visiting. Currently, it is one-to-one work in the privacy of people's homes that forms the essence of health visiting and this is likely to continue. This basic approach is supplemented, particularly by clinic work and, to a varying extent, by work with groups. Increasingly, community-based health initiatives are playing an important part. It is proposed that the three basic models are also applicable for the wider 'community' approach and this will be demonstrated on a real life example. The models are seen as a conceptual rather than a 'checklisting' aid.

Individual *and* community work

The success of some health visitors' work with

groups and community-based health projects has led a number of people to infer that this could provide the solution to all problems. However, work with individuals and individual families has the advantage of providing personalised and private care.

Earlier chapters have explained how individual care can help prevent the occurrence, development and deterioration of problems. For example, the Child Development Project (1984) shows the value of personalised antici-patory guidance on promoting health. Tele-vision reaches into most people's homes, but according to Holmes (1984) it is unable on the whole to provide health education which has more than a brief influence on people's behaviour. Early discovery of problems can depend on being able to follow up families at home. For example, this may be necessary because a family has been invited to a clinic screening session but has been unable or unwilling to attend, or because there is an indication that a problem is too sensitive to be discussed in a clinic. Most of a health visitor's supportive care is reliant on privacy, at least initially, so that people can feel free to speak frankly. Home is usually the best place.

Visiting individual families also enables health visitors to become aware of trends amongst the families seen, for example the emergence of health problems amongst the young unemployed or particular difficulties for single parents. These trends can then form the basis of new preventive health inititatives, which in turn may include group or other community-based work. It is another case of a symbiotic relationship between two countervailing aspects of our work, this time between the individual and community approaches.

Community activity can be very important, particularly for health visitors working in areas where problems abound. Gradually it will probably be seen rather less as 'political activity' but, increasingly, as a practical way of helping people in the locality to become more self-dependent.

The relatively small initial 'catalytic' involve-ment of the health visitor can enable people

in difficulty, or potentially so, to find a way to discover their own solutions. It helps give people courage to seek and make use of the resources that are already available to them. For example, there are funds such as Urban Aid of which they are probably unaware or, perhaps, too self-effacing to take up.

Community activity and the models

It is probably easiest to demonstrate the way the three models can be used to provide an outline and a way of marshalling thought about health visitor community-based activi-ties, by using a real example of this sort of work. Sue Phillips (1986) started work in a south London housing estate as a newly qualified health visitor (see pp. 221–222 and Ch. 9, p. 166). Box 12.1 outlines some of the features affecting family health that struck her so forcefully. This is the 'what-problems' and 'what-particular-health-needs-there-are' model. Child safety and develop-

Box 12.1 Family health needs model for Sue Phillips' community activity

Environmental factors	Physical and mental health	Social aspects of health
Poor and inadequate housing: high rise flats with frequent problems of access as lifts out of order	High incidence of depression amongst young parents	A great deal of isolation, especially amongst single parent families
Housing estate on the edge of two local authorities and allotted low priority by both	Marked level of developmental delay, especially delayed speech	No centre for community activities
No safe play area	Above average level of suspected and actual child abuse	No holiday play schemes
Miles from nearest local authority nursery (waiting list = 200)		No mother and toddler group
Child health clinic very small: no room for group work		

Table 12.1 Prevention model for Sue Phillips' community activity

Aspect of prevention	Through
Prevent occurrence of problems	Self-help support groups for young parents, especially single parents Safe play area
Prevent development of problems	Care of parental mental health and facilities for safe play to improve levels of developmental attainment, especially in speech Regular day care facilities
Prevent deterioration of established problems	Self-help support groups for depressed and lonely parents, especially single parents Day care facilities

mental progress, potential child abuse and maternal mental health were some of the particular concerns.

Miss Phillips started a project aimed at enabling a family centre to be set up. The model in Table 12.1 draws out the three aspects of preventive health care inherent in this work. It gives the 'why-it-needs-to-be-done' and 'how-it-might-be-achieved' perspective. Concerns here are for features such as a safe play area and child care facilities, meeting places and support for parents and for stimulation for the children.

The third model, seen in Figure 12.1, highlights the sources and sort of information that led to the project being undertaken and outlines a view of 'how it is planned and

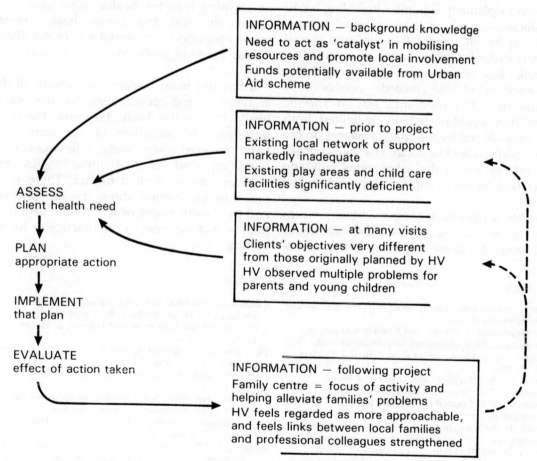

Fig. 12.1 Health visitor cycle model of Sue Phillips' community action.

monitored'. The model draws attention to, for example, what was learned in training, the clients' viewpoint and the results of the project.

Not for everyday tabulation

Demonstrating Sue Phillips' work in this form is not to suggest that she either did, or should have, listed these thoughts and observations. The models proposed in this book are merely ways of thinking about and approaching the work and are tabulated in this book in order to help explain them and for teaching purposes.

It is probable that it would be counter-productive to use these models in everyday health visiting in the form of complex charts or as multifactorial checklists for written records or planning schemes. Providing broad classifications, such as 'environmental factors', 'physical health', 'mental health' and 'social aspects of health' is no better than providing a blank piece of paper, and merely makes the presentation of the records unnecessarily complicated. If turned into lists of specific items, they would necessarily be limited, both conceptually and by the space available on the page. Sadly, checklists can channel concern and interest on to the listed items only and encourage an over-simplistic approach to the work.

Reality is extremely complex. Health visitor training and subsequent practical experience and study gradually build up a breadth of understanding and a wide-ranging knowledge of factors affecting health and welfare. The models provide a variety of ways of looking at the work. Whilst they remain simply a conceptual tool, they are likely to provide the means for creative thinking. This is by being able to be used in many individual ways to highlight and draw attention to important basic issues within the complexities of health visiting.

These models have been used throughout this book to classify and clarify various aspects of the work. Each has a particular perspective, and looking at them all within one example shows even more clearly the special contribution each can make.

This chapter has taken a look at recent influences and at some current challenges, debates and initiatives within the profession. It has rounded up a basic message of the book by showing how the health visitor cycle, the prevention and the family health needs models provide a very useful way of describing a wide range of health visiting concerns.

It has not been possible to include all the arguments and possibilities in preventive health care in this book. However, the basic purposes and objectives of our work have been covered, and many references have been included so that these topics and debates can be studied further. There is so much to be learned about the perspectives and the health needs of the infinite variety of people that we meet in the practice of health visiting.

REFERENCES

Barratt L 1985 Generic versus specialist—the way ahead? Health Visitor 58:155

Child Development Project 1984 Child development programme. Early Childhood Development Unit, Senate House, University of Bristol, Bristol BS8 ITH, pp. 25–28

Council for the Education and Training of Health Visitors 1977 An investigation into the principles of health visiting. Council for the Education and Training of Health Visitors, London, page 7

Council for the Education and Training of Health Visitors 1980 The investigation debate. A commentary on an investigation into the principles of health visiting. Council for the Education and Training of Health Visitors, London

Council for the Education and Training of Health Visitors 1982 Health Visiting. Principles in Practice. Council for the Education and Training of Health Visitors, London

Davidson N 1979 Spread so thin they vanish. Health and Social Services Journal LXXXIX: 1241

DHSS 1979 Nurses, Midwives and Health Visitors Act, 1979. HMSO, London

DHSS 1986 Neighbourhood nursing—a focus for care. Report of the Community Nursing Review. Department of Health and Social Services HMSO, London (Chairman, Mrs Cumberlege)

Dowling S 1983 Health for a change. The provision of preventive health care in pregancy and early childhood. Child Poverty Action Group, London

Downham M A P S, White E McC, Moss T R 1980 A study of childhood morbidity and mortality in relation to the provision of child health services in Newcastle upon Tyne, 1975 and 1976. Health Trends 12: 96–98

Drennan V 1984 A new approach. Nursing Mirror HVA Supplement 159, 14: x–xi

Farmer R D T, Miller D L 1983 Lecture notes of epidemiology and community medicine. Blackwell Scientific Publications, Oxford

Fitton J M 1983 Policy constraints on HV practice (letter). Health Visitor 56:229

Fitton J M 1984a Health visiting the elderly: nurse managers' views. One. Nursing Times Occasional Paper No 10 80, 16: 59–61

Fitton J M 1884b Health visiting the elderly: nurse managers' views. Two. Nursing Times Occasional Paper No 11 80, 17: 67–69

Gray J A M 1983 Role dilemma of health visiting (letter). Health Visitor 56: 83–84

Grierson S 1983 Caring for the carers (letter). Health Visitor 56:44

Health Visitor 1981 Meetings, conferences and reports. Radical Health Visiting. Health Visitor 54:406

Health Visitor 1984 Accept responsibility for 'professional politics'. Health Visitor 57:360

Holmes P 1984 Down the tube? Nursing Times 80, 31:21

Jackson M 1981 Diabetes mellitus: the health visitor's role. Geriatric Medicine 11, 6: 42–45

Jepson M E, Taylor E M, Emery J L 1983 Identification of failures in the child health services by means of confidential enquiries into infant deaths. Maternal and Child Health 8, 1: 26–31

Knight B, Hayes R 1981 Self help in the inner city. London Voluntary Service Council HMSO, London

McCarthy M 1982 Epidemiology and policies for health planning. King Edward's Hospital Fund for London, London

McCarthy M 1985 Understanding health needs. Health and Social Services Journal XCV:133

MacFarlane of Llandaff 1982 Responsibility for future development of health visiting. Health Visitor 55: 273–277

Madeley R J, Latham A 1979 Management aspects of high risk strategies in child health. Community Medicine 1: 36–39

Mills M, Pound A 1986 Mechanisms of change: the Newpin Project. Changes 4, 2: 199–203

Nicoll A 1983 Community child health services—for better or worse? Health Visitor 56: 241–243

Nursing Times 1981 Baroness looks for new role for the HV. Nursing Times 77:1867

Nursing Times 1983 Nurse diabetes specialist. Nursing Times 79, 37:23

Dopson L 1986 Getting in on the Act. Nursing Times 82, 9:64

Orr J 1982 Health visiting in the United Kingdom. In: Hockey L (ed) Primary care nursing. Churchill Livingstone, Edinburgh

Orr J 1983 Is health visiting meeting today's needs? Health Visitor 56: 200–203

Owen G 1983 The development of health visiting as a profession. In: Owen G (ed) Health visiting, 2nd edn. Baillière Tindall, Eastbourne, p. 5

Phillips S 1986 A centre for change. Nursing Times Community Outlook 82, 7: 15–17

Richards I G D 1980 The epidemiology of disease in childhood. In: Mitchell R G (ed) Child health in the community, 2nd edn Churchill Livingstone, Edinburgh

Robinson J 1983 The role dilemma of health visiting. Health Visitor 56: 22–24

Robinson S E, Roberts M M 1985 A women's health shop: a unique experiment. British Medical Journal 291: 255–256

Schofield J 1984 A health visitor's dilemma. Nursing Times 80, 23:21

Smith C 1982a Directory of community health initiatives. National Council for Voluntary Organisations, London

Smith C 1982b Community based health initiatives. A handbook for voluntary groups. National Council for Voluntary Organisations, London

Tyler M, Barnes S 1986 The group approach to living with stress. Health Visitor 59: 14–16

Townsend P 1982 The policy implications of a positive approach to health. Health Visitor 55: 97–101

Waters W E, Cliff K S 1983 Community medicine: a textbook for nurses and health visitors. Croom Helm, London

Watson E 1984 Policies for child health in inner cities. Maternal and Child Health 9: 123–128

While A 1982 Primary health care in the inner city: time for a new approach? Health Visitor 55: 116–117

While A 1986 The value of health visitors. Health Visitor 59: 171–173

Wood T 1985 Formal and informal support systems for mothers with newborn. Midwife Health Visitor and Community Nurse 21: 42–49

World Health Organisation 1982 The place of epidemiology in local health work: the experience of a group of developing countries. World Health Organisation, Geneva

Author Index

Subject Index